Nature's Prescriptions

Foods, Vitamins, and Supplements That Prevent Disease

Nature's Prescriptions: Foods, Vitamins, and Supplements
That Prevent Disease

This book is for information only and is not intended to be a medical guide for self-diagnosis or self-treatment. It does not constitute medical advice and should not be construed as such or used in place of your doctor's medical advice. We recommend in all cases that you contact your personal doctor or health care provider before taking or discontinuing any medication, or before treating yourself in any way.

While every attempt has been made to assure that the information in this book is true and accurate, errors may occur; and it is not possible to cover every condition and treatment. The publisher and editors disclaim all liability in the connection with the use of the information in this book.

> Is there any such thing as Christians cheering each other up? Do you love me enough to want to help me? Does it mean anything to you that we are brothers in the Lord, sharing the same Spirit? Are your hearts tender and sympathetic at all? Then make me truly happy by loving each other and agreeing wholeheartedly with each other, working together with one heart and mind and purpose.
>
> Phillipians 2:1-2 (TLB)

CONTENTS

CONDITIONS

SUPER FOODS

VITAMINS AND SUPPLEMENTS

INTRODUCTION

Nature's best prescriptions

Mark Twain once said, "The only way to keep your health is to eat what you don't want, drink what you don't like, and do what you'd druther not." Well, that might have been true a hundred years ago, but today, it is easier and more fun than ever to stay healthy. You can make up your own mind about the "doing" part, but eating and drinking for health is certainly no chore with today's choices. In fact, some of the healthiest meals you'll ever whip up can be the most delicious. All it takes is good information, a little planning, and a willingness to change some not-so-healthy habits.

If you want to feel well, stay active, and live longer, you've got to think about nutrition. It's actually hard not to think about it, nowadays. Every time you open a newspaper, read a magazine, or turn on the television, there's some new health drink, diet pill, or wonder cure on the market. But most experts will tell you that there is no substitute for a good, balanced diet.

That means you should eat a variety of whole foods to get something that packaged, processed, prepared, and preserved foods can't give you: a blend of all the natural nutrients your body needs, even the ones scientists haven't named yet. It may come as a surprise that we don't know everything, but there are elements in plant foods that experts know are beneficial, but haven't yet identified. That's why you will never get quite the same result from a supplement. So, let's talk about supplements for a moment.

There will always be good reasons for taking a vitamin or mineral supplement. A good example is a woman approaching menopause. It may be hard for her to get the recommended dose of calcium strictly through foods. Yet it's necessary to boost her calcium in order to lower her risk of developing osteoporosis. This is a good time to take a supplement. You will see that many of the other conditions covered in this book will call for a short-term dose of one vitamin or another to bring your system back into balance.

The danger, however, lies in relying on a supplement instead of eating a proper diet. You shouldn't try to fill the gaps left by poor eating habits this way. If you are deficient in vitamin B6 and aren't eating green, leafy vegetables ... well, you should start.

In the past, people suffered from a long list of diseases caused by a lack of proper nutrition, in many cases the lack of one single vitamin. Pellagra was caused by too little niacin; beriberi by a lack of thiamin; scurvy, not enough vitamin C; goiters from too little iodine; anemia; rickets; the list goes on and on. All these sometimes-fatal conditions are preventable by diet.

Today, thanks to advances in nutritional science, these conditions are almost unheard of in most countries. But now you face a different set of risks from a poor diet. Americans are eating too many processed and "fast" foods and skipping meals. This brings a host of other illnesses into the picture; diseases with longer names and sometimes more frightening consequences: diverticulosis, atherosclerosis, angina, and cancer.

Thankfully, just as the diseases have become more difficult to diagnose and treat, our technology has kept pace. Scientists are now able to analyze tiny changes that individual nutrients cause in your body, changes that can impact the course of a disease. This has opened the door to a new era in nutrition.

This modern way of looking at illness and nutrition gives every person the opportunity for more control over his own health. No matter what the condition, no matter how serious or slight your disorder might be, you just feel better about your recovery if you know YOU can do something about it. And when that treatment involves eating fresh, healthy foods, what more could you ask for?

Most doctors know what you've already heard: that diet plays an important role in preventing disease. Unfortunately, they just treat the outcomes of poor nutrition. Most of them don't know enough about nutrition to give their patients good advice. A recent poll of over 3,000 doctors revealed that only 9 percent talked to their patients about how to eat the proper foods. So where does that leave you? Unless you have a book like this one, you are pretty much stuck taking the medicines you are prescribed and doing little more than hoping you'll get better. Not much of a sense of control over your situation. But with *Nature's Prescriptions: Foods, Vitamins, and Supplements That Prevent Disease,* you can finally take an active role in disease prevention, treatment, and recovery.

Vitamins and minerals make up the smallest part of the foods you eat, but they may be the most important. To stay in tip-top condition, your body needs just the right balance of all the vitamins and minerals. A deficiency in any one can mean trouble. When you are ill, that balance is upset and you must adjust your diet in order to bring your body back into balance. That is what this book is all about.

The largest section of *Nature's Prescriptions* covers the most common illnesses and disorders, everything from arthritis to ulcers. Each of these condition chapters, listed alphabetically, discusses in detail the role of diet in the treatment and prevention of that disorder.

Next, there is a section describing each of the major vitamins and minerals, how your body uses them, and which foods are high in that nutrient. Here, you will also find the Recommended Dietary Allowances (RDA), deficiency information, and warnings.

The last part of the book focuses on what we call "super foods." This is a list of foods that nutrition experts recommend over and over again for their high nutrient content. They are proven fighters of various illnesses and disorders. You will learn what these foods contain that make them super and what conditions they are best at defeating.

It shouldn't come as a surprise that many of the recommended foods in the Conditions section, and many of the Super Foods, are either fruits or vegetables. Studies have proven that people who eat fruits and vegetables every day live longer, healthier lives. They suffer from fewer heart attacks and strokes, cut their risk of many cancers by half, have lower blood pressure, and have fewer ulcers. But wait, there's more.

Just by eating strawberries, spinach, broccoli, and yams, you can boost your antioxidant level, save your eyesight, strengthen your immune system, and fight off infectious diseases. Not bad work for one trip to the salad bar.

So why aren't more people eating fruits and vegetables? The National Cancer Institute (NCI) researched that very question and came up with several answers.

Excuse: Fruits and vegetables are too expensive.

Answer: Actually, many snack and dessert foods you buy instead of fruits and vegetables are more expensive and contain fewer nutrients. For instance, the researchers at NCI priced a serving of potato chips at 25 cents and a serving of packaged chocolate chip cookies at 24 cents. In contrast, a banana costs only 17 cents, and an apple 13 cents.

You can save even more money by choosing produce that is in season. It will not only be fresher and more plentiful, the price will be lower, too. Use coupons, check for sales, and buy generic or store brands of canned or frozen fruits and vegetables.

Excuse: Fruits and vegetables take too long to prepare.

Answer: Many grocery stores offer shortcuts for busy people. There is often an aisle in the produce section filled with vegetables that are pre-cut, pre-washed, pre-chopped, or pre-sliced. Everything from salad greens to cabbage, carrots, and broccoli. All you have to do is open and enjoy. Even some fruits come hassle-free. Vacuum-packed fresh pineapple that has already been peeled and cored is a real time-saver. And many months out of the year you'll find colorful and delicious melon balls all ready to go.

Your grocery store may have a salad bar or deli with fresh raw vegetables and ready-made fruit and vegetable salads. Here you can choose your own combinations and amounts.

Fresh is best, but canned or frozen fruit and juices still give you important vitamins. And it's super easy to open a can or grab a bag from the freezer.

To save time later, take a little extra time once a week and cook up a pot of dried beans. That way they'll be ready and waiting for you to add to a soup or serve cold on a salad. Lots of fresh veggies can be cooked or cut up ahead of time and stored for later use.

Excuse: Fresh fruits and vegetables spoil too quickly.

Answer: On your weekly shopping trip, buy fresh produce to use immediately, and canned or frozen items for later in the week. Along the same lines, buy some ripe bananas or tomatoes to enjoy right away as well as some green ones to eat after they've ripened.

Just don't forget you've got a reserve tucked away. Keep them in a pretty bowl on the counter, if you can, or at least visible in the front of your refrigerator.

Excuse: Fruits and vegetables contain harmful pesticides.

Answer: The FDA strictly regulates the kind and amount of pesticides used in the United States. They are very confident that consumers are not at risk from any pesticide residue that may be on fresh fruits and vegetables. If you are still worried, you can remove outer leaves, peel the skin, or lightly scrub your fresh produce.

This book will explain alternative methods of treating and preventing disease through your diet. You may find sections on herbal remedies and even aromatherapy as well. Be sure to follow the warnings and safety guidelines when using any of these remedies.

You should always tell your doctor when you decide to try an alternative remedy, even if he disagrees with that practice. Don't try experimenting with the unknown; take only recommended doses of supplements and herbs, and remember that some herbs take a few weeks to become effective. Be careful with essential oils — they are up to 70 times more powerful than the original plant. Never eat or drink them. Always dilute them in water or massage oil before applying them to your skin, and watch out for allergic reactions.

If you follow these guidelines, you don't need to be afraid of these types of treatments. They may be different from what you are used to, but if you are uncomfortable or in pain, what have you got to lose?

Nature's Prescriptions is full of good nutrition information, timely medical tips, and delicious recipes. You can go straight to a condition of particular interest or browse through it for ways to improve your overall health. Keep it handy when you make up your shopping list and when friends and relatives come to call. Most of all, use this book for natural ways to add vitality and health to your diet and to your life.

Health is the thing that makes you feel that now is the
best time of the year.

Franklin P. Adams

CONDITIONS

ALCOHOLISM

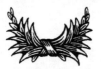

A+ protection from antioxidants

Drinking alcohol can do more than give you a terrible headache the morning after. According to a recent study, alcohol robs your body of important antioxidant vitamins, giving free rein to the free radicals that can damage your organs.

The people in the study were tested to find out how much vitamin E; beta carotene, a form of vitamin A; and selenium, a trace mineral, they had in their blood.

Because of liver and muscle damage from alcohol, the alcoholics in the study had lower levels of the antioxidants than people who weren't alcoholics. It's a vicious cycle, since damaged muscles and liver cause more loss of antioxidants, and this, in turn, causes more damage.

To help repair some of the damage, the researchers recommend giving up alcohol and taking supplements of vitamin E and selenium. Ask your doctor for his guidance in determining how much to take.

Adding foods to your diet that are rich in vitamin C and beta carotene might also help decrease the damage caused by alcohol abuse. Beta carotene is found in dark green and orange fruits and vegetables, such as spinach, carrots, winter squash, sweet potatoes, and cantaloupe. Citrus fruits, sweet red pepper, strawberries, broccoli, and brussels sprouts are good sources of vitamin C.

Warning: when to shun shellfish

Watch out for that slimy little shellfish. He may be packing more than a delicious flavor. If you have liver disease or a weak immune system, or if you are an alcoholic, do not eat raw oysters. They may carry a type of bacteria, called Vibrio vulnificus, that can cause serious illness or even death.

Being an alcoholic means you probably have some stage of liver disease. This makes you 200 times more likely to die from this bacterial infection than healthy people. If you decide to eat oysters, make sure they are cooked. Slurping them from the half shell isn't worth the risk.

Hidden epidemic in the elderly

Your elderly Aunt Sarah isn't the person she used to be. She seems confused much of the time, she's having more trouble with her diabetes, and the paramedics have been to her house twice in the past month to pick her up after a fall. You assume it's Alzheimer's or the signs of old age, but it could be alcoholism.

An estimated 3 million elderly Americans are alcoholics or problem drinkers. Grief and loneliness can often cause older people to seek comfort in alcohol. For many of them, the problem goes unnoticed, even by their doctors or family members.

As the body ages, it produces less of the enzyme that processes alcohol. It also has a lower water content. So, an elderly person can be an alcoholic while drinking relatively small amounts. The daily glass of wine or two that didn't seem to bother Aunt Sarah in her 60s can cause problems in her 80s.

Some clues to alcoholism are depression; confusion; incontinence; insomnia; frequent falling, bruising, or broken bones; bad reactions to medication; and lack of self-care. If your elderly friend, neighbor, or loved one has any of these symptoms, check beyond the obvious. The problem could be alcohol.

ALLERGIES

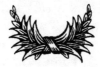

Outwit allergies naturally

Whether caused by heredity, a hormone imbalance, stress, or your environment, an allergy is nothing more than a breakdown in your immune system. Your body is rejecting something that shouldn't give it problems.

Taking care of your immune system is the first step in keeping your allergies under control. Be sure to get sufficient rest and plenty of exercise to keep your immune system in top form. Eliminate alcohol and tobacco — two old pros at breaking down a healthy immune system — and make sure you pay attention to what you eat. Smart eating might be the easiest and most affordable strategy in fighting allergies. Make sure you're getting these nutrients in your diet.

Vitamin C. Vitamin C is one of the best allergy fighters. Not only does it give your immune system a boost, it helps relieve allergy symptoms by reducing the amount of histamine your cells release. Numerous studies show that low levels of vitamin C mean high levels of histamine. Studies also show that taking vitamin C supplements is an effective way to fix this problem. Although dozens of delicious foods are packed with vitamin C, many people prefer using the powdered form. For maximum benefit and improved taste, mix the powder with a citrus-flavored carbonated beverage.

B vitamins. Vitamins B6 and B12 are both known for offering relief from various allergy symptoms. Vitamin B6 is particularly effective at controlling reactions to monosodium glutamate, also known as MSG, the flavor enhancer used by many Chinese restaurants. Research shows that taking B12 supplements for as little as four weeks can improve the symptoms of bronchial, skin, and food allergies. Bananas, potatoes, and wheat germ are good sources of B6. Try some spinach or cottage cheese for a natural source of B12.

Niacin, another member of the B-vitamin complex, helps relieve seasonal allergy symptoms, according to recent studies. Niacin helps put the brakes on allergies by preventing your cells from releasing histamine.

To raise the amount of niacin in your diet, add more lean meats, fish, and beans. If you're thinking of taking supplements, check with your doctor first. Although they are widely available, some forms of niacin supplements can cause serious side effects in high doses.

Calcium, magnesium, and zinc. These three minerals are essential to keep your allergies at bay. A deficiency of calcium, magnesium, or zinc can make your allergic reactions much worse. You should be able to get enough of these nutrients from a well-balanced diet, but if not, supplements are available for all three. Foods such as rice, broccoli, and skim milk are rich in calcium and magnesium. Zinc can be found in liver, oysters, and some lean white meats.

The buzz on local honey

A growing number of allergy sufferers swear that eating locally produced honey can reduce, and even eliminate, the symptoms of hay fever. The idea is the same as using bee pollen — developing an immunity by consuming pollen from the plants you are allergic to — but it seems to work much better. One beekeeper in California claims that her honey has helped locals with allergies ranging from acacia to poison oak.

With honey, you are getting a much smaller and safer dose than you would by consuming pollen itself, so the chance of a serious reaction is much less. Drastic results have been reported from eating as little as one teaspoon of local honey per day. And by eating the honey of local bees, you can be sure that the pollen in the honey comes from plants near your home — the exact plants you are trying to combat. Just make sure the honey was made during the pollination period of your particular allergen, and it hasn't been processed or heated.

Although honey has not been clinically tested as an allergy fighter, the widely reported success of this remedy might be proof that medical researchers can still learn a thing or two from old folk remedies.

Blow away hay fever with natural remedies

Many doctors believe that a natural problem calls for a natural solution. Some over-the-counter antihistamines are effective, but almost all of them will make you drowsy. Experts are constantly searching for new and better ways to treat your allergies without drugs. Try some of these natural remedies if you need allergy relief ... and want to stay awake to enjoy it.

Grasp the nettle. Stinging nettle is a stubborn weed that can give you a nasty, prickling rash if you rub against it in the garden. Take it internally, however, and you have another story. The extract of the nettle leaves, which is processed into capsules, is widely available in health food stores. Several studies show that the extract can relieve hay fever symptoms quickly.

The quercetin question. Quercetin can often control the onset of hay fever by regulating the membranes in your body that release histamine, the same thing commercial antihistamines do. Quercetin is obtained from buckwheat and citrus fruits. It is available in pill form, and the supplements work best if taken twice a day between meals, starting a few weeks before allergy season and continuing through the end of the season.

The coffee cure. Is coffee the answer to your hay fever blues? The results of one UCLA study suggest it may be. In the study, people who took caffeine tablets that equaled about three cups of coffee showed over a 50 percent improvement in their hay fever symptoms. Caffeine is also helpful for people with asthma by relaxing bronchial spasms in the lungs.

Before you load up on coffee, though, be sure your body is ready for the jolt. If you have heart disease or high blood pressure, ask your doctor how much caffeine you can safely have.

4 faulty folk remedies

The quick fix is not always the best fix. Some natural and alternative remedies can do more harm than good. Here are some popular allergy remedies that might be harmful.

Chamomile is thought of by many as a sort of cure-all. Unfortunately, its soothing qualities can backfire for people with allergies. Because chamomile contains allergens, including pollen, it can cause severe allergic reactions. For this reason, people with hay fever and similar allergies should not use teas, extracts, or other chamomile products.

Eyebright is a flowering plant that has been used for years for all sorts of eye irritations, such as those caused by allergies. It has been used on everything from dry eyes to red eyes to runny eyes, and yet its effectiveness and safety have not been documented in any controlled study. What's worse, putting any nonsterile substance in your eye carries a high risk of infection. Until it is more closely studied and produced, eyebright should be considered a folk remedy with potentially disastrous side effects.

Ephedra and its active component ephedrine have been hailed as natural decongestants, but they can cause dangerous side effects, like dizziness and high blood pressure. Although this herb can offer relief from discomfort, most herbal experts don't recommend using it.

Bee pollen has been getting a lot of attention as an allergy remedy. Some people think consuming pollen from the plants you are allergic to will help you develop an immunity to them, but there is very little evidence to support this claim. In fact, doctors strongly warn against taking bee pollen if you have a history of hay fever. Severe allergic reactions have occurred in people with allergies taking as little as one tablespoon of pollen. Best to stick to conventional wisdom, and avoid the source of your allergy.

ALZHEIMER'S DISEASE

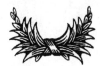

Asian remedy holds promise for Alzheimer's

The key to beating Alzheimer's disease may lie in a type of moss grown in the mountains of China. For centuries, the Chinese have used tea brewed from the *huperzia serrata* moss to treat memory loss in the elderly. Scientists have now isolated a compound found in the moss and turned it into the drug huperzine A. They are testing "hup A" in the fight against Alzheimer's.

A natural brain chemical called acetylcholine is vital for normal memory and thinking. People with Alzheimer's disease have a lack of acetylcholine, which affects their brain function. Huperzine A works by fighting the enzyme in your body that destroys acetylcholine.

Large medical trials in China have had good results, with few side effects, using huperzine A against Alzheimer's disease. U.S. scientists are getting ready to study this new drug, but they already suspect it may be more effective than existing treatments. It also holds promise for treating other brain disorders such as stroke and epilepsy.

You may be able to find the herb that is used to make huperzine A in your local health food store. It is combined with other ingredients, such as ginkgo, in a product called Food for Thought. In this form, the herb may be called *hyperizia serrata*.

Ancient plant protects your brain

The dried leaves of the ancient ginkgo tree have a potent effect on your body's blood flow. Better blood flow to your brain means clearer thinking and better memory power, both of which are gradually lost to people with Alzheimer's disease.

Although it's still a controversial treatment, several studies show that ginkgo has a positive effect when given to people with Alzheimer's. While it can't reverse the ravages of the disease, taking it may improve your thinking, emotional well-being, behavior, and sleeping habits. The studies showed few, if any, side effects.

It's important to choose a good quality extract of ginkgo biloba if you decide to take it. Gingkoba and GinkGold are supplements that contain pure ginkgo. They come in liquid, capsule, or tablet form. Amounts used in the studies varied from 120 to 160 milligrams (mg) of ginkgo a day up to 240 mg. For people with Alzheimer's, these large doses seem more effective than smaller doses of 40 mg you might take to boost memory power.

Natural brain builders

Juicy peaches, crunchy carrots, mouthwatering melons, sweet ears of corn. If you've loved fruits and veggies since you were a kid, you're smarter than you know. An ongoing study at an Ohio university is finding that people who eat lots of fresh fruits and vegetables over the course of a lifetime seem less likely to get Alzheimer's disease. The study shows it's especially important to eat tomatoes and dark green and yellow vegetables containing a combination of vitamin A, beta-carotene, and vitamin C.

By fighting free radicals that can damage your body, these antioxidant vitamins may just keep your brain in top working order.

The evidence for E

Inexpensive, widely available vitamin E supplements show great promise for slowing down the progress of Alzheimer's disease. In a recent study, people with moderate cases of Alzheimer's were given 2,000 international units (IU) of vitamin E a day. As a result, the people with Alzheimer's who were treated with vitamin E were able to care for themselves an average of seven months longer than those who didn't take the vitamin.

While the research looks promising, most doctors aren't ready to recommend taking large doses of vitamin E. Megadoses of vitamin E can cause bleeding problems and should be used only under a doctor's supervision.

Finger foods fill a need

A dietician at an Ohio nursing home found a solution that prevents unwanted weight loss and makes life easier for a person with Alzheimer's and his caretaker. The simple idea is to use more finger foods — morsels that can be picked up easily and eaten without utensils. When the menu at the nursing home was adapted to include more finger foods, people ate more and maintained a healthy weight.

To make the change to finger foods, try these substitutions:

Instead of:	Try:
poached eggs	hard-boiled eggs
cereal	French toast sticks
roast turkey	chicken strips
mashed potatoes	tater tots
pies	brownies
baked fish	fish sticks
salad with dressing	cucumber slices

ANEMIA, IRON-DEFICIENCY

Give iron-poor blood a boost

Residents of a small town in Georgia have long been in the practice of eating kaolin, a white clay substance found a foot or so beneath the surface of the earth. These peculiar eaters display a behavior called pica, a hunger for things that aren't normally considered food. Bizarre eating habits, such as ice chewing and clay eating, often point to a common nutritional deficiency like anemia. Nutritionists estimate that 20 percent of adult women and 3 percent of adult men are affected by this condition.

Iron-deficiency anemia can be caused by blood loss, problems with your body's absorption of iron, or not getting enough iron in your diet. If you have iron-deficiency anemia, it's important for your doctor to find out why your iron is low. Recent studies show that low iron levels can lead to heart disease and even death, especially in older people.

Symptoms of low-iron include fatigue, difficult breathing, weakness, headache, fainting spells, and depression. You also might notice a paleness to the color of your skin, nail beds, and lower eyelids. In its later stages, anemia can cause rapid pulse, irregular heart rate, and chest pains. Women may notice abnormal menstruation. Men can experience loss of sex drive and impotence.

If your anemia is caused by too little iron in your diet, here are some ways to boost your iron naturally.

- **Eat some meat.** The best food for replacing iron is red meat, particularly organ meats such as calf liver and kidney. For lighter fare, you might try poultry or seafood. The type of iron found in meat, fish, and poultry is more easily absorbed into your body than other types of iron. A good rule of thumb is — the darker the meat, the greater the iron content. Dark meats are also rich in vitamin B12 and zinc, important nutrients in preventing anemia.

- **Don't forget the peas and beans.** Since the best natural source of iron is red meat, a strict vegetarian diet can lead to iron deficiency. But with all that fat and cholesterol, you might be shy about loading up on liver. A simple solution to this problem is to eat white poultry with legumes, such as peas or dry beans. Studies show that the animal protein in the poultry helps your body absorb iron from the veggies.

- **No meat? No problem.** If you think you need meat to get your iron, think again. Iron that doesn't come from meat sources is usually less concentrated and less easily absorbed by your body, but it still helps the fight against anemia. Some good alternative sources are eggs, dairy products, grains, and legumes. If you're a fan of soy, try tofu or any number of other soy products. Dried fruits, nuts, and blackstrap molasses are also good sources of iron.

- **Think green and leafy.** One of the best ways to make sure you get the iron you need is by eating your green leafies. While green leafy vegetables don't contain much iron, they do contain a lot of folic acid and other nutrients. Folic acid plays a key role in helping your body absorb iron and the equally important vitamin B12. So don't forget the greens.

- **It isn't just for breakfast anymore.** Everyone loves a tall glass of orange juice, but did you know it can also chase away anemia? Vitamin C makes it easier for your body to absorb iron. It is so important, in fact, that a lack of vitamin C can sometimes cause anemia. Some nutrition experts say you should get at least 500 milligrams (mg) of vitamin C every day, while others claim you can safely take up to 20 times that amount. Ask your doctor what's best for you.

- **Round up some iron allies.** Iron may be the key to keeping your blood cells up and running, but just getting enough iron won't do much good unless you eat a healthy diet. Vitamin A, vitamin E, thiamin (B1), riboflavin (B2), and copper are important ingredients for healthy blood. Foods rich in these vitamins and minerals help your body hold on to the iron it gets. Liver, dark green vegetables, and dairy products are great sources of riboflavin and vitamin A. Shellfish, nuts, cereals, and legumes are good providers of copper and thiamin, and for extra vitamin E, try some wheat germ.

Fire up the skillet

For an extra boost of iron in your diet, why not shut off the microwave and get out the pan? Research shows that foods cooked in cast-iron skillets are higher in iron.

Anemia alert

While many foods help you get the iron you need to prevent anemia, certain foods decrease your body's ability to absorb it.

- **Schedule your coffee breaks.** If you're going to drink coffee or tea, it's better to do it before you eat. Research shows that drinking these beverages during or after a meal reduces your body's absorption of some types of iron, while drinking an hour before your meal does not. While this does not affect absorption of the type of iron found in meat, it does affect iron from vegetable and dairy sources. It also reduces absorption of the type of iron contained in almost all iron supplements.

- **Don't overload on fiber.** Although it's a necessary part of everyone's diet, eating too much fiber can lessen the amount of iron absorbed from other foods. In addition, too much fiber can cause constipation and gas.

- **Beware of certain foods.** Strangely enough, some of the same foods that contain iron, like milk and egg yolks, can actually slow down your body's absorption of it. Spinach and rhubarb also contain elements that make it harder for your body to absorb iron. The best solution? Get your iron from a variety of sources.
- **Give the Rolaids a rest.** Antacids also present a problem if you are trying to boost iron consumption. Doctors report that a lack of hydrochloric acid in the stomach is a big cause of iron deficiency, especially as people get older. This acid helps the digestive system break down and absorb nutrients like iron. Antacids, like Rolaids and Tums, rob your body of this essential acid, which can leave you iron-poor.

Leave iron pills to the pros

In some cases, your doctor might decide that changes in your diet won't be enough to reverse your anemia, and he may prescribe iron supplements. Most iron supplements come in 325 mg tablets, taken one to three times a day. It is usually best to take the tablets with meals. Although this makes the treatment work more slowly, it helps cut down on side effects.

Even though iron tablets might seem like the easiest solution, your problem might not be with your diet. If you suffer from difficulties in absorption, no amount of food or supplements will correct your condition.

Treatment for any type of anemia should focus on the underlying cause of the condition. Your doctor will be able to find the cause and recommend a therapy program that will do you the most good.

ANGINA

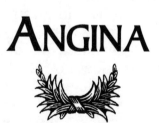

Ease the squeeze of angina pain

Pain is never pleasant, but when the pain is in your chest, it can also be very scary. However, chest pain doesn't always mean you're having a heart attack. Sometimes recurring chest pain is due to angina.

Angina occurs when the blood flow to your heart is temporarily restricted and your heart can't get all the oxygen it needs. When this happens, you feel a pressing or squeezing type pain, usually in the area just under your breastbone. However, the pain can sometimes spread to your shoulders, neck, jaws, arms, or back.

Angina attacks most often occur after exercise but can also be set off by stress, extreme heat or cold, heavy meals, alcohol, or cigarette smoke.

These things are only triggers, however. The root cause of this heart problem is atherosclerosis, or narrowing of the arteries. Your heart is unable to pump as much oxygen-rich blood through these narrow arteries, and the result is chest pain. The condition usually is relieved by resting or by taking medicine prescribed for angina, such as nitroglycerin.

Fortunately, unlike a heart attack, angina usually causes no permanent damage because blood flow is only partially cut off. In a heart attack, the blood supply to part of your heart is blocked completely, damaging your heart muscle beyond repair.

If you have angina, consider yourself fortunate in one respect. This condition may serve as a warning to take better care of your heart and your health to prevent more serious heart problems.

- **Boost vitamins C and E.** Keeping up your C and E intake might take some pressure off your chest. One study found that men who had low levels of vitamins C and E were more likely to have angina. Another small study found that men with active angina had the lowest levels of vitamin E, and when some of them received vitamin E supplements, they had a significant decrease in their angina attacks.

- **Moderate alcohol for angina.** Many publicized studies have touted the heart-protecting effects of alcohol, particularly red wine. One large study, the Physicians' Health Study, examined more than 22,000 male doctors. This study found that moderate drinking may indeed protect against angina and heart attack. Compared to men who drank less than one alcoholic drink per day, men who drank one drink per day were less likely to experience angina or have a heart attack. However, moderation is the key, because the same study also found an increased risk of cancer among men who consumed two or more drinks a day.

- **Eat small and light.** You may not think digesting your food is a difficult chore, but it does make your heart work harder. That increases its need for blood. Heavy meals and rich foods can strain your heart, making you more likely to have an angina attack after meals. Try eating smaller, lighter meals, and take some time to relax afterward.
- **Trim fat and trim down.** Excess weight can aggravate your angina. The more weight you carry around, the harder your heart has to work. Excess fat can also clog up your arteries, so even if you're not overweight, you should eat low-fat foods to keep your arteries clear and your chest pain free.

Angina does not have to control your life. If you take sensible precautions and follow your doctor's advice, you can live a normal, relatively pain-free lifestyle for years to come.

When to call 911

You've had angina attacks before, but this one is almost unbearable. Should you just grimace and endure the pain or head for the hospital? Here are some signs that you should seek emergency medical attention:

- Extreme pain or discomfort that gets worse and lasts longer than 20 minutes.
- Pain or discomfort along with weakness, feeling sick to your stomach, or fainting.
- Pain or discomfort that does not go away when you take three nitroglycerin tablets.
- Pain or discomfort that is worse than you have ever had before.

If you are experiencing any of these symptoms, call an ambulance or have someone drive you to the hospital. Do not attempt to drive yourself.

3 'unstable' symptoms

You know a stable job is better than an unstable one, and a stable personality is more desirable than an unstable personality. It only makes sense that stable angina is better than unstable angina, but what's the difference?

Stable angina usually follows a pattern. The pattern is different for different people, however. Some people may tend to have attacks after exercise, while emotional stress may be more likely to set off angina in others. Usually, the pain of stable angina goes away in just a few minutes.

Symptoms of unstable angina include:

- Angina pain while resting, or pain that wakes you up.
- Sudden moderate to severe angina pain in someone who has never had it before.
- Significant increase in frequency or severity of angina in someone with previously stable angina.

Unstable angina is more serious than stable angina because it means you're more likely to have a heart attack. Watch for these symptoms, and get medical attention if you experience any. Your doctor will be able to tell you how serious your condition is and what can be done for it.

Possible angina trigger

Carbon monoxide is a colorless, odorless gas that may go undetected as an angina trigger. Doctors recently screened 104 people who had been admitted to the hospital with angina pain. Three people had definite carbon monoxide poisoning, and five others had signs of exposure to carbon monoxide. The three people with serious levels of carbon monoxide had all been exposed to faulty kerosene heaters.

If you suffer from angina, you may want to invest in an inexpensive carbon monoxide detector. The U.S. Consumer Product Safety Commission says every home should be protected by at least one detector outside each sleeping area. For angina sufferers, it could be an important warning signal of an impending attack.

ARRHYTHMIAS

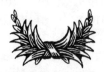

How to steady your heartbeat

You have probably experienced occasional periods when your heart seems to flutter or beat slower or faster than normal. Most arrhythmias, or irregular heartbeats, fall into this "once in a blue moon" category. These heartbeats are usually harmless, and they don't require treatment.

In some cases, however, arrhythmias can be life-threatening, causing your heart to stop beating altogether. Although some arrhythmias are unexplainable and unavoidable, the following tips may help keep your heart ticking like a trusty clock.

- **Balance your electrolytes.** Your heart depends on electrical impulses to control its rate and rhythm. Two minerals, potassium and magnesium, are particularly important to your heart's electrical activity. These minerals, also known as electrolytes, conduct electrical activity from one location to another. An imbalance of these minerals can affect your heart's rhythm. One study found that increasing daily intake of potassium and magnesium by 50 percent reduced some types of arrhythmias.

- **Take care of your heart.** Some arrhythmias are caused by heart disease. In these cases, it is the heart disease that should concern you. The arrhythmias are just a warning that you should take care of your heart. For heart-healing hints, see the *Heart attack* and *High blood pressure* chapters.

- **Moderate your calcium intake.** An irregular heartbeat can be a symptom of too much or too little calcium in your blood. Your muscles, including your heart, need calcium to contract. Make sure you get plenty of calcium from your diet. If you take supplements, don't overdo it.

- **Oil up your blood vessels**. You know too much fat can clog your arteries and damage your heart. But did you know if you replace the saturated fats in your diet with polyunsaturated fats, like the kind found in sunflower seed oil and fish oil, you may help your heart keep a steady beat. Studies have found that sunflower seed oil and fish oil decreased the severity and frequency of arrhythmias in animals, but researchers aren't sure if they have the same effect in humans. Since polyunsaturated fats are healthier for your heart anyway, why not try sautéing your veggies in a little sunflower seed oil or throw some salmon on the grill. The oil might steady your heartbeat, but the taste may just make your heart skip a beat.

Mondays are hazardous to your health

Many people dread Monday mornings, and now they have a good reason. A recent study found that Mondays can be hazardous to your health, even after you've retired. A deadly type of arrhythmia that can cause sudden cardiac death occurs more often on Monday mornings than any other time. Another smaller peak occurs on Friday. You are least likely to experience arrhythmias on Saturday or Sunday. Researchers speculate that the pressure of going to work on Monday increases your production of stress hormones that may trigger arrhythmias. This establishes a pattern over the years that doesn't just disappear with retirement.

Can you do anything to prevent this Monday morning phenomenon from striking you? Unless you're wealthy enough to avoid working for a living, the only answer may be to relax and remember that another weekend is always just around the corner.

ARTHRITIS

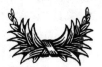

4 winning ways to attack arthritis

If you think painkillers are the only way to relieve your arthritis symptoms, you need to think again. According to recent research, several vitamins and minerals can provide natural relief from your pain.

- **Get plenty of antioxidants.** Arthritis may have a powerful enemy in antioxidants. One study in Boston found that people with osteoarthritis of the knee who had a high intake of antioxidants were less likely to have the disease progress any further. The people who had the highest intake of vitamin C, a major antioxidant, were three times less likely to have their arthritis get worse. Vitamin C helps build and repair all the connective tissues in your body. This includes the ligaments, tendons, and cartilage that surround and cushion your bones. In some forms of arthritis, the cartilage between your joints becomes frayed and worn, leaving a painful bone-grinding connection. Vitamin C may help keep your joints comfortably cushioned.

  The antioxidants vitamin E and beta-carotene also helped, though not as much as vitamin C. Another study found that people with low levels of vitamin E, beta-carotene, and selenium were more likely to develop rheumatoid arthritis.

  Eat plenty of fresh fruits and vegetables every day to get lots of anti-arthritis antioxidants.

- **Add some B vitamins.** A recent study found that people who received a daily supplement containing 6,400 micrograms (mcg) of folic acid (B9) and 20 mcg of cobalamin (B12) had as much gripping power in their hands as people who used NSAIDs like aspirin and ibuprofen. They also had fewer tender joints.

  To get the most effective dose of these pain-killing B vitamins, ask your doctor for a prescription. You'll pay less for them, and your doctor will be able to monitor any side effects.

- **Delight in some D.** Vitamin D is vital to building healthy bones. That may explain why one large study found that some people with osteoarthritis were three times less likely than others to have their disease get worse. These people took in at least twice as much vitamin D as the study participants who were getting less than the recommended dietary allowance (RDA). If you think you are not getting enough vitamin D, go soak up some sunshine or eat plenty of vitamin D-rich foods like milk and eggs.

- **Check your iron.** Your body needs iron to build healthy blood, but some people have trouble maintaining a healthy iron level. If you have arthritis, you may not have enough of this important mineral. Arthritis sufferers who take aspirin or other nonsteroidal anti-inflammatories (NSAIDs) on a regular basis may have a tendency to bleed more freely. This loss of blood can lead to iron deficiency anemia, a condition that can usually be corrected easily with supplements or iron-rich foods like meat, poultry, fish, and eggs.

Let your doctor decide if you need iron supplements. Taking too much iron can cause iron overload, a serious condition that can damage your liver.

Feast on fish for pain-free joints

Does your rheumatoid arthritis make you feel like you've been sleeping in a sardine can when you wake up in the morning? Eating sardines for dinner occasionally might relieve some of that morning stiffness. According to researchers, people with rheumatoid arthritis who eat fish containing omega-3 fatty acids have fewer tender joints and less morning stiffness. Adding fatty fish like salmon, sardines, tuna, or herring to your diet regularly may not cure your arthritis, but it could be a delicious way to loosen up your joints. If you choose to take fish oil capsules instead, the effective amount is 3 to 5 grams daily.

Veggies ease arthritis symptoms

If you don't already love broccoli and spinach, the pain of arthritis may make them seem more appealing. Studies show that many people with rheumatoid arthritis benefit from a vegetarian diet. Researchers aren't sure why vegetarian diets help, but they think it could be because meat affects the types of fatty acids in your blood. Your immune system uses these fatty acids to make substances that can cause inflammation.

If you decide to avoid meat, make sure you get enough protein from other sources. Soy is a healthful meat substitute. For more information about soy, see the *Super foods* section.

Super supplement hailed as arthritis cure

You may have heard about a new wonder supplement that rebuilds joints and reverses arthritis. Featured in the book, *The Arthritis Cure,* and widely marketed by health food companies, glucosamine sulfate is touted as a superior form of arthritis pain relief.

Its most sensational feature is its ability to rebuild tissue you've lost in your joints. Sound too good to be true? Maybe not.

Glucosamine is a natural compound of glucose and amino acids. It forms the main ingredient for most of the connective and cushioning tissue in your body. It is the breakdown of these tissues — such as cartilage and synovial fluids — that causes the pain and immobility of osteoarthritis.

The theory behind glucosamine supplements is that if you replace this important building block, your joint tissue will start to build up again. And it looks like the theory might work.

When combined with a sulfate, glucosamine apparently stimulates your cartilage to regrow. At the same time, it reduces swelling in your joints and eases the painful symptoms of arthritis. In clinical tests, glucosamine sulfate supplements consistently showed better results than both traditional arthritis remedies and placebo groups.

In one Portuguese test that involved more than 1,200 arthritis sufferers, 95 percent of those who took glucosamine showed a positive response to the supplement. All of them had significantly less pain while resting, standing, and exercising.

In other studies, glucosamine has increased patient mobility, reduced joint swelling, and provided better and longer-lasting pain relief than ibuprofen. Many doctors, however, are reluctant to recommend glucosamine because most of the studies have been relatively short-term, usually lasting four to eight weeks.

According to the authors of *The Arthritis Cure,* glucosamine sulfate supplements should be taken as part of an anti-arthritis regimen that also includes exercise and a well-balanced diet. These doctors recommend a dosage between 1,000 and 2,000 mg per day, depending on your weight. You should take the supplements several times throughout the day, preferably with meals. The authors also stress getting enough vitamin C and manganese in your diet, as these important nutrients can increase the effectiveness of the supplements.

Glucosamine supplements are classified as a "dietary supplement," and, therefore, are not regulated by the government. That means they are not approved by the Food and Drug Administration. Although the supplement appears to be safe and may be effective in treating osteoarthritis, this lack of regulation means you can't be sure of the quality and purity of the product you buy.

As always, it's best to check with your doctor before taking any supplements, particularly large amounts. As part of a balanced program, glucosamine supplements may help you stem arthritis pain and feel more like your old self again.

Exotic oils soothe joints

You may have heard that fish oil is good for arthritis symptoms, but according to recent studies, some unusual oils may also reduce joint inflammation in people with rheumatoid arthritis. These oils include evening primrose, flaxseed, rapeseed, and borage seed oils. They contain a fatty acid similar to omega-3 called gammalinolenic acid (GLA). Because these oils aren't found in foods you normally eat, you have to get them from supplements. The effective dose is 1 to 2 grams daily.

Water down your joints

If you have arthritis, relaxing in a bathtub full of warm water may ease your aching joints, but drinking a glass of cool water may also help. Water helps cushion and lubricate your joints. You should drink at least eight glasses of water a day to help keep your joints gliding smoothly along.

Foods that make you ache

If you eat tomatoes and then have a joint-aching flare-up of arthritis, that probably doesn't mean the tomatoes caused your pain. Although the percentage of people who have allergic reactions to foods is very small, many people believe some foods can trigger bouts of arthritis symptoms. If you think certain foods may be making your arthritis worse, try eliminating them from your diet one at a time until you see an improvement. Just remember that arthritis symptoms tend to come and go, and the relief you feel after eliminating a particular food could be a coincidence. Try eating the trouble-making food again to see if it causes symptoms. The foods most often thought to aggravate arthritis include milk; shrimp; wheat products; certain meats; and nightshade vegetables like tomatoes, potatoes, eggplant, and bell peppers.

Gout: avoiding a royal pain

Wise old Ben Franklin once said, "Be temperate in wine, in eating, girls, and sloth; or the gout will seize you and plague you both." This warning not to overdo food and alcohol was sound advice. In

Ben's day, gout was thought of as the "disease of kings." It seemed to strike mostly wealthy men who indulged in the rich food and alcohol that poor people couldn't afford.

Gout is a form of arthritis that begins when you have too much uric acid in your body. This excess acid forms needle-like crystals that can lodge in or around a joint, causing inflammation and extreme pain. Although gout can affect many areas of your body, your big toe suffers the pain of gout most often.

Researchers now know that the tendency to develop gout is partly genetic, but eating certain foods, being overweight, and bingeing on alcohol can make you more likely to get the condition. Over half of the people with gout are overweight, so your best strategy for avoiding this condition may be to maintain a healthy weight. The following suggestions might also help.

- **Pass on the purines.** If you would like to help control your gout naturally, avoid foods that contain purines. Purines are substances that can increase the amount of urate in your body, which can cause uric acid crystals to form in your joints. Meat, especially organ meat, yeast, beans, peas, spinach, asparagus, and cauliflower are high in purines.
- **Limit your alcohol.** If you down too many double martinis or bottles of beer, a hangover may be your reward. But if you have gout, too much alcohol can make your joints, as well as your head, throb with pain. Alcoholic beverages increase the amount of uric acid in your blood. Binge drinking, in particular, may bring on a painful attack of gout.
- **Wash it away with water.** Drinking alcohol may be a no-no for a person with gout, but other fluids, especially water, are a definite yes. Drink six to eight glasses of water daily to help flush uric acid out of your body before it can set off painful inflammation in your joints.

You don't have to be rich for gout to strike you, but take some of Ben Franklin's advice — go easy on the food and alcohol. It may help you avoid the "disease of kings."

Ginger takes ache out of arthritis

Recent research suggests that ginger may work as a natural anti-inflammatory, reducing the redness, pain, and swelling that often accompanies arthritis. A 2-1/2-year study conducted in Denmark of 56 people who suffered with arthritis or muscle pain found ginger relieved muscle discomfort, pain, and swelling in three-quarters of the study participants.

The people who experienced relief with ginger took an average of 5 grams of fresh ginger or 1 gram of powdered ginger daily. Some people in the study decided to take extra ginger and took up to 4 grams of powdered ginger a day. The lead researcher, Krishna Srivastava, Ph.D., noted that the more ginger people took, the greater their relief.

Another study of seven people with rheumatoid arthritis found that ginger provided substantial pain relief while the conventional drugs they were taking only provided partial or temporary relief. Six of the participants in this study took 5 grams of fresh ginger or 0.1 to 1 gram of powdered ginger daily. One participant consumed 50 grams of lightly cooked ginger each day. All of the people in this study reported better joint movement and less pain, stiffness, and swelling.

None of the people in the study reported any serious side effects from taking ginger.

A natural remedy for arthritis is welcome news to people who regularly relieve their pain with nonsteroidal anti-inflammatory drugs (NSAIDs). NSAIDs, such as aspirin and ibuprofen, are notorious for causing ulcers, which lead to thousands of deaths each year. All of the 200 drugs currently used to relieve arthritis pain have side effects.

ASTHMA

Cures from your kitchen

Enjoy a bowl of chicken soup. Your asthma is kicking in. You can feel your chest tightening. You start to wheeze. Mucus seems to clog your lungs. Wouldn't it be comforting to find a bit of relief in something as natural and satisfying as mom's homemade chicken soup?

You know that expectorants can ease the after-effects of an asthma attack and soothe your cough. That's because these products help thin and loosen the phlegm in your chest. Scientists have now proven that hot liquids, especially chicken soup, also help break up congestion and nasal mucus.

Inhaling the warm vapor definitely helps, but that apparently is not the only benefit. Chicken soup seems to have some unique characteristic that works either through its scent or its taste to thin the phlegm in your chest and head. Mom always knew that old-fashioned chicken soup was more than just old-fashioned good.

Feast on cold-water fish. From the cold oceans beneath the northern lights comes help for asthma sufferers. A study of Eskimo, Japanese, and Dutch populations links a diet high in omega-3 fatty acids, or fish oil, to low instances of asthma.

Small amounts of fish oil over a long period of time seem to give the best results. This strategy makes it easier for the average person to work it into their normal diet. The best natural sources are mackerel, salmon, striped bass, lake trout, herring, lake whitefish, anchovy, bluefish, and halibut. If you'd like to try fish oil supplements, check with your doctor first.

Pour yourself a cup of coffee. You still have your morning coffee or daily soda in spite of all the bad press on caffeine. Well, now you can feel better about it if you have asthma. Scientists report that caffeine can actually help some asthma sufferers by relaxing and expanding the air passages in the lungs. But don't overdo it. Too much caffeine can increase your blood pressure and heart rate and cause insomnia. A moderate amount, especially during an asthma attack, may feel like a breath of fresh air.

Clear the way for easier breathing

Researchers have discovered that people with asthma have lower than normal levels of several important nutrients. In several studies, when the asthma sufferers took supplements of these nutrients, their symptoms improved. Doctors are still exploring exactly why this is so, but they do know that a careful balance of nutrients keeps the body's systems working in harmony. When you don't have enough of any single nutrient, it can affect every process.

Breathe easier with vitamin C. A test group of asthmatics took supplements of 1 to 2 grams of vitamin C, a natural antihistamine. In the majority of cases, breathing symptoms improved.

Try to get as much vitamin C as possible from natural sources like citrus fruits and juices, strawberries, broccoli, brussels sprouts, and sweet red peppers.

Before taking large doses of any supplement, check with your doctor. Too much vitamin C in your body can cause diarrhea and other side effects.

Lower your risk with E. Low levels of vitamin E may put you at a higher risk of developing asthma, while getting more E may offer some protection. Vitamin E is a powerful antioxidant, which means it protects your cells from damage by free radicals. Some healthy food sources are baked sweet potatoes, sunflower seeds, and fortified cereals.

If you're watching your fat intake, you may want to take a supplement, since many foods high in vitamin E are also high in fat. Although vitamin E is relatively safe, large doses — over 400 international units (IU) — taken over a prolonged period of time may cause blurred vision, diarrhea, dizziness, headaches, nausea, or unusual fatigue.

Consider selenium. Several studies show that asthmatics tend to have low levels of selenium, a mineral that functions much like vitamin E in the body. When a test group of asthmatics took 100 micrograms (mcg) of sodium selenite, a selenium supplement, their breathing abilities improved.

You can add selenium to your diet naturally. Good sources include liver, kidney, and seafood. If you want to try supplements, talk it over with your doctor. Too much selenium can be toxic.

Open airways with magnesium. A diet rich in magnesium may help your lungs and airways fight the muscle spasms of asthma attacks. In fact, one form of the mineral, magnesium sulfate, has been used by doctors to help asthma sufferers breathe easier.

It's best to get the magnesium you need from natural food sources, since this spreads its absorption throughout the day. Eat nuts, legumes, soybeans, seafood, and dark green vegetables to be sure you're getting the recommended dietary allowance (RDA) for magnesium — 280 to 350 milligrams (mg).

The healing power of ginkgo

You have probably heard of ginkgo helping just about every ailment known to man. While that may not be quite true, it certainly seems to have many healing qualities. One is its ability to prevent bronchospasms, a sudden narrowing of the main air passages from the windpipe to the lungs. If you have asthma, a bronchospasm feels like a tightening or squeezing in your chest that makes it difficult to breathe.

Ginkgo biloba extract, or GBE, is sold as a food supplement. While no serious side effects have been reported, some people taking ginkgo experience headaches or digestive problems.

How to head off attacks

Most asthma attacks are triggered by allergens, substances that can cause you to have an allergic reaction. With a little foresight, you can keep most of these allergens under control.

Know what foods to avoid. If you have a food allergy, you may not have asthma, but if you have asthma, you could have a food allergy. Confused? It's not surprising. What this really means is that if you have asthma, you could have an allergic reaction to certain foods, which would then bring on an asthma attack.

The most common allergic triggers are shellfish, soy, wheat, nuts, eggs, fish, chocolate, and milk. Other foods could also cause a reaction. That's why it's important to notice what you eat and how your body responds.

Go easy on processed foods. Much of the food you eat is processed. This means that flavorings, preservatives, sweeteners, conditioners, and artificial colors are added to make the products look or taste better and last longer on the shelf. Amazingly, very few people react to the more than 2,000 FDA-approved additives that are routinely added to food. But there are exceptions.

- FD&C yellow No. 5 is used in cake mixes, chewing gum, ice cream, cheese, and soft drinks. Some people will have an asthma attack after eating one of these artificially colored products.
- MSG stands for monosodium glutamate. It's a flavor enhancer that can bring on severe asthma attacks in people sensitive to this additive.
- Sulfites are used to preserve food and to sterilize the bottles used for alcoholic beverages, like wine. They often trigger attacks in sulfite-sensitive asthmatics. Foods high in sulfites are dried fruits, except dark raisins and prunes; bottled lemon and lime juice; beer, wine, and wine coolers; pickled foods; molasses; dried potatoes; sparkling grape juice; wine vinegar; gravy; and maraschino cherries. A common place to find sulfite-treated foods is at a salad bar.

When you're grocery shopping, make sure you read food labels. When you dine out, ask your waiter to find out if the restaurant uses any of these additives.

Watch what you eat before exercising. If you have a condition called exercise-induced asthma (EIA), you know that vigorous activity can set off a chain reaction in your airways that leaves you dizzy, tired, and wheezing. It's a common problem for asthma sufferers, affecting 80 to 90 percent of them.

But did you know that eating certain foods even two hours before you exercise can trigger an episode? Doctors have discovered that shrimp, celery, peanuts, egg whites, almonds, and bananas are the most common causes of food-related EIA attacks. In some cases, the typical asthma symptoms become worse than usual, even resulting in collapse.

So, if you find that even the stairs are giving you trouble, you may have EIA. Watch your diet before you head to the tennis courts, and leave the banana behind.

Beware of royal jelly. Royal jelly is a substance honey bees produce as food for their larvae. It can reportedly boost your energy, your immune system, and improve other aspects of your health. But for some people, it can mean a sudden life-threatening asthma attack or allergic reaction. Allergists and immunologists believe that royal jelly contains something that triggers a reaction in certain people. If you plan on taking royal jelly, watch out for signs of an allergic reaction — coughing or itching on the roof of your mouth, on your palms, or on your feet.

Kitchen culprit doubles your risk

If you can't stand the heat ... get out of the kitchen, but only if you have a gas stove. Researchers say if you cook with gas, you are at least twice as likely to develop breathing problems, especially the wheezing and shortness of breath associated with asthma.

They believe the cause is nitrogen dioxide, a pollutant produced by gas cooking. Using an exhaust fan doesn't seem to help since it only removes cooking odors and water vapor, not cooking fumes. So, the next time you plan dinner, think about not only what you cook, but how you cook it.

Iron out your asthma

Iron is essential to life. It's found in hemoglobin, the part of your blood that carries oxygen throughout your body. Without oxygen, your body dies. But, while too little iron can cause problems like anemia, researchers now think too much iron may cause asthma. If you take an iron supplement, make sure you don't take in more than the recommended dietary allowance (RDA). The RDA for adults over 50 is 10 mg a day. This is one case where more is definitely not better.

Break this startling link to asthma

You probably never thought suffering from heartburn could make it hard to breathe, but doctors have discovered an amazing link between gastroesophageal reflux disease (GERD) and asthma. Studies show that up to 80 percent of asthma sufferers also have GERD, a condition where stomach acid backs up into the esophagus, causing heartburn.

If your breathing problems didn't start until you were an adult and there's no history of asthma in your family, heartburn could be causing your symptoms. Other signs are wheezing or coughing at night or after exercise or meals.

If you treat your reflux disorder, you may find asthma relief at the same time. Talk it over with your doctor and follow his advice.

For more information about reflux, see the *Heartburn and indigestion* chapter.

ATHEROSCLEROSIS

Healthy eating = healthy arteries

The thought of eating healthy, low-fat foods seems like a good idea until you think of your favorite creamy dessert or a big, juicy cheeseburger. But switching your preferences to a lucious piece of fruit or a casserole made with wholes grains and vegetables can make the difference between healthy arteries or blood vessels filled with plaque.

Fat combines with cholesterol and builds up in your arteries. The result — atherosclerosis, a clogging and hardening of the arteries that frequently leads to heart attacks, strokes, and other health problems. Making a few simples changes in your diet could protect your heart and your arteries from disease.

Think fruits, veggies, and grains. Plan more of your meals around fruits, vegetables, and grains. For example, dishes that combine beans and rice are filling and high in protein. You might replace some of the meat protein in your diet with soy-based foods like tofu. Whole-grain breads and cereals and fruits and vegetables have a lot of fiber, which helps lower LDL "bad" cholesterol, and it may even raise HDL "good" cholesterol. Fruits and vegetables also contain the antioxidants vitamin C, vitamin E, beta carotene, and selenium. Antioxidants prevent harmful free radicals from damaging your arteries.

You don't have to cut out meat altogether — just choose lean cuts and eat smaller portions. Fish and skinless turkey and chicken are lower in fat than beef and pork. And don't stop eating calcium-rich dairy products. Just pick low-fat or fat-free varieties.

Choose healthy fats. Eating foods high in saturated fat can increase your cholesterol level. Saturated fat is found in animal products like meat, egg yolks, milk, cream, butter, and cheese. Several vegetable fats, such as coconut oil, palm oil, and hydrogenated vegetable oils, are also high in saturated fat. Saturated fats are usually hard or solid at room temperature.

Studies show that foods high in polyunsaturated fats, like safflower oil and sunflower oil, lower bad LDL cholesterol, but they may also lower good HDL cholesterol. According to experts, foods high in monounsaturated fats, like olive oil and canola oil, lower bad cholesterol but not good cholesterol.

The American Heart Association recommends you limit your fat to 30 percent of your calories. Less than 10 percent of your calories should come from saturated fat. But remember, these guidelines are for healthy adults. If you have high cholesterol or heart disease, follow your doctor's advice.

Add some omega-3 fatty acids. These fatty acids help lower LDL cholesterol and raise HDL cholesterol. Fish that live in cold, deep waters, like salmon, tuna, and sardines, are rich sources of omega-3. If you don't like fish, oat germ; walnuts; soybean products; flaxseed; several kinds of dry beans; and purslane, a type of lettuce used in soups and salads in Mediterranean countries also contain omega-3, but generally in smaller amounts than fish.

If you avoid saturated fat and cholesterol and eat more fruits, veggies, and grains, you'll help your arteries and your heart. To lower your risks even more, exercise, maintain a healthy weight, and stop smoking.

For more information, see the *High cholesterol* chapter.

'B'eef up your defense

Beans and green vegetables should be a regular part of your diet. They contain B vitamins that help you fight another enemy of healthy arteries — homocysteine. This substance, a byproduct of protein metabolism, damages and narrows your arteries, which can lead to heart attacks and strokes. Homocysteine may even be more harmful than cholesterol, especially if you smoke or have high blood pressure.

This was clear from a study of 750 people with atherosclerosis. The people who had the highest levels of homocysteine were at a greater risk of death than those with high cholesterol. Smokers and people with high blood pressure had an even greater risk.

Folic acid (B9) works with two other B vitamins, cobalamin (B12) and pyridoxine (B6), to keep homocysteine from damaging your arteries. Folic acid is plentiful in pinto and kidney beans, avocado, spinach, asparagus, and broccoli. Beef liver, oysters, salmon, cottage cheese, and milk are good sources of vitamin B12. You can find B6 in baked potatoes with their skins, bananas, avocados, and chicken.

Some people, especially the elderly, are deficient in B vitamins. If you feel you need more than you can get from your diet, talk it over with your doctor before taking supplements. Getting too much of one or more of these vitamins can cause serious side effects.

Coffee lovers take heart

If you drink coffee and smoke, watch out for clogged arteries. A study in Norway found that coffee drinking raised cholesterol and homocysteine levels, especially in smokers. Both of these substances can lead to the buildup of plaque, which clogs arteries and causes heart attacks and strokes. This was true of people who drank filtered, boiled, and instant coffee but not decaffeinated.

The study also showed that people who got plenty of folic acid, from fruits and vegetables or vitamin supplements, were protected from the bad effects of coffee drinking. There was also a mild connection between tea drinking and lower levels of homocysteine, probably because tea contains small amounts of folic acid.

Another study reported on the long-term use of unfiltered coffee made by the plunger method called cafetière. People who drank five to six cups of coffee made by this method increased their risk of a heart attack by 12 to 20 percent. The risk decreased, however, when they switched to filtered coffee.

Unclog your arteries with vitamin C

When you look at your plate and find steamed broccoli and tomato slices, and maybe some cantaloupe on the side, you'll see a good helping of vitamin C. And what you see is good for your blood vessels and good for your heart, especially if you have atherosclerosis.

In a recent study at Boston University, a single dose of vitamin C opened up the clogged blood vessels of the people in the study. According to the researchers, vitamin C's antioxidant effect seemed to be responsible for the healthy improvement.

Vitamin C also lowers your cholesterol and reduces the buildup of plaque in your arteries. These are good reasons to include a lot of heart-healthy fruits and vegetables in your diet.

Nature's spicy blood clot buster

Ginger is a versatile herb. It not only adds flavor to your meals, it does double duty when it comes to keeping the blood flowing smoothly through your blood vessels. Ginger works as an antioxidant to fight the buildup of plaque that hardens and clogs arteries.

And it keeps blood from clotting by reducing the stickiness of blood platelets. Ginger also improves the digestion of fats, which lowers the amount of cholesterol in your blood.

A study done in India showed that 5 grams of ginger a day reduced the stickiness of platelets, making blood less likely to clot, even after a high-fat meal. Although that doesn't mean you can eat all the fat you want just by adding ginger to your diet, it's good to know ginger is a helpful weapon in your battle against atherosclerosis.

Just a word of caution — if you are taking heart medicine, talk with your doctor before using ginger. Ginger might intensify the effects of certain heart medicines, which can be dangerous.

Optimism could save your life

If you have atherosclerosis, being hopeful about the future can protect you from a stroke. That seems to be the message coming from a study in Finland.

Researchers studied the degree of hopelessness in 942 men who had atherosclerosis in their carotid arteries. These large arteries, located in the neck, provide blood to the brain.

Four years after the original testing, researchers did a follow up. Again they measured the thickness of the men's carotid arteries, an indication of the risk of stroke.

The men who expressed the strongest feelings of hopelessness at the beginning of the study showed the most thickening of their carotid arteries.

Researchers hope to determine why hopelessness increases the risk of stroke. If you have atherosclerosis, it's a good idea to eat a low-fat diet, stop smoking, maintain a healthy weight, get plenty of exercise, and lower your high blood pressure. Taking charge of your life will help remove the feelings of hopelessness. So keep the faith. Where there's hope, there's life.

Healthier arteries the Mediterranean way

In the early '60s, scientists noticed that the people of Greece lived longer and had less heart disease and some other diseases than people of most other cultures. This prompted researchers to take a look at their diet, and here's what they discovered.

Greeks eat lots of antioxidant-rich fresh fruits and vegetables, as well as whole-grain breads and pastas. Fish and chicken are eaten only a few times a week and red meat only several times a month. They also consume large amounts of olive oil, a monounsaturated fat that may lower cholesterol. Wine is also a normal part of a Greek meal. Two glasses of wine a day for men and one glass for women may lower the risk of heart disease, according to some studies. The Greeks eat very little dairy products, except for cheese and yogurt. Fresh fruit is served for dessert instead of sweets.

This heart-healthy diet might help you live longer. In one study, people with atherosclerosis who followed a Mediterranean-style diet showed a whopping 76 percent reduction in their risk of heart attack, stroke, and heart failure.

BRUISING

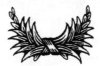

Beat bruises with vitamins

If you smack your shin into the corner of your coffee table, you probably expect to have a bruise the next day. However, when bruises appear for no apparent reason, the cause may be your diet rather than your clumsiness. A vitamin deficiency can sometimes cause unexplained bruising.

- **Keep up your vitamin K.** Vitamin K is responsible for producing substances that help your blood clot. Your body makes vitamin K from bacteria in your intestines, although you can also get it from food sources. If you take antibiotics or have a liver disorder or ongoing diarrhea, you may become deficient in vitamin K. Because a deficiency in vitamin K reduces your blood's ability to clot, it can lead to unexplained bleeding or bruising. Pump up your vitamin K intake by eating leafy green vegetables, egg yolks, vegetable oil, cheese, and liver.

- **Get your fill of vitamin C.** Vitamin C helps your body make collagen, which is needed for healthy skin, bones, teeth, and blood vessels. When you don't get enough of this vitamin, your blood vessels can weaken, causing bruising or bleeding under your skin. Vitamin C is easy to get in your diet. It is found in fruits, particularly citrus fruits like oranges and grapefruits. Green leafy vegetables, green peppers, and strawberries are also good sources of vitamin C.

CANCER

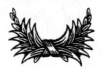

Vitamins that vanquish cancer

In 1900, diarrhea killed more people than cancer. Today, people rarely die from diarrhea, but cancer has become the number two killer disease. Why has cancer become so widespread? The answer may be on your dinner plate. About 40 percent of cancers in men and 60 percent of cancers in women are associated with diet. That's because some foods, or the way you cook them, may actually put you more at risk for cancer.

If you get enough of certain vitamins, however, you may give yourself a fighting chance against this disease. Vitamins are a vital part of a healthful diet, and research finds that some vitamins may protect you from one of today's most dangerous killers.

- **Beat the "big C" with vitamin C.** Cancer may sometimes be referred to as the "big C," but its biggest enemy could be vitamin C. Many large studies have found vitamin C to be an effective cancer preventive. The protective effect of vitamin C is particularly strong for cancers of the stomach, esophagus, mouth, and pancreas. Adding some vitamin C to your diet may also save you from cancers of the rectum, breast, and cervix. It may even help protect you from lung cancer. Getting enough of this cancer-crushing vitamin isn't difficult. It can be found in most fresh fruits and vegetables, particularly citrus fruits like oranges.

- **Elevate your vitamin E.** If you eat a high-fat diet, you may also have a high chance of getting cancer. When your body tries to break down certain fats, it can produce cancer-causing chemicals. Vitamin E may help by stabilizing those fats and helping to rid your body of toxic chemicals. However, the main sources of vitamin E are fats, so if you want to prevent cancer, you have to be careful what form of vitamin E you get. Olive oil and wheat germ oil are good sources, and supplements are also an option.

- **Add some vitamin A and beta carotene.** Munch on mangos and chew on carrots, because fresh fruits and vegetables are brimming with beta carotene. Beta carotene is a precursor to vitamin A, which just means that it is turned into vitamin A in your body. Although studies show that foods high in beta carotene may protect against lung cancer, some studies have found that smokers who took beta carotene as supplements were actually more likely to get lung cancer. However, beta carotene from natural sources like spinach, broccoli, and apricots should reap nothing but good health for you. You can get vitamin A from dairy products and liver, but high dose supplements can be toxic and should not be taken without your doctor's advice.

- **Be sure to get this B vitamin.** Women who don't get enough of the B vitamin, folic acid, may have a higher risk of precancerous changes in the cervix. You'll have an even higher risk of cervical cancer if you also smoke, use oral contraceptives, or have numerous sexual partners. To get plenty of folic acid and help make sure your next pap smear comes back normal, eat folate-rich foods like spinach, beans, and broccoli.

- **Mix and match antioxidants.** Every breath you take may be creating cancer-causing free radicals. As your body processes oxygen, it also creates unstable molecules called free radicals. These maverick molecules can damage your cells, making you more likely to fall prey to cancer. Luckily, your body uses substances called antioxidants to wipe out free radicals. Some of the best antioxidants are vitamin E, vitamin C, and beta carotene. Several large studies have given a mixture of antioxidants to people to see if they help fight cancer. One study in China found that people who took a combination of vitamin E, beta carotene, and the mineral selenium were 13 percent less likely to die from cancer. Natural antioxidants in foods may prevent cancer better than those found in supplements.

Dirt-cheap mineral rich in cancer protection

Selenium, a mineral found in the soil, may substantially slash your risk of prostate, colon, and lung cancer. Don't dish up dirt for dinner, however. Food grown in that soil also contains selenium and is probably much tastier.

Studies have found that selenium may lower your risk of several types of cancer. Unfortunately, the soil in some parts of the country contains low levels of this important mineral. One study found that cancer rates were higher in such areas. Luckily, since selenium's health benefits have become known, some farmers have begun to include it in fertilizer.

Good sources of selenium include brazil nuts, brewer's yeast, broccoli, cabbage, garlic, chicken, mushrooms, radishes, and seafood. Getting plenty of selenium from foods may be wise, but taking supplements may not be. Too much selenium can cause serious side effects. The American Cancer Society does not advise taking selenium supplements, because the difference between a safe amount and a toxic amount is so small.

Slash cancer risk with Asian secret

Exotic, mysterious Asia may help unravel some of the mysteries of cancer. Many types of cancer that plague the rest of the world are uncommon in Asia. These include cancers of the breast, prostate, and colon, which are all strongly associated with dietary risk factors. What dietary delights do Asians dish up that keep them safe from cancer? Researchers have investigated some possibilities in the hopes that Asia might help the rest of the world lower cancer rates.

- **Serve up some soy.** If you want to avoid breast, uterine, or prostate cancer, perhaps you should start your day with a refreshing glass of soy milk, or end it with some soothing tofu. Some researchers believe that soy is responsible for the low rates of these cancers in the East. Soybeans provide a large portion of protein in the Japanese diet. Other Asian countries also enjoy soy products on a regular basis. Researchers think plant chemicals called "phytoestrogens" are responsible for the soybean's protective effect. They act like weaker versions of human hormones. A recent study found that women who ate the highest amount of phytoestrogen-rich foods were less than half as likely to get uterine cancer. Soy is one of the strongest providers of phytoestrogens.

- **Enjoy grains and vegetables**. A high-fiber diet can help lower your risk of cancer, and Asians get plenty of fiber daily. Grains like rice are present at nearly every meal, and fresh vegetables form a large part of the Asian diet.
- **Cut the fat in cooking**. Steam or stir-fry your supper, and you may keep cancer away. People who eat high-fat diets are more likely to get cancer, and much of the fat in your diet may come from your cooking methods. Asians could have lower cancer risks because they are more likely to stir-fry food in soy sauce instead of deep-frying in oil like many Americans. Rural Chinese get only about 14 percent of their daily calories from fat. Most Americans, on the other hand, get about 37 percent of their calories from fat.
- **Try tasty tea.** Tea could hold the key to locking out cancer. The green tea that is so popular in Asian countries may lower your risk of stomach, esophageal, gastrointestinal, liver, lung, and pancreatic cancers. Just one daily cup may cut your risk of esophageal cancer in half.

Asia may provide the rest of the world with other clues for avoiding cancer. Some of the herbs and flavorings used in cooking, such as onions and garlic, may provide cancer protection. Asians are less likely to overeat and become obese, which can increase your risk of many cancers. Most Asians also get more exercise than people in many other parts of the world, because they walk or bicycle instead of relying on cars.

Although Asians are less likely to get most types of cancer, they tend to have higher rates of stomach and esophageal cancers. Scientists think regular use of pickled and smoked food causes these higher cancer rates. Overall, however, low cancer rates in the Orient give the rest of the world reason to adopt many Asian eating habits.

Best drink for healthy breasts

You may have had your first taste of an effective breast-protector at your mother's breast. Researchers have discovered that milk may help prevent breast cancer. A recent study followed more than 4,000 women for 25 years. Researchers found that women who drank the most milk had the least chance of getting breast cancer. Other dairy products didn't have the same protective effect. Since you already know that milk helps keep your bones strong, drink up for healthy bones *and* healthy breasts.

Detect breast cancer early to save lives

Did you know that in one year, almost as many Americans die from breast cancer as were killed during the 12 years of the Vietnam War? To keep from becoming one of the casualties in the war on breast cancer, follow these American Cancer Society guidelines:

- **Age 20 to 39:** Do a breast self-exam monthly, have a doctor's exam every three years, and get your first mammogram by age 40.
- **Age 40 to 49:** Continue your monthly self-exams, have a doctor's exam every year, and get a mammogram every one to two years.
- **Age 50+:** Monthly self-exams are still important. Have a doctor's exam and a mammogram yearly.

Cancer-causing food you should quit

You know that cigarette smoke contributes to cancer, but did you know that smoked foods can also raise your cancer risk? Foods that are smoked, salt-cured, or salt-pickled may make you more likely to get cancer of the stomach or esophagus. The heat from smoking may create carcinogens in the food, and salt cured or pickled foods contain nitrates that may become carcinogens in your stomach.

Fiber-filled diet fends off cancer

Fill up with fiber every day, and you may fend off cancer. A high-fiber diet can especially lower your risk of colon and rectal cancer. Fiber speeds food through your digestive tract so your body gets less exposure to carcinogens that may be in the food.

The National Cancer Institute says most people need to double their amount of daily fiber. It recommends 20 to 30 grams a day rather than the 11 grams the average person takes in. However, to avoid side effects, such as excessive gas, don't get more than 35 grams a day.

To take advantage of this easy cancer-thwarting strategy, eat more whole-grain breads, pastas, and cereals; and add some extra fruits and vegetables to your diet.

A matter of fat

Face the facts. People don't like fat on their bodies, but most people love fat in their mouths. Buttery biscuits and fried burgers may be tasty, but they might cause more than just a pot belly or thunder thighs. Dietary fat may also contribute to the development of cancer.

Studies find that a high-fat diet may raise your risk of cancer of the colon, rectum, prostate, and endometrium (lining of the uterus). Although fat has long been thought to contribute to breast cancer, new studies are finding that may not be the case. There may, however, be a relationship between a high-fat diet and lung cancer, the number one cancer killer. One study found that women who ate high-fat diets were five times more likely to get lung cancer than women who ate low-fat diets.

Even though fat may raise your risk of cancer, scientists don't consider it a carcinogen, or cancer-causing substance. However, if you have been exposed to a carcinogen, a high-fat diet can help cancer get started in your body and grow.

According to the American Cancer Society, the average American gets about 37 percent of his calories from fat. It recommends you cut your fat intake to less than 30 percent of your total daily calories. For example, if you normally eat 1,800 calories a day, you shouldn't get more than 540 calories from fat.

Dietary tips to avoid cancer

The American Cancer Society works hard to find ways to help prevent cancer. Through extensive research, it has come up with the following dietary recommendations:

- Choose most of the foods you eat from plant sources.
- Limit your intake of high-fat foods, particularly from animal sources.
- Be physically active. Achieve and maintain a healthy weight.
- Limit consumption of alcoholic beverages, if you drink at all.

Olive oil — your bosom buddy

You've thrown out your usual bottle of cooking oil to cut calories and protect yourself from cancer. What can you use to fill the gap? Try some olive oil. While most fats may contribute to cancer risk, olive oil may help protect you from at least one — breast cancer.

Harvard researchers studied Greek women to find out if their low breast cancer rate might be the result of their high use of olive oil. They found that women who consumed olive oil more than once a day were less likely to get breast cancer than women who ate it once a day or less.

Olive oil is also a good natural source of vitamin E, which may provide additional antioxidant protection against cancer.

Cancer-smart alcohol consumption

You don't have to be an alcoholic to suffer side effects from alcohol consumption. Even a moderate intake of alcohol is associated with a higher risk of cancer of the breast, rectum, and pancreas. In larger amounts, alcohol may make you more likely to have cancer of the mouth, esophagus, and larynx. Excessive drinking also can damage your liver and increase your risk of liver cancer.

However, you may have heard that an occasional glass of wine is good for your heart, and a recent study suggests that it may help prevent cancer, too. The study found that red wine contains resveratrol, a strong cancer inhibitor. The resveratrol in wine comes from the skins of grapes. While wine may be enjoyable, eating grapes or drinking grape juice should provide you with cancer-fighting resveratrol without the possible added risks.

Though no one is sure about a link between alcohol and cancer, experts suggest that if you don't drink, don't start. If you do drink, limit your intake to less than one ounce of pure alcohol a day. That equals about two cans of beer, two glasses of wine, or two average cocktails.

Flavorful cancer fighters

Add some flavor to your food, and you could be doing your body a favor. Some familiar flavorings may help prevent cancer.

- **Garlic and onions.** Smelly breath may be a small price to pay for cancer protection. People who include lots of onions and garlic in their food, like the Chinese and Italians, may not always have kissably fresh breath, but they do have lower rates of stomach cancer. These aromatic vegetables contain flavonoids, plant compounds which may protect against cancer.

- **Basil.** Fresh basil may add more than zesty flavor to your foods. It can help your body increase production of glutathione, a substance that helps rid you of toxic, cancer-causing chemicals. Further studies need to be done to confirm basil's cancer-fighting abilities. In the meantime, it can be a delicious, healthful addition to your favorite dishes.
- **Rosemary.** To cut the fat in your cooking, you may be adding extra herbs and spices to replace the flavor. If rosemary is one of those herbs, you might be getting cancer protection as well. Rosemary is a strong antioxidant, and studies are finding that it may help prevent breast cancer.
- **Curry.** If your favorite restaurant serves spicy Indian food, count yourself lucky. It could be giving you extra cancer protection. Turmeric, the main ingredient in curry, contains a substance called curcumin that gives turmeric its yellow coloring. Turmeric can also be found in yellow rice. According to new research, curcumin may also help prevent the growth of colon tumors.

A grilling cancer risk

Some celebrations just wouldn't be the same without a cookout. Whether it's burgers, chicken, or steaks, cooking on an outdoor grill can add fun and flavor to your food. But be careful — it may also give your food extra cancer-causing potential. Smoke, flame, and high temperatures can create carcinogens in your food.

You don't have to give up grilling, however. Just take steps to protect yourself. Cook foods slowly, raise them as far away from the fire as possible, and wrap them in foil. Then you can enjoy your cookout without cancer worries.

Fruits and veggies weigh in against smoking

If everyone in the United States stopped smoking, the cancer rate would probably plummet. However, if everyone ate more fruits and vegetables, it could reduce the cancer rate even more. Studies find that people who eat lots of fruits and vegetables are about half as likely to get cancer. The American Cancer Society recommends that you eat at least five servings of fruits and vegetables daily.

According to a recent survey, 48 percent of the population believe that fruits and vegetables can lower their cancer risk. Apparently, knowing is only half the battle since only 9 percent of those surveyed eat the minimum recommended amount.

Although smoking may raise your risk of cancer more than not eating your veggies, the vegetable-avoiders outnumber the smokers. Cancer rates could drop drastically if people would put down their cigarettes and pick up some broccoli, oranges, or squash instead.

Turning the tide against cancer

The tide is slowly turning against cancer. In the years between 1971 and 1990, death rates from cancer climbed steadily. However, between 1991 and 1995, deaths from cancer were down for all segments of the population.

Former killer diseases like smallpox and polio were conquered through the discovery of effective vaccines. The victories against cancer have so far been smaller and not quite as dramatic. However, these small advances add up to fewer people dying from this dreaded disease.

Studies find that cancer often can be prevented through diet and lifestyle changes. Something as simple as the foods you eat every day may help determine whether you are struck by this devastating illness. Your daily diet gives you the power to fight this deadly disease, so take advantage of this power, and use it wisely.

Does coffee + chocolate = colorectal cancer?

If you're a chocoholic or a caffeine fiend, you may be more likely to get colorectal cancer. A recent study found that people who drank more than four cups of coffee a day were four times more likely to get colorectal cancer, and people who ate a candy bar every day were twice as likely to get it.

So if you drank four cups of coffee and ate a candy bar every day, would you be six times as likely to get colorectal cancer? The math may not add up, but if you want to avoid this type of cancer, maybe you should try subtracting some chocolate and caffeine from your diet.

Prostate protection from tomatoes and sunshine

If you want to avoid prostate cancer, perhaps you should stretch out on a lawn chair and order a pizza. Studies have found that vitamin D and tomato products may make you less likely to get this form of cancer.

- **Soak up some vitamin D.** A recent study found that men with a certain gene that helps them absorb vitamin D were less likely to get prostate cancer. This finding supports other studies that suggest the "sunshine vitamin" may help prevent the disease. For example, one study found that men who lived in areas with less sunlight were more likely to get prostate cancer. Since your body manufactures vitamin D from sunlight on your skin, the high rate of prostate cancer may have been due to lower levels of vitamin D. Of course, you can also get vitamin D from your diet. Some foods that are high in vitamin D include butter, egg yolk, liver, and fatty fish like tuna, salmon, and herring. Fortified cereals and dairy products are also good sources.

- **Take two tomatoes and call me in the morning.** A ripe, red tomato, fresh off the vine, looks delicious. The substance that gives tomatoes that inviting red color could help protect your prostate from cancer. Studies find that lycopene, a carotenoid found in tomatoes, may ward off prostate cancer. It may also help you avoid cancer of the pancreas and stomach. One large study on the effects of foods on prostate cancer found that three of four prostate-protecting foods were tomato products. They were tomatoes, tomato sauce, and pizza. Men in this study who ate 10 or more servings of tomato products a week were 45 percent less likely to get prostate cancer.

You may also get prostate protection from your diet by cutting the fat and adding some fiber instead. Early studies suggest that a low-fat, high-fiber diet can lower your risk of prostate cancer. It may also lower your weight. So when you order that prostate-protecting pizza, make sure you get it with low-fat cheese.

Clip colon cancer risk with calcium

If colon cancer runs in your family, run to the nearest grocery store and stock up on calcium-rich foods. Colon cancer has strong hereditary connections, but few cases can be blamed on genetics alone. Some extra calcium in your diet may help you avoid this disease.

A recent study at Loma Linda University found that calcium could reduce your risk of colon cancer. Calcium seems to slow down the rate at which colon cells multiply, making it less likely those cells will become cancerous.

Not for women only

The breast of a man is different from a woman's. It's one of the things that sets the two sexes apart. When it comes to breast cancer, there are also differences. The vast majority of breast cancer cases occur in women. However, men are not totally safe from this disease. About 1,400 cases and 260 deaths from breast cancer can be expected in men in one year. Even though that is less than 1 percent of the cases, men should be aware that it can happen to them. Regardless of your sex, report any changes in your breast to your doctor immediately.

CANKER SORES

Natural therapy for soothing sores

Are painful canker sores making you feeling cantankerous? These unpleasant sores usually erupt inside the lip or cheek, or on the tongue, making life miserable. Fortunately, they are not contagious and generally heal within a couple of weeks.

In the meantime, try not to fan the flames. Cool down hot foods before eating them. Avoid anything acidic, salty, spicy, or sugary like tomato sauce, pickled peaches, hot peppers, and lemon pie. Watch out for sharp edges of foods like potato chips that can further irritate the sores. Use a straw to avoid contact if you drink carbonated beverages.

Cold and creamy beats the heat. During an outbreak, cold milk can soothe the pain of eating with canker sores. Just swish a mouthful around, and swallow from time to time during your meal.

You may be able to prevent cankers by eating from four table-spoons to two cups of plain live-culture yogurt a day. Be sure to buy the kind that contains *Lactobacillus acidophilus,* a bacterium that keeps your immune system healthy.

Treat with tea and "E." A quick fix for the pain of a canker is as easy as a cup of tea — without the cup. Simply hold a wet tea bag in your mouth over the canker sore. Adjust the bag from time to time for comfort, but keep it over the sore for at least 10 minutes. The tannin in black tea is an astringent that will help dry up and heal the sore. Dandelion tea may also heal cankers and prevent their return.

For early treatment, punch a hole in a vitamin E capsule and squeeze the gel directly on the ulcers as soon as they appear. This can be repeated from time to time until they are healed.

Swish away pain. A good gargle can work wonders, too. Some studies suggest that certain bacteria in your mouth make it easier for sores to form. A solution of three parts water to one part hydrogen peroxide can help keep your mouth clean and make it harder for bacteria to grow. You might want to try a few of these herbal mouthwashes as well.

- **Goldenseal,** known for its ability to kill certain bacteria, can soothe and heal canker sores. Make a mouth rinse by mixing six grams (two teaspoons) of goldenseal in a cup of boiling water. After it cools you can rinse your mouth with it several times a day.
- **Myrrh** is another antibacterial substance that usually comes in an alcohol solution. You can use it directly on the sores or rinse your mouth with it. To make a mouthwash, mix five to 10 drops of the myrrh solution in a glass of water.
- **Sage** makes a good mouthwash for canker sores because it has both antiseptic and anti-inflammatory qualities. Add two teaspoons of finely cut sage to a cup of boiling water, mix, and cool before using.
- **Geranium and lavender oils,** one drop of each mixed with a half cup of water, make an aromatic mouthwash that can be used four times a day.
- **Deglycyrrhizinated liquorice mouthwash,** a mouthful to say, was tested in India on 20 people with canker sores. Fifteen subjects found a 50 to 75 percent improvement within one day, and their sores were completely healed within three days. The glycyrrhizine is removed from this form of licorice. That ingredient can cause serious side effects, especially for

people with high blood pressure and heart problems. Would sucking a piece of licorice candy do just as well? Probably not. Most so-called licorice candy made in this county is actually flavored with anise.

'Beef' up protection against canker sores

Allergies crank 'em up. Certain foods and drinks often trigger canker sores in some people. Among the most common are chocolate, seeds, nuts, gelatin, alcohol, and anything spicy or acidic.

In one study of 21 people with canker sores, 20 had food allergies. After being told what to avoid, 18 subjects reported an improvement in their condition. To prevent canker sores, try to figure out if you're allergic to certain foods. You may see an improvement in your own condition as well.

Sensitive to cinnamon? This spice is one of the worst culprits when it comes to causing canker sores. You may have already dropped red-hot candies, cinnamon-flavored chewing gum, and cinnamon buns. But it also hides in foods like cookies, cereals, and chili recipes, or flavored teas and coffees. And it's sometimes added to mouthwashes, toothpastes, and breath fresheners to make them taste better. To avoid an unpleasant surprise, it's a good idea to check the label for this hot ingredient in any product you put in your mouth.

Canker sores usually appear in places that come in direct contact with the cinnamon. People who frequently suck on hard candies tend to get them on one side of the tongue or cheek. Cinnamon tea drinkers, on the other hand, are more likely to get them throughout the mouth.

"B" alert and iron out deficiencies. What if you've given up everything that has any flavor and still suffer from painful sores? Maybe you're not getting enough iron and B vitamins, especially folic acid and B12. A lack of these seems to be a main cause of recurrent canker sores.

Eating lots of beef liver is one way to get enough of all three, but there are other, perhaps more tempting, alternatives. Good sources of iron and folic acid include green leafy vegetables and soybeans. To get both vitamin B12 and folic acid, try chicken livers. Another good source of B12 is fish, especially sardines, herring, and salmon.

Other missing B vitamins may lead to canker sores as well. You may be low in B1 (thiamine), found in brewer's yeast, beans, nuts, egg yolks, and fruits and vegetables; B2 (riboflavin), found in fish, poultry, milk, and green vegetables; or B6, (pyridoxine) found in avocados, bananas, chicken, turkey, and sunflower seeds.

Zero in on zinc. Your canker sores could be caused by a zinc deficiency. One study involved a 15-year-old boy who suffered with canker sores for six years. He was treated with a variety of medications, but the sores kept coming back. When doctors found he was deficient in zinc, they gave him 50 milligrams (mg) of zinc sulfate by mouth three times a day. After three months, the canker sores disappeared and did not come back for a year.

Before taking high doses of zinc, have your blood tested to see if you have a deficiency. The recommended dietary allowance for a healthy male is 15 mg. Most experts suggest that 50 mg per day is the most you should take even to restore a deficiency.

The best food sources of zinc are beef, oysters and other seafood, poultry, beans, and whole grains.

Do cankers lead to cancer?

If you're a canker sore sufferer who loves beer and hot dogs, you may want to rethink your choice of refreshments.

Beer and hot dogs contain nitrites, and research has shown that nitrites can turn into nitrosamines and cause cancer. Studies also show that people who get canker sores and eat a lot of nitrites are seven times more likely than average to get cancer of the esophagus.

But the good news is black tea and vitamin C seem to prevent nitrites from breaking down into cancer-causing nitrosamines. So you may want to drink iced tea or lemonade with those hot dogs instead of beer.

Nitrites are also found in smoked fish and processed meats like ham, bacon, sausage, and luncheon meats. You can also balance your nitrites with extra vitamin C by having a glass of orange juice with your breakfast bacon or sausage. Put lettuce and tomato on a ham sandwich. Keep a shaker of vitamin C sprinkles handy and add them freely at the table.

Vegetables contain nitrites, too. But they have other substances that prevent the breakdown of nitrites into nitrosamines. In fact, eating fresh vegetables actually seems to lower the risk of getting cancer.

Chances are, canker sores won't increase your risk of cancer. But eating more fresh vegetables and fewer processed meats is a healthy habit in any case.

CARPAL TUNNEL SYNDROME

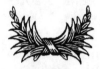

'B' aware of nutrition connections

If you work in an assembly plant, use a computer, do needlework, or pursue any job or hobby that involves repeating the same movement of your hands and wrists, you're a prime candidate for carpal tunnel syndrome. The problem often arises because you push yourself beyond the point where common sense tells you to stop. Frequent, brief breaks to stretch your hands could be enough to prevent the problem. But nutrition might play a part, too.

Vitamin B6 link? Several studies have investigated the link between vitamin B6 and carpal tunnel problems. The answer is still controversial. Some say a lack of vitamin B6 might cause carpal tunnel syndrome, and taking B6 supplements should improve it. Other studies show that supplements have no effect, and taking them may be unsafe. So how do you know if you have a B6 deficiency and whether you should treat it?

It's rare to have a true deficiency of vitamin B6. You are more likely to have a borderline case. If you are elderly, vitamin B6 is naturally in shorter supply in your body, so you are more at risk. Also, certain prescription drugs, including birth control pills, can keep you from absorbing B6.

Signs of a vitamin B6 deficiency include numbness, tingling, and pain in your hands and feet. Unfortunately, these are the same symptoms of a B6 overdose. If you don't know which you have, you could harm yourself by taking a supplement. With a deficiency, your symptoms will go away with treatment; but with an overdose, they may become permanent. Therefore, you should let your doctor decide whether a supplement is necessary.

Usually you get enough vitamin B6 in the foods you eat every day. Protein foods, such as chicken, pork, fish, and dried beans, are rich in vitamin B6. So are whole grains, wheat germ, potatoes, and bananas. By eating a variety of healthy foods, you'll keep up your body's stash of vitamin B6 and guard against the carpal tunnel connection, if there is one.

Diet may be critical. Sometimes other factors can affect your likelihood of developing carpal tunnel syndrome.

- **Obesity.** Being overweight makes you a target for a number of health problems, including carpal tunnel syndrome. Overweight people often have swollen hands and feet because of an imbalance in their bodily fluids. If you gain weight quickly, it can also throw off this delicate balance. That's why carpal tunnel syndrome is sometimes a problem during pregnancy. If you're overweight, follow a healthy eating plan to erase the excess pounds. You might find you no longer have that pain and numbness in your hands and wrists.

- **Diabetes.** Having diabetes puts you at higher risk of carpal tunnel syndrome. Diabetes can affect your heart, blood vessels, and circulation. It can also damage nerves such as the median nerve, the focus of pain in this condition. If you have diabetes, keep tight control of your diet. This will minimize the risk of carpal tunnel syndrome along with the other negative effects of diabetes.

If you watch your diet and get enough vitamin B6, you may be able to control the painful symptoms of carpal tunnel syndrome. However, nutrition alone cannot correct this condition. See your doctor for advice on the best treatment course to follow.

CATARACTS

Ante up some antioxidants

We all prize light and clarity in the world around us, especially when it comes to vision. But a cloudy haze of cataracts can throw up a smokescreen between you and the things you want to see. Before your eyes ever get to this point, however, you can choose foods and nutrients to help keep your vision clear and strong.

Exposure to light and oxygen can damage your eyes by producing harmful molecules called free radicals. Antioxidants are vitamins, minerals, and other substances that counteract this damage. Recent studies show that taking antioxidant supplements may cut your risk of cataracts in half. Simply by eating fruits and vegetables and taking a daily multivitamin that contains antioxidants, you can lower your risk of cataracts. Take advantage of the way specific antioxidants can protect your eyes by following these helpful hints.

- **Corral some C.** Increase your intake of vitamin C to help fend off cataracts. You can get this vitamin from food, supplements, or both. Some experts believe vitamin C supplements are safe if you take up to 2,000 milligrams (mg) a day. Actually, a supplement of 200 to 500 mg is probably all you need. To get more vitamin C from food, look for the freshest fruits and vegetables. Some of the highest in vitamin C are oranges, lemons, tangerines, strawberries, cantaloupe, broccoli, brussels sprouts, and sweet red peppers.
- **Enhance your E.** If you have enough vitamin E in your diet, your risk of cataracts is about half the risk of people with low vitamin E. To get more of this health-enhancing nutrient in your diet, add a little wheat germ oil, sunflower seeds, or dried almonds. Instead of white flour and white rice, eat whole wheat, oats, and brown rice. Some researchers suggest you can safely take up to 400 international units (IU) of vitamin E daily, but don't exceed that amount. Vitamin E supplements from natural sources may be slightly better for you than the synthetic kind.
- **Add some A.** Vitamin A is good for your eyes, but don't take large doses since it can build up in your body and become toxic. You're better off just getting the recommended dietary allowance for vitamin A (4,000-5,000 IU) from a multivitamin and supplementing your diet with foods rich in carotenes. Carotenes or carotenoids are substances in food that are converted to vitamin A in your liver. Add a fresh carrot or half a baked sweet potato to your daily diet, and you've safely doubled your intake of vitamin A.
- **Count on a combo.** The antioxidants selenium and glutathione form a powerful team to protect your eyes from cataracts. A high level of these nutrients must be present in your eyes to counteract free-radical damage. To get more selenium in your diet, cut back on sugar, choose whole grains instead of refined ones, and cook your vegetables lightly. Boiling vegetables reduces their natural selenium content. Broccoli, cabbage, celery, cucumbers, and lean meats should give you a good supply of selenium.

To add more glutathione to your diet, eat plenty of fruits and vegetables, but make sure they're fresh, not canned. Processing cuts way down on the amount of glutathione in foods. To get the highest amount of glutathione naturally, eat fresh asparagus, raw avocado, potatoes, and raw spinach. If you prefer a supplement, you should take glutamine, an amino acid that your body converts into glutathione. This seems to work better than taking glutathione directly.

- **Turn up the turmeric.** Curcumin is a natural antioxidant found in the spice turmeric. In a recent study, rats fed curcumin proved to be much more resistant to cataracts than those who didn't get the spicy treat. Researchers suspect that this might work in humans, too. Turmeric is a spice often used in Indian dishes that contain curry. So, if you develop a taste for spicy Indian food, you might be protecting your eyes while you tickle your palate.

Ferret out fat and salt

You know that too much fat and salt can be harmful to other parts of your body. There's also a connection with your eyes. A recent Italian medical study found that people who eat the most salt and fat have a higher risk of developing cataracts.

Too much salt in your diet can cause your blood pressure to rise and interfere with the blood vessels in your eyes. Most people should limit their intake of salt to 2,400 mg a day. If you have high blood pressure, don't get more than 2,000 mg. To limit your salt intake, don't add salt to food when you cook it or when you sit down to eat it. Avoid fast foods and be careful of processed foods by reading the sodium content on labels.

You already have important reasons to limit the fat in your diet — to avoid obesity, heart disease, and cancer. Protecting your precious eyesight is yet another good reason to eat healthy, low-fat fare. Keep your daily fat calories to 30 percent or less by limiting the amount of fat you cook with; avoiding fried foods; and watching for hidden fat in meats, dairy products, baked goods, and other prepared foods. Emphasizing a diet of fresh fruits, vegetables, and whole grains will automatically help you eat less fat.

CHRONIC FATIGUE SYNDROME

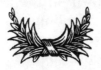

5 tips to chase away chronic fatigue

Most people love a good mystery. Trying to figure out "who-dunit" can be fun and relaxing. However, when the mystery is "why am I so tired all the time?" and not even your doctor has the answer, it is neither fun nor relaxing.

Everyone feels tired sometimes, but if you have persistent fatigue that lasts more than six months, and your doctor has ruled out other causes, you may have chronic fatigue immune dysfunction syndrome (CFIDS). Other symptoms of this mysterious disorder include mild fever, tender lymph nodes, sore throat, headaches, confusion, and muscle aches.

Diseases similar to chronic fatigue have baffled doctors for over a century. Each generation has had different names and different possible causes for these disorders. They have been called neurasthenia, the yuppie flu, shirkers syndrome, and chronic EBV (Epstein Barr Virus.) Possible causes have included anemia, allergies, low blood sugar, yeast infections, viruses, and mental disorders.

CFIDS often begins after an illness like a cold, bronchitis, or mononucleosis. Researchers still have not established a definite cause for CFIDS, but most now believe it is caused by some type of virus or by a malfunctioning immune system. Although CFIDS has no tried and true treatment or cure, researchers and people with the disorder have found some strategies that may help.

- **Amino acid advice.** Some people with chronic fatigue syndrome have found that certain amino acids help ease their symptoms. Lysine is an amino acid that fights the herpes virus that causes cold sores and mouth ulcers. The same virus may play a role in CFIDS. L-carnitine may also be helpful. It is a combination of lysine and methionine, another amino acid. Natural sources of lysine include eggs, fish, lima beans, red meat, potatoes, milk, cheese, and yeast. If you choose to take supplements, the recommended dosage is 1 to 2 grams daily. Another amino acid, arginine, can undo lysine's hard work, so steer clear of it. Don't take any supplements that contain arginine, and try to limit your intake of arginine-rich foods like chocolate, nuts, raisins, whole wheat, and brown rice.

- **Vitamins and minerals add energy.** With any chronic illness, your body's supply of essential vitamins and minerals can become drained. Magnesium levels seem to be particularly low in people with CFIDS, and supplementation with magnesium has improved symptoms in some people. A multivitamin/mineral supplement may help give you energy and keep your nutrient levels on an even keel.

- **Herbal energy boosters.** Echinacea, a colorful flowering plant, was first used as medicine by Native Americans. Early settlers soon began to use this healing plant as treatment for problems ranging from dizziness to rattlesnake bites. Although echinacea's medicinal use declined after the discovery of antibiotics, modern research has found that echinacea can provide natural help for a sluggish immune system. And anything that gives your immune system a boost might boost your energy levels as well.

  Ginseng, a root used as medicine for centuries in the Far East, may help pick you up and get you moving. Ginseng has reportedly been used to cure almost any illness you can imagine. Studies show that ginseng increases energy, improving athletic performance by helping your muscles work longer and more efficiently. Research also finds that ginseng helps your immune system produce more of the cells that attack infections.

  One recent study tested the effects of echinacea and ginseng on people with chronic fatigue syndrome. Both herbs significantly increased the immune function of cells.

  If you decide to try these herbal supplements, look for standardized ginseng supplements that contain 4 to 7 percent ginsenosides. The recommended dosage is 100 mg daily. Echinacea is most commonly sold as a liquid extract. Experiment with dosage to find what works best for you, but for immune system boosting try 10 to 25 drops of extract or one to two capsules a day. If you take echinacea for an extended period of time, it loses its effectiveness, so try taking it for three days on and three days off.

- **Try a little Coenzyme Q10.** Every cell in your body needs Coenzyme Q10 to produce energy, so a shortage of this substance might contribute to chronic fatigue. While no studies confirm this, you might try taking it for a few weeks to see if it helps. Experts recommend 90 to 200 mg daily. Since supplements are expensive, you should stop after six weeks if you see no improvement.

- **Fatty acids.** Omega-3 and omega-6 fatty acids may be the end of the tired, aching muscles of CFIDS. These fatty acids may help reduce inflammation, pain, and flu-like symptoms. You can find these acids in evening primrose oil (omega-6) and fish oil (omega-3).

If these nutritional tips don't help your chronic fatigue, don't despair. CFIDS sometimes disappears just as mysteriously as it appeared. In the meantime, rest, eat right, and exercise as much as you can. And who knows? Research may soon uncover the solution to this medical mystery.

COLD SORES

Fight cold sores before they pop up

It's embarrassing. Right before an important meeting, a painful red sore pops up and makes a home on your lip. If you've ever had a cold sore, you're certainly not alone. Each year more than 100 million cold sores pop up, and that's just in the United States.

Cold sores, also called fever blisters, look and feel a lot like canker sores. Unlike canker sores, however, they are caused by a contagious virus called herpes simplex. There is no cure for herpes, and once you have the virus, you may experience outbreaks of cold sores from time to time. But don't give up ... there are ways you can fight back.

- **Try some *Lactobacillus acidophilus*.** This may sound like a long-extinct dinosaur, but it's not. It's alive and well and living in your yogurt. Some studies suggest that this live culture may be the key to preventing outbreaks of cold sores. If yogurt is not your thing, the culture can be taken as a supplement. In fact, some experts say that the capsule form available at health food stores is the most effective way to take it. Remember, the culture must be alive to do you any good, so make sure you buy your capsules refrigerated, and keep them that way.

- **Eat a well-balanced diet.** Good nutrition is essential for keeping your immune system strong. The virus that causes cold sores can flare up more easily when your body's defenses are weakened. Particularly important are vitamins C and E, folic acid, and zinc.
- **Dab on some sunscreen.** Sunscreen can protect more than just your skin these days. Wearing it on your lips can prevent cold sores, experts say. Some researchers estimate that about 25 percent of flare-ups are caused by exposure to the sun. For the best protection, use a sunscreen with an SPF (sun protection factor) of 15 or greater. You can buy lip balm with SPF 15 protection at most grocery stores and drugstores.

5 easy ways to stop the sting

You feel a cold sore coming on. What should you do? There may be no cure for cold sores, but that doesn't mean you're at their mercy. You can sit back and wait for the stinging to start, or you can take action. The choice is yours.

Harness the power of protein. If you've had a cold sore before, you often know when you're about to get another one. To prevent a budding cold sore from forming, dip the corner of a cloth napkin or handkerchief in milk, and then apply it to the sore spot. Hold this compress in place for five seconds, then remove for five seconds. Keep this up for five minutes, then repeat the process every few hours. This also works for sores that have already developed. Some experts think the protein in the milk helps speed along the healing process.

Put your pain on ice. As soon as you feel a new cold sore, head for the freezer. An ice cube held to the sore soon after it appears may make it go away faster, and the ice will also help numb the pain of the sore. Hold the ice directly over the cold sore for about 15 minutes. If direct contact becomes too chilling, drinking cool liquids or sucking on frozen treats can have a similar soothing effect.

Watch what you eat. Avoid foods and activities that will bother your sores. Citrus fruits and juices, tomatoes, and other foods high in acid can irritate your mouth. Also, steer clear of sharp and coarse foods that can aggravate the tender spots in your mouth and slow the healing process. Try to eat mostly soft, bland foods and dine with caution.

Think zinc. Getting enough of this important nutrient in your diet can help prevent cold sores, but if you've already got one, zinc can still help. Many sore throat lozenges contain of zinc. For faster healing, place a lozenge directly on your sore and allow it to dissolve slowly.

Cover the culprit. Certain oils can soothe and protect cold sores as they heal. Vitamin E oil, applied directly to the sore, can speed healing. A few drops of echinacea oil, available at health food stores, may protect a cold sore by fighting germs. Covering your sore with petroleum jelly creates a protective coating against irritants and further infection. Applying some witch hazel may help dry up your cold sore.

Relax your cold sores away

Outbreaks of cold sores can be triggered by stress. Stress weakens your immune system, leaving you defenseless against the virus. According to researchers, one of the best things you can do to keep away these painful sores is relax.

Some experts suggest relaxation techniques and breathing exercises to reduce the risk of cold sores. Others prefer daily meditation to preserve mental and emotional wellness. And exercise, of course, is always a great stress-buster. Perhaps the best recommendation is to do whatever works best for you to keep the stress in your life under control.

Lysine to the rescue

Amino acids to prevent cold sores? Sounds a little strange, but if you get cold sores a lot, this might be your best bet for protection.

According to doctors at Indiana University Medical School, an amino acid called L-lysine can prevent recurrence in many chronic cold sore sufferers. And even though some of the people developed cold sores again, they had fewer outbreaks, and the sores went away faster. If you have frequent flare-ups, they say, it is best to take a small dose of about 500 milligrams (mg) per day, then boost up to 3,000 mg per day during an outbreak.

Your body doesn't make lysine, so if you want to experience its healing power, you have to go out and get it. Lysine is available in pill form at many health food stores, but it's also found in some foods. Wheat germ, poultry, pork, and ricotta and cottage cheese are all high in the helpful amino acid.

Researchers warn that people who use lysine should check their cholesterol levels first. Some studies suggest that lysine can cause the liver to produce too much cholesterol.

Lysine comes with another warning, too. To get the protective benefits, you must avoid foods containing arginine, a substance that prevents lysine from working. Lay off such favorites as peanuts, seeds, whole grains, rice, and gelatin.

COLDS

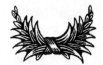

Kicking colds naturally

Man has searched for a cure for the common cold since the first caveman came down with the sniffles. Colds are probably the most common illness in the world, affecting almost everyone sooner or later. Despite our best efforts, we still haven't found a cure. However, research has discovered ways to help you get rid of a cold more quickly or make you less likely to catch a cold in the first place.

- **Clobber colds with vitamin C.** The question of whether vitamin C can cure or prevent the common cold has bounced around among experts for years. In the 1970s, Professor Linus Pauling claimed vitamin C could prevent and cure colds and the flu. He became famous after writing a book about vitamin C's therapeutic uses. Many other doctors and researchers disagreed with him, and the debate continued.

  However, a recent summary of modern research shows that, while vitamin C may not prevent your cold, it can shorten your symptoms by about 21 percent. Studies also find that if you take large doses of vitamin C when your cold starts, your symptoms will be less severe.

  Most research has studied the effects of regular daily intake of vitamin C, not large therapeutic doses. Although vitamin C is not toxic like some vitamins, large doses may cause side effects like diarrhea.

- **Think zinc.** Although a miracle cure for colds still hasn't been discovered, zinc may at least offer some relief. Recent

studies have found that people with colds who use zinc gluconate lozenges recover from their cold symptoms more
quickly than others. Zinc significantly reduces the amount of
time people suffer from nasal congestion and drainage, sore
throat, hoarseness, and headache.

If you decide to try zinc lozenges, look for a form called
zinc gluconate-glycine, because the zinc is easily released
when you suck on the lozenge. Be warned, however, that
these lozenges may look like candy, but they don't taste like
candy. Side effects include bad taste and nausea. If you think
a quicker end to your cold symptoms is worth the unpleasant
taste, think zinc and get relief.

- **Herbal prevention and treatment.** If you'd like to stop that
cold before it starts, try some herbal protection. Echinacea, or
purple coneflower, is a member of the daisy family that may
help you avoid the misery of a cold. It works by giving your
immune system a boost to help fight off germs that cause colds.

   If you don't manage to prevent that cold, some herbs offer
relief from cold symptoms. Goldenseal helps your runny
nose and respiratory tract by soothing your mucous membranes. It's often combined with echinacea for a strong, cold-
reducing remedy.

   Eucalyptus can help cleanse your lungs and ease congestion. Breathing in the vapors of hot eucalyptus tea can dry up
a stuffy nose. Eucalyptus oil added to water in a vaporizer
works well, but never put eucalyptus oil directly on your skin.

   Ginger can soothe a sore throat and eliminate mucus. For
years the Chinese have used tea made from fresh ginger root
to treat colds, coughs, and flu. Simmer three or four thin slices
of fresh ginger root in a pint of water for 10 to 30 minutes for
a warm, tasty tea that could curtail your cold symptoms.

   Chamomile can help clear your stuffy nose and sinuses.
Pour hot water over a handful of chamomile flower heads in
a bowl, place a towel over your head, lean over the bowl, and
breathe in the steam. You can also gargle with a cup of tea
every hour to soothe a sore, scratchy throat.

Natural cough quieters

A noisy cough can be painful for you and annoying for those
around you. If you want to quiet your cough without gulping bottles
of expensive cough syrup, try some natural home remedies.

- **Chicken soup for the cougher.** Almost any mother will be glad to tell you about the healing powers of chicken soup. Modern research seems to agree with "Dr. Mom." One study found that even when chicken soup was diluted 200 times, it still interfered with the substances that can trigger colds. Other studies find that hot soup can break up congestion and thin out mucous secretions.
- **Herbal relief.** If you enjoy hot herbal tea, try some hyssop the next time you have a cough and scratchy throat. Hyssop tea mixed with honey is thought to be especially effective at loosening phlegm. Horehound lozenges from your health-food store may also bring soothing relief.
- **Go bananas.** If a chronic cough is driving you bananas, maybe you should try eating some bananas. Heartburn is responsible for one in 10 chronic coughers, and research finds that eating bananas may bring relief from heartburn and the cough it causes.
- **Drink up.** If your cough is caused by a cold or the flu, drink plenty of warm liquids and plain water. This will loosen mucus in your lungs, keep down a fever, and help flush germs out of your body.

Unstop sinuses with spices

If you suffer from clogged sinuses that make your head pound and invite infection, try adding some spice to your life. Chew some horse-radish root, or sip some soup made with garlic. Hot and spicy foods like these can help open your nasal passages and unclog sinuses.

CONGESTIVE HEART FAILURE

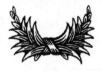

Pump up your heart

Congestive heart failure is a serious condition, but it isn't quite as bad as it sounds. Heart failure occurs when your heart fails to pump enough blood to meet your body's needs.

Among the first symptoms of heart failure are fatigue and weakness. If your condition continues, you may experience breathing difficulties and your legs, feet, and ankles may swell. This swelling is where the "congestive" part of heart failure comes in. It is caused by blood backing up into your veins, forcing fluid out of your blood vessels and into surrounding tissues. This backup of fluid can also cause your liver and other internal organs to become enlarged.

Fortunately, congestive heart failure is a very treatable condition. It may even serve to wake up some people to their heart's plight. Congestive heart failure may give you a second chance to take proper care of your heart. By following these tips, you'll be well on your way to a healthier heart.

- **Put down the salt shaker.** Sodium causes your body to retain fluid, and this can make your swelling worse. Too much sodium may also contribute to high blood pressure, which can lead to congestive heart failure. Try to keep your sodium intake under 3,000 mg daily.

- **Give up alcohol.** In congestive heart failure, your heart isn't pumping at its full capacity. Alcohol can cause your heart to pump even slower and weaker, but it may not be the only type of drink you should skip. Limiting your intake of beverages, in general, may help reduce the build up of fluid in severe heart failure.

- **Think thiamin.** A severe deficiency of this B vitamin can lead to beriberi, a disease that causes symptoms ranging from mental disturbances to paralysis. Heart failure can also be caused by this disease. Alcoholics and elderly people who are undernourished are at high risk for this type of heart failure. Make sure you are getting enough thiamin in your diet by eating nuts, beans, seeds, and avocados.

- **Watch your weight.** Keeping your weight down may help prevent you from getting heart disease in the first place, but if you already have congestive heart failure, you may want to watch your weight on the scales every morning. Rapid weight gain, more than a pound a day for three consecutive days, can be a warning signal that you're retaining too much fluid. Weigh yourself after you've gone to the bathroom, but before you've had breakfast. If you notice a significant gain, call your doctor.

- **Add some potassium and magnesium.** This dynamic duo may work to keep your heart pumping strongly. A deficiency of these minerals can cause arrhythmias, or an irregular heartbeat. Magnesium can help relax narrow blood vessels, making it easier for your heart to pump blood through them. Potassium supplements may help reduce fluid build-up.

- **Catch up on chromium.** Early studies indicate that chromium, a mineral that helps your body use insulin effectively, might also help treat congestive heart failure. Some researchers think that chromium may help widen constricted blood vessels and help your heart burn oxygen more efficiently. More studies need to be done on the effects of chromium on heart disease, but in the meantime, you can get chromium from fresh fruits and vegetables.

- **Fill up on fish oil.** A fishy solution to your heart problems may be as easy as one-two-three ... omega-3, that is. Fish oil contains heart-healthy omega-3 fatty acids, which can benefit your heart in several ways. Omega-3 helps relax blood vessels and makes your blood less sticky. This helps it flow more easily, so your heart doesn't have to work as hard to push it through your blood vessels. Fish oil also helps lower blood pressure, prevents arrhythmias, and may help prevent fatty deposits from accumulating on your artery walls. All these factors add up to a heart that beats a little easier.

Easy does it on salt substitutes

If you have congestive heart failure or high blood pressure, your doctor may have advised you to cut back on your sodium intake. You love the taste of salt, so you turn to a salt substitute. Before you shake freely, read the label. Many salt substitutes contain sodium, just in smaller amounts than regular table salt. If you add more to get the salty taste you love, you may be getting as much sodium as before. Many salt substitutes also contain potassium chloride. This can be harmful in large amounts, particularly if you have kidney problems or if you are taking medication for heart failure or high blood pressure.

Coenzyme Q10: the cellular spark plug

Every cell in your body needs energy, particularly the hard-working cells in your heart. It is no coincidence that Coenzyme Q10 is present in every cell of your body. This vitamin-like substance is required to produce energy in your cells, which is why it is sometimes referred to as "the cellular spark plug."

Fortunately, you can manufacture this important substance in your body, but it's a complicated process. It requires adequate amounts of several vitamins and minerals. According to a leading CoQ10 researcher, if you become deficient in any of these nutrients, which include several B vitamins, you will also be deficient in CoQ10.

Some researchers believe that a deficiency of CoQ10 might contribute to heart disease, particularly congestive heart failure. Although more studies need to be done, several studies support the benefits of CoQ10 for people with heart disease.

- **Congestive heart failure.** The most widely accepted benefit of CoQ10 involves congestive heart failure. People with congestive heart failure have significantly lower levels of CoQ10 in their blood than healthy people.

    In one study, 81 percent of the people who took CoQ10 had significant reductions in heart rates, blood pressures, and respiratory rates after just three months. They also experienced improvements in other symptoms of heart failure including insomnia, swelling, dizziness, skin discoloration, breathing difficulty, sweating, and heart palpitations.

- **Angina.** In one study, researchers gave CoQ10 to people with chronic stable angina for seven days. The people were then studied to see how long they could exercise without setting off an episode of angina pain. The exercise time in the CoQ10 group increased significantly.

- **High blood pressure.** Studies find that people with high blood pressure have low levels of CoQ10. One small study found that CoQ10 lowered blood pressure in four out of 17 people. While this might not seem significant, it means CoQ10 might help certain people who are deficient in CoQ10 lower their blood pressures.

- **Heart surgery.** CoQ10 may help hearts heal more rapidly after surgery. Recent studies have found that people treated with CoQ10 before surgery had better heart function after surgery.

- **Arrhythmia.** Animal and human studies suggest that CoQ10 may be able to reduce irregular heartbeats in some people.

Coenzyme Q10 may not be a miracle cure for all heart problems, but research results so far are promising. You can beef up your CoQ10 levels naturally by eating liver, sardines, mackerel, peanuts — and beef.

Talk with your doctor before taking supplements. If you decide to give supplements a try, take them with foods that contain fat. This will help increase absorption because CoQ10 is a fat-soluble substance. Most studies on CoQ10 have used doses ranging from 3 mg to 150 mg daily. According to researchers, very few side effects have been reported.

CONSTIPATION

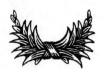

How to get moving again, naturally

You are considered healthy if you have a bowel movement anywhere from three times a day to three times a week. Too often though, you can get preoccupied with the notion that once a day, after breakfast, is the proper routine. For most people, that just isn't so. If you feel that you truly are constipated, consider perhaps the most important influence on your intestines — your diet

Fiber is the critical ingredient you need to control constipation. Mother Nature has given you a wide variety of healthy ways to add fiber to your diet, starting with fruit. Eating lots of raw fruit, including the skin and pulp, is a delicious way to keep your body healthy. Remember that cooked foods such as applesauce, and dried foods like apricots, prunes, and raisins, are also full of natural fiber.

Raw vegetables have plenty of fiber, and they also serve as natural laxatives. They get things going in your intestines while they fill your body with lots of key vitamins and minerals. For maximum fiber, try broccoli, cabbage, carrots, cauliflower, celery, lettuce, and spinach.

If you prefer cooked vegetables, stick with broccoli, spinach, string beans, potatoes, turnips, peas, corn, brussels sprouts, asparagus, cauliflower, squash, or rhubarb. Unlike some produce, these delicious vegetables will give you lots of fiber even after they've been cooked.

Although fiber is good for you, it's best to start eating it gradually. Believe it or not, you could suffer more constipation as your digestive system struggles to cope with the added roughage. The solution is to add fiber to your diet slowly, about 10 grams each day until you're eating between 20 and 35 grams daily. Good sources include whole-grain cereals, bran muffins, brown rice, and whole-grain breads.

Add small amounts of unprocessed bran, also called miller's bran, to baked goods, cereals, and fruit. This isn't necessarily the same type you'll find in high-fiber packaged cereals, so read your labels. Unprocessed bran might cause bloating and gas when you first start using it, but if you gradually adjust your diet over a few weeks, you should have no problems.

Just like the plumbing in any house, your body needs its system flushed out on a regular basis, even more so when it's loaded with fiber. To do this, drink lots of liquids; health professionals recommend one to two quarts every day. Many find that milk is constipating, however, so go easy on the moo juice.

Herbal relief

Do you like the idea of brewing your own natural remedy? If so, one of these herbal blends may be just your cup of tea for easing constipation.

Senna and cascara sagrada are both stimulant laxatives. This means they relieve constipation by getting your bowels moving. They are good, short-term remedies, but not recommended for use over a long period of time. Side effects can include cramping, vomiting, electrolyte disturbance, fat malabsorption, fat-soluble vitamin deficiency, and dependence. A combination of senna and fiber that was tried in one study worked better than senna alone.

Psyllium seeds are a bulk-forming laxative, which means you take them with liquid, and they expand in your intestines, forcing a bowel movement through pressure. This type of laxative is considered safer for long-term use. One or two times a day, stir two teaspoons of seeds or one teaspoon of husks into water or juice and drink it down quickly. Remember to take this and any other type of bulk-forming laxative with large amounts of fluid. One drawback is that it can cause excess gas, but the good news is that it may lower cholesterol.

Danger in the medicine drawer

Using an artificial laxative may seem like a quick, easy solution to a bothersome problem, but you need to be cautious. Laxatives can be habit forming, and once your intestines start relying on them, your body won't do the work on its own. Remember that diarrhea is a side effect of too many laxatives and can be even more dangerous to your system.

Mineral oil has been used for many years as a laxative since it lubricates the stool, making it easier to pass. But it can take vitamins and calcium with it on the way out. Talk to your doctor before using mineral oil, especially if you take an anticoagulant (a drug that prevents blood clots). It could affect the performance of this drug.

Magnesium salts are present in many over-the-counter saline laxatives and health aids, including Milk of Magnesia. Because it works so quickly, this type of laxative is a favorite with older adults. What isn't so popular are the side effects: cramping, watery stools, dehydration, and the possibility of magnesium intoxication.

It would take a great deal of a saline laxative to bring you to this danger level, but it's a very real concern if you have kidney problems and continually overuse laxatives. The American College of Gastroenterology recommends that saline laxatives containing magnesium only be used in special, severe cases and not as a long-term solution for constipation.

What's all the buzz?

For some people, a prescription for constipation is as close as your honey pot. A small European study explored the age-old remedy of drinking a mixture of one to three tablespoons of regular honey and water to get the bowels moving. They found that if you are not suffering from irritable bowel syndrome, you just might have a honey of a cure.

DEPRESSION

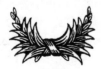

2 cups a day keep the doctor away

If you're looking for a fast, easy way to lift your spirits, try a jolt of java or a touch of tea. In a 10-year study of female nurses, caffeine seemed to make a big difference in the rate of serious depression.

Healthy women who drank two to three cups of coffee a day had the lowest reported rates of suicide. Too much caffeine can make you jittery and keep you awake at night, so you don't want to overdo it. But if your mood needs a boost, try a little caffeine.

To feel better, go fish

If a recent study is correct, our finned friends could hold the key to beating depression. Cutting back on the fat in your diet is a good idea, but if you cut out the fat in fatty fish, you may be missing the boat. Fish oil is rich in DHA and EPA, two omega-3 fatty acids that help develop, protect, and heal your brain. Medical studies show that eating food rich in DHA may combat depression. Dark, oily fish are high in omega-3 fatty acids, especially salmon, sardines, mackerel, bluefish, and tuna. Add them to your weekly diet to help beat depression.

Pack protein for a positive attitude

Do you live for sugary snacks and white-flour confections? Do you move through the day waiting for your next junk-food fix? If this is your eating style and you're constantly feeling a little down, maybe it's because you're not getting enough protein. A German study found that people were more unhappy after they began low-protein diets to treat kidney disease.

When you eat simple carbohydrates without adequate protein, such as a slice of birthday cake without milk, your blood sugar swings wildly up and down. The effects of flucuating blood sugar levels can leave you tired and depressed.

To get your blood sugar back on an even keel, eat plenty of fresh fruits, vegetables, and complex carbohydrates such as whole grains, rice, and pasta. Then add about 50 grams of protein per day if you're a woman and about 63 grams daily if you're a man. A five-ounce portion of lean meat, chicken, or fish contains about 35 grams of protein. Two cups of skim milk have 16 grams of protein, and one cup of nonfat yogurt has 12 grams. One serving of meat, two of milk, and one of yogurt will provide your protein for the day.

Between meals, stick to healthy snacks that contain a little protein, too. Choose fresh fruit with a bit of low-fat cheese or whole grain crackers with skim milk and you'll banish those high-sugar blues and help keep depression away.

Helpful herb may heal the blues

Sometimes folk medicine turns out to be good medicine. Such is the case with St. John's wort, a common flowering herb used to treat depression. In Germany, it's used extensively to treat anxiety, depression, and insomnia. Now a recent study supports its use as a natural anti-depressant. More studies need to be done to establish exactly how St. John's wort works, but so far researchers have found it a safe alternative for people with mild depression.

Herbal expert Dr. Varro E. Tyler recommends making an herbal tea by pouring one cup of boiling water over one to two heaping teaspoons of dried St. John's wort and letting it steep for 10 minutes. You would probably need to drink one or two cups of this tea each day for at least four to six weeks before you notice any benefits. You should be able to find St. John's wort at your local health food store.

The right vitamins to lift your spirits

Keeping yourself physically healthy is important for staying emotionally healthy, too. This includes getting the right food and nutrients, including the right vitamins. Certain vitamins play an even more important role than others in beating back the blues. Two vital ones are vitamins B and C.

Build up your B vitamins. If you are feeling depressed, you could be deficient in vitamin B. The vitamin B complex is actually made up of several B vitamins with different properties, but they all work together in your body. You need enough thiamin, niacin, riboflavin, folic acid, and B6 for your emotional health. A lack of any of these vitamins can leave you feeling depressed.

To replace B vitamins naturally through the food you eat, rely on lean meat, liver, brewer's yeast, yogurt, beans, and leafy green vegetables. If you want to replace B vitamins with a supplement, it's easier to keep a good balance by taking B complex, rather than singling out one B vitamin. If you are ill, elderly, or under a lot of stress, you might benefit from a supplement.

Center on vitamin C. Depression is one of the first symptoms of a vitamin C deficiency. Even a slight lack of C can rob you of your feeling of well-being. To get more vitamin C in your diet, eat plenty of fresh fruits and vegetables, especially citrus fruits, broccoli, cantaloupe, and sweet red peppers. If you feel you need supplements, you can find them at any grocery or drugstore.

DIABETES

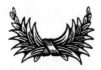

Nature's armor combats diabetes

Mother Nature has some tricks up her sleeve to outsmart diabetes. Several plants, including herbs, can help prevent some of the problems associated with diabetes. The following natural remedies can be found at grocery stores or health food stores.

Ginseng is often considered a wonder drug, but it's really a wonder herb. It helps diabetics control their blood sugar levels.

In addition, ginseng is known for improving mental alertness, mood, and psychological well-being. This could lead to better diet choices, a more active lifestyle, and more effective weight loss.

Prickly pear cactus also might help diabetics maintain normal blood sugar levels. According to researchers, diabetics who eat nopal, also called the prickly pear cactus, on an empty stomach can lower their blood sugar levels almost 25 percent. Keep in mind, however, the nopal must be fresh. Processed and dried nopal does not produce the same benefits.

Gurmar, a vine that grows in the rain forest, means "sugar destroyer" in Hindi. When eaten, the leaves of this vine take away your ability to taste sweetness. It also seems to lower blood sugar levels and reduce the amount of insulin needed by people with diabetes. This regulating effect helps to smooth out the rise and fall of a diabetic's blood sugar level.

Gurmar also lowers cholesterol, heals damaged pancreatic cells, and improves insulin production in laboratory animals.

Grapeseed extract is a natural source of PCO, a nutrient found in small amounts in peanuts, cranberries, apples, and onions. As well as being a strong antioxidant, PCO helps your body use vitamin C and improves circulation. By strengthening your capillaries, including those that bring blood to your eyes, PCO helps to prevent retinopathy, the leading cause of blindness in diabetics.

The most commonly available PCO supplement in America is made from the bark of pine trees, but it's worth it to look a little harder. Grapeseed extract PCO is more potent and costs about half as much.

Bitter melon is a small fruit that looks like a shrunken cucumber. It has been used for many years in other cultures to improve glucose tolerance without increasing insulin levels. Bitter melon is also called balsam pear, bitter gourd, and bitter cucumber. Look for this exotic fruit in Asian food stores.

Fenugreek, an oddly named plant, has powerful seeds. Fenugreek seeds may reduce fasting blood sugar levels when taken with meals, and researchers think they can also lower your risk of heart disease by fighting cholesterol and preventing artery damage.

Flax is a grain that works many wonders. Flax and flaxseed can improve your cells' glucose tolerance, control cholesterol, and help guard against heart disease. In addition, some research shows that flax can give a boost to your kidneys. One of the best things about flax is that the little grain works its glucose magic just as well taken as a supplement as it does when eaten in foods. Most health food stores carry a variety of flaxseed products, including flour, meal, and oil.

Amazing minerals tame diabetes

While minerals are essential to every diet, certain minerals seem to help keep diabetes away. The best way to get your minerals is through a healthy diet, but sometimes supplements are necessary. Check with your doctor.

- **Chromium.** This mineral helps your blood deliver and use insulin, guarding your body against insulin resistance and hypoglycemia. In test after test, scientists found that people who get more chromium have greater control over their blood sugar levels and are less likely to suffer from diabetes.

  Good sources include beef, liver, seafood, mushrooms, whole grains, asparagus, and nuts. Potatoes and apples are also rich in chromium, but make sure you eat the skin, too.

- **Magnesium.** Diabetes is linked to a deficiency of magnesium in several ways. First, people with low levels of magnesium are more likely to develop diabetes. Second, diabetics who take insulin often develop a magnesium deficiency, which increases their risks of complications. Greater insulin resistance, lower insulin production, high blood pressure, and heart and blood vessel problems have all been linked to low levels of magnesium.

  Good natural sources of magnesium are beans, broccoli, corn, shellfish, and skim milk. Since magnesium is easily stripped from foods during processing, it is best to look for fresh and unprocessed food items.

- **Zinc.** Diabetics almost always have low levels of zinc. A recent study revealed that only 6 percent of the diabetics tested were getting enough zinc. Research shows that low zinc levels can damage your retinas and even cause blindness.

Red meat, shellfish, and lima beans are your best bets to get more zinc naturally.

4 vitamins that defeat diabetes

Eating a well-balanced diet is essential to preventing and controlling diabetes. Although it is important to cover all your nutritional bases, some vitamins are more important than others.

Vitamin A plays a vital role in insulin control. The more effective your insulin is at controlling blood sugar, the less likely you are to develop diabetes. In one recent study, researchers learned that higher levels of vitamin A in a person's diet makes insulin more effective in controlling blood sugar.

Good sources of vitamin A and beta-carotene, a form of vitamin A, include milk; liver; and deep orange and dark green fruits and vegetables like sweet potatoes, carrots, and spinach. Vitamin A can be toxic in large amounts. To prevent getting too much, it's best to get vitamin A from food sources instead of supplements.

Vitamin C not only helps your body control its blood sugar level it also can help lower blood cholesterol and improve circulation. As an antioxidant, vitamin C helps to neutralize free radicals that damage the cells of diabetics more easily than those of other people. Vitamin C also improves insulin sensitivity in people who are overweight.

Grapefruit, orange juice, broccoli, sweet red pepper, and brussels sprouts are good sources of vitamin C.

Vitamin E is another valuable antioxidant in the fight against diabetes. Studies show that people with low levels of vitamin E have an increased risk of developing diabetes. Vitamin E may protect you from diabetes by destroying cell-damaging free radicals in your body.

Vegetable oils, such as safflower, canola, and corn oils; wheat germ; sunflower seeds; sweet potatoes; and shrimp are good sources of vitamin E.

Biotin, a relatively unknown B vitamin, may be able to reduce the amount of insulin your body needs. In various tests, blood sugar levels in diabetics were cut in half, while insulin levels were not affected. You can get biotin from liver, egg yolks, and cereals, but supplements seem to be just as effective.

The latest 'miracle' food for diabetics

There's a new bean in town that many diabetics are calling a miracle. It's called chana dal, an Indian bean that looks a lot like the chickpea. In various tests, this little wonder was rated as low as a 12 on the glycemic index. It is a sweet bean that can be used in many recipes, and it retains its firmness when cooked. Like other legumes, chana dal is high in protein and fiber. It also contains a small amount of monounsaturated fat, which is now recommended as part of a healthy diet by the American Diabetes Association.

Chana dal can be found at most Indian markets. If you like to shop by mail, you can get this bean through a company called Phipps Ranch. To place an order or receive a catalog, call Phipps Ranch at (800) 279-0889.

Exercise to avoid diabetes

The good news about Type II or noninsulin-dependent diabetes is that even if you inherit a tendency to get this disease, you usually need a trigger, like obesity, to develop it. Other factors that put you at risk are age, high blood pressure, smoking, and lack of exercise.

For all these reasons, your most powerful weapon for preventing Type II diabetes is exercise. It is also the factor over which you have the most control. It's no coincidence that 80 percent of all diabetics are overweight. Many doctors consider proper weight even more important than the calorie makeup of your diet, and exercise is the key to any effective weight-loss program. Regular exercise is so effective, some doctors say, that it can actually reverse diabetic symptoms even after they've started.

If you are diabetic, you need to exercise with caution. It is better not to exercise right before bedtime. Exercise can change the rate at which your body uses insulin. These changes in your metabolism could cause low blood sugar during sleep, which can be very dangerous.

Fiber helps maintain blood sugar level

Soluble fiber, like that found in grains, fruits, and vegetables, helps your digestive system break down food and keeps your blood sugar level stable.

Researchers at Harvard recently found that women who eat a diet high in fiber and low in sugar are much less likely to develop diabetes. In addition, the researchers reported that it is important to get your fiber from the right sources. The less processed or refined the fiber is, the better it is at preventing diabetes.

Foods such as whole-grain breakfast cereal, broccoli, and apples are less processed, so the fiber remains in its natural form. This is the type of fiber your body needs. White bread, white rice, and french fries are highly refined foods that lack fiber.

Add fiber to your diet, but don't go overboard. Eating too much fiber can cause gas and constipation and get in the way of a healthy diet by sacrificing other vital nutrients.

Caffeine sounds low blood sugar alarm

Here's some good news for diabetics and coffee lovers. Recent tests show that caffeine can help diabetics recognize the beginnings of low blood sugar. The stimulating effect of caffeine seems to help heighten sensation and, therefore, intensify the early warning symptoms of low blood sugar.

According to the study, the caffeine in two to three cups of coffee should be enough to produce the desired effect in your body. But if you have heart disease or have had a stroke, talk with your doctor before drinking more than a cup of coffee a day.

The best thing you can do to maintain proper blood sugar levels at all times, experts say, is to recognize symptoms early and then fight off attacks by eating something.

Problem foods you'd never suspect

If you think pizza is your friend, recent findings suggest you better think again. One study of diabetic volunteers who ate pizza for dinner showed much higher blood sugar levels during that night's sleep, even though levels were controlled after the meal. Researchers aren't sure what ingredient in the pizza caused this blood sugar increase. Because of this danger, the delicious pie is probably a better choice for lunch than dinner.

Oysters-on-the-half-shell are another favorite treat, but they can be deadly. Shellfish like oysters, clams, and mussels feed by straining water through their systems, which makes them more likely to pick up dangerous bacteria in the ocean. These bacteria can cause food poisoning and even blood poisoning when shellfish are eaten raw. This is dangerous for anyone, but it poses a special threat for diabetics. Fortunately, these bacteria are killed when shellfish are cooked thoroughly.

Wondering about sushi? Raw fin fish can contain its own kind of parasites and bacteria. Freezing kills the parasites, but only thorough cooking kills all the bacteria. Because of the special risk, diabetics should never eat raw or undercooked seafood of any kind.

Another problem for diabetics is eating too much protein. Meat and dairy products contain an abundance of protein. While protein is a necessary building block for the growth and repair of your body, too much of a good thing can be dangerous. Any protein your body can't use has to be eliminated, and this means extra work for your hard-working kidneys.

Also, because many sources of protein are high in saturated fat and cholesterol, people who eat excess amounts of protein are at higher risk of heart disease.

Ask your doctor how much protein you should eat every day and follow his advice carefully.

The best way to control your weight

Because of the current war against fat, lots of people are trying to lose weight by removing fat from their diets. To make matters worse, these fat calories are often replaced with simple carbohydrates like sugar and honey. Low-fat diet foods are notorious for putting taste back into fat-free snacks by loading them up with sugar. Don't be fooled.

Even though fat is under attack, calories still count. And pound for pound, simple sugar calories stimulate the most insulin production in your body. The best way to safely control your weight and guard against diabetes is to eat a well-rounded diet, complete with foods rich in polyunsaturated fats, such as sunflower oil or safflower oil, or monounsaturated fats, such as olive oil, canola oil, avocados, and nuts. Instead of loading up on sweets, round out your diet with foods high in complex carbohydrates like fruits and vegetables.

Simple test helps determine diabetes risk

Over 16 million people in the United States are afflicted with some form of diabetes, but only half of them know it. Sometimes the onset of the disease is so gradual, you could be suffering permanent damage from diabetes for years before you realize you have it. How can you tell if you are diabetic or are in danger of becoming diabetic? Take this simple test by answering true or false to the following statements:

- I am older than 40.
- I am 20 percent or more overweight.
- I am a woman who has had a baby weighing more than 9 pounds at birth.
- I have a sister or brother with diabetes.
- I have a parent with diabetes.
- I get little or no exercise during a normal day.

If you answered "true" for three or more of these questions, you are probably at significant risk of developing Type II diabetes.

The symptoms of diabetes include an increase in thirst and the need to urinate more. You may lose weight despite feeling hungry more often. You might also notice tingling or complete loss of feeling in your hands or feet or blurred vision. If you have any of these symptoms, see your doctor.

DIARRHEA

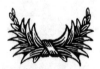

Sweeteners can sideswipe your system

Just when you think you're doing something good for your body by going sugar free, you find out it's causing your diarrhea. Sorbitol, a popular sugar substitute found in many sugar-free candies, gum and dietetic foods, may be the culprit behind your discomfort. It doesn't take much of this little sweetener to cause gas and bloating. A few more grams and you could feel cramping and diarrhea.

If you find you are sensitive to this product, make sure you check labels. Sorbitol is also used in vitamin supplements, over-the-counter drugs, and some prescription medications.

4 steps to recovery

When you have diarrhea, your body loses a lot of liquids and nutrients very quickly. Food passes through the intestines so fast that your bloodstream has no time to absorb vitamins or minerals. This presents two very clear dangers: dehydration and malnourishment.

- **Renew, refresh, restore.** When you lose body fluids, it is important to replace "electrolytes," the salts and minerals normally found in your blood, tissue fluids, and cells. For an easy, do-it-yourself recipe, mix one teaspoon of salt and four teaspoons of sugar into one quart of water. Drink two cups of this every hour. Many underdeveloped countries use an inexpensive but effective brew to treat diarrhea, which you can try as well. They simply drink the cooled water left in the pot after cooking rice. This liquid contains a lot of starch and nutrients left from the boiled rice.
- **Drown your sorrows.** While you suffer from diarrhea, you have to keep your system "in the drink." This means downing at least eight to 10 glasses of liquid each day. Water, caffeine-free sodas, popsicles, herbal tea, broth, or gelatin are good choices.
- **Baby your body.** After things have returned to normal, eat soft, bland foods, such as cooked cereal, rice, eggs, custard, bananas, yogurt, soda crackers, toast, skinless baked potatoes, or chicken.
- **Recovery no-no's.** For several days after experiencing diarrhea, stay away from fruit; alcohol; caffeine; milk; gassy foods like beans, cabbage and onions; and spicy, greasy, or fatty foods.

Herbs from the healing garden

Man has been healing himself for centuries with simple herbs from the forest and garden. Today, you don't even have to own a garden to get the benefit of years of herb lore. You only have to visit your local health food store. To relieve diarrhea, try one of these age-old remedies.

The taste of chamomile may be bitter, but the plant itself has a strong, fresh scent, much like the smell of apples. People in the Middle Ages planted chamomile in their garden paths so that when they stepped on them, the crushed leaves would give off a pleasant fragrance. Experts recommend chamomile tea for almost any digestive disorder. Try a cup if you have cramping or diarrhea.

You can combine two diarrhea remedies by mixing one to two tablespoons of carob powder into applesauce for fruity relief. This should be taken three to four times daily.

Maybe your best memories of camping are of the marshmallows you roasted over the open fire. You may be surprised to learn that marsh mallow is actually a plant people used long ago for food as well as healing. The marsh mallow root was made into a sweet paste and prescribed for a cough or sore chest. Today our marshmallows contain no part of the plant at all, just a combination of flour, eggs, and sugar. However, parts of the marsh mallow are still used as a natural healer. For diarrhea, you can take 1000 mg of marsh mallow root two to three times daily.

Acidophilus is a natural, "friendly" bacteria you have in your intestines. Sometimes, a poor diet or a course of antibiotics can affect how much acidophilus is alive and active in your colon. If you have too little, you could suffer from all kinds of digestive problems, from diarrhea to constipation. By taking supplements, you can restore the balance of good and bad bacteria. Follow label directions carefully.

Spicy hot cinnamon is not only wonderful to have in the kitchen but handy in the medicine cabinet as well. You may get some relief from diarrhea by using cinnamon's essential oil. Follow the directions on the bottle.

Betony, a member of the mint family, has long been used in medicine. Steep the leaves to make a tea helpful in treating diarrhea.

Herbs have a long tradition of healing digestive problems. The next time you suffer from diarrhea, try one of these natural remedies and see if it makes a difference.

'Helpers' may do more harm than good

Using anti-diarrhea products may not be as helpful as you think. They slow down your intestines so much that you may not get rid of the diarrhea-causing bacteria in your body as quickly as you would otherwise. You should only take over-the-counter medication if you have mild diarrhea that is not caused by an infection.

If you take an antacid containing magnesium, you may be doing more than relieving heartburn or indigestion. Studies have shown that high doses of magnesium can cause diarrhea, and in severe cases, death. These products are safe only if taken in the recommended doses for a short time.

Are you allergic to gluten?

Your favorite deli order is pastrami on rye, but lately you've noticed it gives you cramps, diarrhea, and maybe a whole host of other problems. Don't blame the pastrami. You may have an allergy to gluten — the mixture of proteins found in wheat, rye, barley, and other grains. This inherited allergy is called celiac sprue disease, and it can severely damage the lining of your intestines. If you think this may be causing your problems, try substituting products made with rice, corn, or soybean flour.

DIVERTICULAR DISEASE

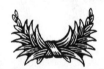

Defeat it with diet

If you are over 60, you probably have already developed small pouches or sacs in your colon, called diverticula. It's a fact of lifestyle and diet. The good news is that most people with diverticulosis never even know they have it.

If, however, you progress to the more serious form of the disease, diverticulitis, you'll certainly develop symptoms. And they're a nasty lot: cramps, abdominal pain, gas, constipation, diarrhea, and sometimes blood in your stool. The trick is avoiding this altogether, and the way to do it is with diet.

You need to make two changes in your eating habits to prevent diverticulosis from ever starting. If you have the condition, these changes also will help keep it from turning into the more critical diverticulitis. What are they? Increase fiber and liquids, and eat less red meat.

It sounds simple enough, but experts have discovered that few Americans get anywhere near the minimum daily fiber requirement of 20 to 35 grams. As part of a modern, industrialized country, we have gotten away from the simple, natural diet of fruits, vegetables, and grains. Processed and refined foods make up the bulk of our meals, and our bodies are paying the price.

Did you know that only plant foods contain fiber? This means you need to get creative in the produce section of your store. Try out different fruits. Combine grains and vegetables for easy one-dish, high-fiber meals. And go wild in the bakery with muffins, bagels, pitas, and breads that are full of flavor and whole grains.

Remember, too, that the more processing a food goes through, the less fiber it has. This can mean deciding to eat a baked potato instead of mashed ones; eating corn on the cob instead of canned, creamed corn; and eating a crunchy sweet apple instead of drinking apple juice.

Raspberries, blackberries, blueberries, pears, acorn squash, brussels sprouts, black-eyed peas, lima beans, kidney beans, brown rice, and oatmeal are all foods high in fiber, and delicious in the bargain.

If your doctor recommends a fiber supplement to mix with water, you'll benefit from an extra 4 to 6 grams of fiber in each 8-ounce glass. A daily drink is an easy way to keep your colon happy and help prevent this painful disease.

E. COLI POISONING

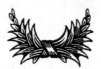

Stop E. coli before it starts

How do you like your steak? Rare, medium, well-done? Most places that serve steak ask for your preference. And if it's not cooked properly, you send it back. But how about your hamburger? If you were served a rare burger, would you mind? You should if you are concerned about food poisoning. A particularly harmful organism, *Escherichia Coli Type 0157:H7 (E. coli)*, lives in the intestines of infected cows and can contaminate meat during slaughter. You can't tell if the meat you buy is infected, since it looks and smells normal.

The good news is that thorough cooking kills off this nasty organism. So cook all your meat well if you want to avoid the abdominal pain, cramping, and bloody diarrhea this infection causes. Ground beef, in particular, needs to be thoroughly cooked. Make sure it is no longer pink, its juices run clear, and the inside is hot.

If you live on a farm, or know someone with dairy cows, you may have the opportunity to drink fresh milk. As natural and healthy as it sounds, this is not a good idea. The *E. coli* bacteria living on cow's udders or on milking equipment can contaminate raw milk. The process of pasteurizing heats milk to a temperature where all bacteria are killed, much like the process of cooking food. Don't take chances when it is so easy to avoid trouble.

A 'berry' good remedy

Fresh blueberry muffins, pancakes, and syrup may make a delicious breakfast, but they won't help the diarrhea you can get from bacterial infections. In fact, fresh blueberries may even act as a laxative.

Dried blueberries, however, are a popular European remedy for treating diarrhea. In the United States, you may have a hard time finding the dried fruit, but it's easy to make your own. Simply spread some fresh berries out in the sun until they wrinkle and shrivel up. Then, either eat about three tablespoons of the berries, or crush them, boil them for 10 minutes, strain, and drink as a tea.

Have you ever heard of a bilberry? It's a variety of blueberry that works just as well on diarrhea. You may find dried bilberries or bilberry extract in your local herb shop.

Yogurt battles bad bacteria

There are many reasons to eat yogurt besides its deliciously creamy taste. You've probably heard that it is full of calcium for your bones and "good" bacteria for your intestines.

All that is true, but there's more. A study out of the University of Minnesota determined that yogurt kills three different strains of *E. coli* bacteria. This is especially good news if you are traveling to areas where *E. coli* infection is common.

But even if you travel no farther than the corner market, a cup of yogurt every day is still an enjoyable way to boost your calcium and give your insides a good infection-fighting treatment.

Ethnic foods that ease digestion

Do you love Indian food? If you do, you may be getting some protection from intestinal troubles. Scientists from universities in Norway and the Netherlands tested the antibacterial effects of curcumin, the yellow pigment in turmeric, a common Indian spice. These scientists discovered that curcumin, under certain conditions, is toxic to *E. coli* bacteria.

Although testing has not yet made its way from the laboratory to the kitchen, it's possible this spice is doing your digestion some good.

If you can get your hands on some traditional Ethiopian herbs, you may have another weapon to fight *E. coli*-related illnesses. Researchers at Addis Ababa University in Ethiopia tested 63 local plants against seven strains of bacteria, including *E. coli*. They found that all of them attacked at least one of the microorganisms.

These herbs may not be items you'll find at your local grocery, but it is encouraging to know that science is continually investigating new, natural ways to combat illness.

A toast to tranquil tummies

If you want to protect yourself against *E. coli* and other intestinal bacteria, perhaps you should have a glass of wine. Studies have proven that both red and white wines contain an antibacterial substance that is more effective against this type of bacteria than even Pepto-Bismol.

It's not the alcohol content that does the job, but rather a compound in the grapes that is released during fermentation. So if you enjoy a glass with dinner, you really are helping your digestion.

A solution from the garden

Is a case of bad breath worth getting rid of tummy troubles? If you're suffering from an unpleasant episode of food poisoning, you may think any price is worth relief.

A group of doctors in China tested several spice plants for bacteria-fighting properties and discovered that both raw garlic and onion controlled the growth of *E. coli* bacteria. They also discovered that all the spices tested were less effective after they had been heated in boiling water.

Look for ways to work these two fragrant vegetables into your meals, uncooked. Mince them into a salad, or add them after other ingredients have cooked. Then pop an after-dinner mint.

EAR INFECTIONS

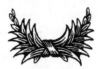

Chew away bacteria

Your chewing gum may chew up bacteria but only if you choose the right kind. Chewing gum that contains a natural sweetener called xylitol has been found to help prevent tooth decay and ear infections.

Most sweeteners promote tooth decay because bacteria feed on sugars like fructose and glucose, creating acids that eat away at your teeth. However, research has found that bacteria cannot live on xylitol like on other sweeteners. One study of preschool children also found that chewing gum with xylitol cut the incidence of ear infection in half.

Researchers think this is because xylitol prevents bacteria from attaching itself to the back of your mouth, where it can later enter your ear and set off an infection.

Children are especially prone to painful ear infections. Maybe they'll be happier about taking their "medicine" if it comes in a stick of gum.

EATING DISORDERS

Top 10 ways to stop an eating disorder

Eating disorders run a range of mild to deadly serious. From binge eating disorder and bulimia to anorexia nervosa and aging-related appetite loss, all take a heavy toll on your body. In fact, eating disorders are deadly for one out of every 10 people who suffer with these problems.

Although eating disorders like anorexia or bulimia nervosa are more common in young people or athletes, anyone can develop an eating disorder at any stage of life. You may start out simply dieting, then begin to binge, eventually develop bulimia nervosa, and even end up anorexic. Worse, once you develop an eating disorder, the imbalance in your body and brain created by your unhealthy diet tends to keep you from breaking that vicious and sometimes deadly cycle.

If you suspect or know that you suffer from an eating disorder, see your doctor. Effective treatment of eating disorders includes a combination of counseling, a healthy diet, and behavior changes. The following tips can also help.

Don't diet. Some researchers suspect eating disorders are triggered by strict diets that have made brain chemicals go haywire. In addition, the deprived feeling many people have on these diets can actually trigger a bout of binge eating.

But there's an even greater incentive to leave these deprivation diets behind. If you binge, you're less likely to lose weight or maintain any weight loss you do have. You're also more likely to have food cravings, especially for carbohydrates.

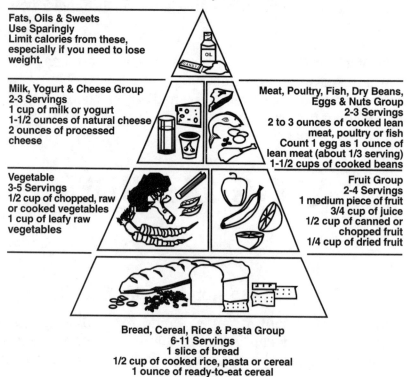

Fats, Oils & Sweets
Use Sparingly
Limit calories from these,
especially if you need to lose
weight.

Milk, Yogurt & Cheese Group
2-3 Servings
1 cup of milk or yogurt
1-1/2 ounces of natural cheese
2 ounces of processed
cheese

Meat, Poultry, Fish, Dry Beans,
Eggs & Nuts Group
2-3 Servings
2 to 3 ounces of cooked lean
meat, poultry or fish
Count 1 egg as 1 ounce of
lean meat (about 1/3 serving)
1-1/2 cups of cooked beans

Vegetable
3-5 Servings
1/2 cup of chopped, raw
or cooked vegetables
1 cup of leafy raw
vegetables

Fruit Group
2-4 Servings
1 medium piece of fruit
3/4 cup of juice
1/2 cup of canned or
chopped fruit
1/4 cup of dried fruit

Bread, Cereal, Rice & Pasta Group
6-11 Servings
1 slice of bread
1/2 cup of cooked rice, pasta or cereal
1 ounce of ready-to-eat cereal

Instead of dieting, follow the suggestions of the food guide pyramid. (See illustration on previous page.) Make sure you don't eat fewer than the recommended number of servings from each category.

Cut caffeine. Caffeinated foods and beverages can worsen feelings of anxiety and depression. They also may increase your risk of going on a binge eating spree.

Divide meals into several smaller ones. Eat them throughout the day. This will help keep blood sugar levels stable and reduce the risk you'll get so hungry you'll stuff yourself later. But be careful not to increase calories unless you need to gain weight.

Record everything you eat. Get a little notebook you can easily carry with you. Note the time you ate, what you were doing, where you were, how much you ate, as well as your feelings before and after eating. Having a written record will help you identify and work on behaviors that contribute to your disorder.

Schedule your meals and snacks. Be sure and stick to your schedule. This will prevent you from becoming so hungry you gorge yourself later.

Eat a nutritious, sugar-free diet. The sooner you start eating a healthy diet again, the sooner you'll be able to kick your eating disorder. In a study of bulimic girls, researchers found that those who switched to a nutritious, sugar-free diet were free from binges after three weeks. The girls who continued their regular diets were not able to break the binge habit.

Include complex carbohydrates with each meal. This will help maintain your body's balance of blood sugar, insulin, and serotonin, which is a brain chemical that influences your feelings of calmness and contentment. Fruits, vegetables, and whole-grain breads fit the bill.

Take a supplement. Generally, vitamin and mineral deficiency is common in people with eating disorders.

Zap eating disorders with zinc. Since most people with eating disorders generally have vitamin and mineral deficiencies, that usually means they have low levels of zinc. In fact, one study found that 54 percent of people with anorexia or bulimia nervosa were zinc deficient.

A lack of zinc interferes with your senses of taste and smell and can cause you to lose interest in food almost entirely. Evidence suggests that low levels of zinc tend to perpetuate the problem. Once you get your zinc levels back to normal, it may be easier to get the rest of your eating disorder under control.

Good sources of zinc include lima beans, oysters, turkey, wheat germ, and yogurt. You may also want to ask your doctor if you would benefit from taking a separate zinc supplement.

Educate yourself about nutrition. This way you'll be better informed about what foods to eat for health and how to eat to lose weight if that's your goal. Although good nutrition alone won't break the cycle of an eating disorder, it is an important part of the journey back to healthy eating habits.

Feel good again with the feel-good food plan

The goal of this food plan is obvious — to help you feel good again. After years or months of an eating disorder, feeling good about yourself and your eating habits may seem as likely as finding the Holy Grail. However, not only is it possible, it's also a lot more likely. Developed by Elizabeth Somer, M.A., R.D., author of *Food and Mood: The Complete Guide to Eating Well and Feeling Your Best,* this plan focuses on a healthy, balanced eating lifestyle. Here are the daily goals:

- Reduce fat in your diet to 25 percent of calories.
- Limit sugars to 10 percent or less of your total calories.
- Limit caffeine to two servings or less.
- Eat at least three servings of fruit, four servings of vegetables, seven servings of breads and grains, and one serving of legumes.
- Divide calories evenly between five or six small meals a day. Eat a meal or snack every four hours.
- Take a vitamin/mineral supplement if you are not eating at least 2,500 calories a day from a variety of nutritious foods.

In addition, she recommends that you always eat breakfast, and drink at least eight glasses of water every day.

Finally, Ms. Somer suggests you'll have a better shot at success if you gradually work your way toward these goals instead of trying to make the changes all at once. Changing your habits slowly will give your body and brain chemicals time to adjust. And that may be just what you need to succeed.

Defeating the devil of desire — binge eating

If you constantly crave chocolate and stuff yourself with sweets, you may be suffering from binge eating disorder.

Binge eating disorder (BED) is a much milder form of the more commonly known eating disorder, bulimia nervosa. They're not the same, although it's easy to get them confused.

People with bulimia nervosa eat huge amounts of food, then rid themselves of the extra calories by vomiting, fasting, exercising excessively, or using laxatives. Those with binge eating disorder also eat large amounts at one sitting but don't attempt to purge their bodies afterward.

Think you may be suffering from binge eating disorder? Although surveys show 55 percent of people binge at least once a week, binge is a tough term to pin down because it means different things to different people.

Some people think any amount of a so-called "forbidden" food, even a cup of ice cream, is a binge. Although many people overeat now and then, binge eating disorder is a different sort of beast.

Do you frequently eat what others would consider unusually large amounts of food? Do you have trouble controlling what or how much you eat, often not stopping until you are uncomfortably full? If so, you may have a problem with binge eating disorder.

In addition to using the suggestions mentioned in this chapter, find a dietitian or mental health professional familiar with BED to help you overcome this problem. BED is not an easy disorder to treat on your own. Many people find that a health professional who teaches behavior therapy can help them learn effective ways to deal with the negative emotions that triggered their binges in the first place.

Dealing with bulimia the diet way

Your best shot at beating bulimia nervosa is to work closely with your doctor and a nutritionist who can help you change your eating habits. You need a structured eating plan as opposed to a restrictive diet, which may actually trigger binges. Here are some other helpful tips that can get you started on the road to recovery.

- Use a food diary to plan meals and snacks. Record what you plan to eat as well as what you actually eat. If you are still having trouble with binges, your food diary may help you see why and how you can correct the problem.
- Stretch your meals and make them more filling by including vegetables, salad, and/or fruit at each one.
- Emphasize foods that have plenty of complex carbohydrates so you'll feel full, with just a little fat to make that fullness last longer. Researchers suspect carbohydrates may help bulimics by increasing serotonin levels. High serotonin levels have a calming effect. Trying to achieve this effect is what leads

many bulimics to binge on carbohydrates in the first place. However, experts suggest you may be able to avoid binges by eating moderate amounts of carbohydrate-rich foods throughout the day. In order to boost serotonin levels, always combine fruit with another food such as nonfat, sugar-free yogurt or a bagel.

- Eat foods that are naturally divided into portions, such as potatoes, fruits, cartons of yogurt or cottage cheese, and frozen dinners.
- Always eat meals and snacks sitting down.
- Use silverware. Avoid finger foods.
- Eat while your food is warm. You'll feel fuller.

How to get cravings under control

Even if you don't have an eating disorder, most people have problems controlling their food cravings now and then. If you're trying to peel off a few pounds, giving into cravings can really wreck your weight loss plan. Here are some tips to help.

Feast on fiber. It may sound totally unappealing, but the truth is that the most satisfying and filling foods are full of fiber, protein, and water.

Food researchers have found boiled potatoes to be especially satisfying. Beans and lentils, because of their high-fiber content and your body's tendency to absorb them slowly, also make you feel fuller longer.

Tell high-fat foods to take a hike. High-fat foods cause more cravings for high-fat foods. Once you get on this crazy carousel, it can be hard to get off.

Munch on mini-meals. Eating five or six small meals, instead of three big ones, will help stabilize your blood-sugar levels. This will keep you from getting so hungry you end up stuffing yourself at the next meal. If you're watching your weight, divide your daily calories among the five or six meals. Just because you're eating more meals doesn't mean you need to eat more calories. You simply need to spread them out better.

Recognize your trigger foods. If potato chips turn you into a munching monster, don't buy them. Also, never go grocery shopping on an empty stomach. The temptation to grab anything and everything off the shelves is too hard to resist.

Down with strict, restrictive diets. Nerve chemicals and hormones go wildly out of whack on quick weight-loss diets. Your cravings will be more uncontrollable than ever.

Curb your craving with a healthy substitute. If you're craving crunchy, opt for pretzels instead of potato chips. Even better, crunch on carrots or an apple. To calm a raging chocolate craving, try some sugar-free cocoa. If you're cruising for anything creamy, good low-sugar, low-fat alternatives include oatmeal, hot cereal, and reduced fat and sugar soups and puddings.

Be prepared. Try to have some healthy alternatives around the house or with you at all times. You're more likely to beat a craving if you don't let it catch you off guard.

Favor complex carbos over simple sugars. Although simple sugars give you a rush, it isn't long before they leave you feeling more tired than ever. Beat the low-blood-sugar blahs with complex carbohydrates, such as whole-grain breads, crackers, cereal, and pastas. Other good choices include brown rice and vegetables.

Perk up with protein. Too many complex carbohydrates can put you to sleep. That's why it's important to include protein in your diet, too. If you want to feel full, yet alert at the same time, try combining a complex carbohydrate with a protein, such as crackers and cheese.

But what happens if a craving just won't let go? If you do find yourself caving in, you can at least control portion sizes. Eat a little and throw the rest away. Your soul will feel satisfied but you won't have to berate yourself for totally losing control.

Axe appetite loss

Appetite loss is not necessarily a sign that you're suffering from an eating disorder. Any number of other causes can contribute to appetite loss including heart or lung disease, cancer, memory loss, depression, and even certain medicines.

However, it's important to find out what's causing your appetite loss and get it under control, especially if you're losing weight when you don't need to. Otherwise you're likely to suffer from increasingly serious problems such as muscle loss, general weakness, tiredness, and even a reduced ability to fight off disease or recover from surgery or sickness.

First, see your doctor to check for underlying problems that may be contributing to your loss of appetite. Often, just getting any medical problems under control will improve your appetite. In addition, try these tips to titillate your taste buds:

Take a multivitamin. A loss of appetite is actually one of the first signs of a vitamin or mineral deficiency.

Spice up your life. Sometimes appetite loss occurs because meals have become boring and bland. Experimenting with new spices, textures, and flavors will often turn on your appetite and take your taste buds to new heights.

Go for some garlic and onions. Marinating foods in garlic and onion-based dressings will add flavor without offensive odors.

Viva variety. If variety can spice up your life, it will certainly do the same for your meals. Try to tempt all your taste buds with a mixture of sour, spicy, sweet, and salty foods.

Enjoy ethnic. Go on an appetite adventure and sample some ethnic and regional foods. This is a good way to find new taste combinations that really rev up your appetite.

Eat with a companion. If you don't have a live-in partner, try to participate in church and community gatherings, and meet family and friends for a meal as often as possible. You may be surprised to find how much your appetite is aroused just by getting out and socializing.

Go for some gravy. If your mouth tends to be dry, moisten your foods with gravy, include soup with your meals, and drink plenty of non-caffeinated liquids.

Soften up. If you have trouble chewing, consider cooking meats in a pressure cooker, or cook meat for a longer period of time than normal to make it extra tender. If you still have trouble chewing, replace whole meats with ground meats or get your protein in the form of egg and cheese.

Knock out nausea. Sucking on hard candy, eating dry bread, or sipping some flat soda are all quick and easy ways to handle a bout of nausea. Don't eat too much at one time, but be sure to eat on a regular schedule. Small, frequent meals are your best bet. Getting overly hungry can increase your feelings of nausea. Don't eat your favorite foods when you're feeling sick. If you do, you run the risk of never liking them again.

Put on pounds to put off poor health

If you suffer from anorexia nervosa or just plain old appetite loss, you're likely to lose a lot of weight. Weighing too little can be just as dangerous as weighing too much. In fact, some studies suggest being underweight may shorten your life. Of course, if you're dramatically underweight, you run the risk of shutting down your whole body system.

If you're underweight, here are some healthy ways to pack on some extra pounds:

Make the most of your favorite meal. Is there one meal you look forward to above all others? Then try adding a few extra foods to this meal to make up for those where you typically eat very little. For example, if you really like breakfast, but normally eat only toast and cereal, try including a piece of cheese and fruit to boost your nutrition and calorie count.

Fill your favorite foods with extra calories. An easy way to get extra calories is to add nonfat dry milk or breakfast powders to cereals, casseroles, and soups. This way, even if you can't eat all the foods you know you should, you'll at least get energy from the extra calories you pack into your favorite foods.

You may also want to try stimulating your appetite before a meal with a high-calorie nutritional supplement, such as a liquid meal drink or even yogurt. A recent study of 16 older men found that the older men ate a heartier lunch than they normally did if they ate some high-calorie yogurt beforehand.

Avoid high-fiber foods. When you're struggling with appetite loss, high-fiber foods can make you feel fuller than you really are and reduce your intake of other foods.

Avoid gassy foods and drinks. Stay away from foods that make you feel bloated. Although these foods vary from person to person, some common culprits include beans, broccoli, cabbage, carbonated drinks, and coffee.

Save drinks for last. If you drink too much too soon during your meal, you may not eat as much food as you should. If you need to take medicine with your meal, wait until you've finished eating if possible.

EMPHYSEMA

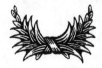

Emphasize nutrition

For people with emphysema, poor nutrition is a real threat. It can weaken the muscles you need to breathe, make it harder for you to exercise, and hurt your immune system. It also makes you more vulnerable to colds, flu, and other illnesses. This can leave you feeling depressed and hopeless. But healthy eating can help.

Meals may be more difficult when you have emphysema, especially if you're on oxygen or must breathe through your mouth to get enough air. You might not know you're short on nutrients, but your body will show it. Make nourishment a priority, and you'll help your emphysema and your overall health. Here are some specific steps to take:

- **Cut some carbohydrates.** When you eat a meal high in starch and sugar, your body has to work harder to get rid of the carbon dioxide that's produced. So make sure the carbohydrates you eat really count. Instead of eating sugar and refined flour, eat more nutritious whole grains, such as whole wheat breads and cereals, brown rice, and unrefined oatmeal. For sweets, rely on the natural sugar in fruits for delicious taste and the most nutrition. Include lots of healthy vegetables, both low-carbohydrate ones such as broccoli and spinach, and high-carbohydrate ones like sweet potatoes and squash.

- **Plan on protein.** You need to get enough protein, but too much can be hard on your body. Taking in around 15 percent of your daily calories in protein should be about right, but your doctor may prescribe more protein if he thinks you're not getting enough. Fish is a good source of high-quality protein, and the fish oil it contains may give you added health benefits, like protecting your heart.

- **Feel OK about fat.** If you have emphysema and have been losing weight, you probably don't need to worry too much about fat. People who must have mechanical help to breathe are sometimes given a mix of foods in which fat accounts for almost 50 percent of calories. Check with your doctor to see what percentage of fat he thinks is appropriate for your diet.

- **Turn up the heat factor.** Feel free to eat hot, spicy foods such as chili peppers, mustard, horseradish, cayenne pepper, garlic, and onions. Besides making your meals more appealing, they help you feel better by opening your air passages.

- **Get your vitamins and minerals.** Make sure you are getting at least the recommended daily allowance, especially of vitamins A, C, and E. Vegetables such as carrots, watercress, and spinach provide these vitamins. Fruits such as grapes, oranges, lemons, and black currants are also good choices.

- **Take a nice long drink.** Although it's not really a food, water is an important part of your daily diet if you have emphysema. Drinking eight to 10 glasses of water or other healthy liquids a day will help thin mucus so it's easier to cough up.

The vitamin C connection

If you have emphysema, chances are you're a smoker or a former smoker. That's where the vitamin connection comes in.

Researchers have found that vitamin C almost completely stops white blood cells from clumping and sticking to the inside walls of blood vessels. This type of blockage is one of the harmful effects of cigarette smoke. The researchers believe that having enough vitamin C in your blood could protect you from the heart and lung diseases caused by cigarette smoking.

Another study checked the respiratory function of 835 men and found that the more vitamin C in their blood the better their lungs functioned. This backs up previous studies showing that vitamin C may protect your lungs from damage and help them work better. Taking in plenty of vitamin C may not reverse the damage of emphysema, but it might slow it down or help keep it from getting worse.

It's easy to get vitamin C in your diet from a variety of tasty fruits and vegetables. Oranges, lemons, grapefruit, strawberries, and tangerines are excellent fruit sources of vitamin C. Broccoli, brussels sprouts, cabbage, collards, kale, spinach, tomatoes, and watercress are vegetables high in C. If you have trouble getting enough vitamin-C-rich foods into your diet, you can turn to supplements. Check with your doctor to see what dose of vitamin C he feels is appropriate for you.

The vitamin A attack plan

Even though you may not be deficient in vitamin A overall, you could lack it in one place that really needs it — your lungs. Smoking damages your lung cells so they can no longer absorb and use vitamin A as they should. Without vitamin A, the cells secrete less mucus. Air passages get narrower, and it's harder for you to breathe.

A recent medical study examined the link between vitamin A and breathing difficulty in people with COPD. Subjects taking vitamin A supplements for 30 days showed significant improvement in their ability to breathe. In a study done on animals, vitamin A actually reversed some of the lung damage of emphysema.

These studies are small, but their findings are promising. Adding more vitamin A to your diet is a simple way to get the disease-fighting benefits of this important vitamin. To do this, you need to eat foods that are high in beta carotene, the substance that is converted to vitamin A in your body. These foods include spinach, broccoli, winter squash, sweet potatoes, carrots, pumpkin, cantaloupe, and apricots.

It's much better to get your vitamin A from foods than from supplements. It's easy to overdose on vitamin A, which can be toxic in large amounts. If you really feel you need a supplement, get your doctor's advice.

Helpful herbs for emphysema

Herbal treatments are as old as civilization and as current as today's news. Scientists are rediscovering the benefits of using herbs to treat many of today's modern ills, including the lung disease emphysema. Two herbs, mullein and elecampane, seem to be helpful in relieving some of the discomfort of chronic lung disease.

- **Mullein**, a common blooming plant in the United States, has traditionally been a treatment for respiratory diseases. Other common names for mullein are candleflower, candlewick, and longwort. It is prized for its soothing effect on throat tissues and is helpful for frequent coughs. Experts recommend making a tea with two teaspoons of dried, crushed mullein flowers or leaves for each cup of boiling water. You should strain the tea before drinking it.

- **Elecampane**, also known as inula helenium, scabwort, or yellow starwort, is an herbal member of the daisy family. Known as a remedy for coughs, elecampane is often added to cough medicines in Europe. It may be especially effective in calming coughs that won't quit, such as asthmatic or bronchial coughs. Herbal experts recommend using the dried, shredded root of the elecampane plant to make a tea. Combine one teaspoon with a cup of cold water and let it steep for eight to 10 hours. Strain the tea, heat it, and drink it up to three times a day to soothe your chronic cough. You'll notice a sweet flavor, since the elecampane root is also used in powdered form to make a sugar substitute for diabetics.

FIBROCYSTIC BREAST DISEASE

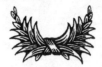

5 ways to 'bust' painful breasts

Fibrocystic breast disease is a benign breast disorder, which means it's not harmful. The term "fibrocystic breast disease" is misleading and, frankly, scary. That's why many medical professionals now call this condition "fibrocystic change."

If you suffer from painful, fluid-filled cysts in your breasts, don't assume you have a benign breast disorder. Just to rule out anything more serious, see your doctor and have a breast exam including a mammogram.

Once your doctor has ruled out a serious condition, there are things you can do to help yourself. One of the easiest is looking at your diet and making some changes.

Remember your B vitamins. When you think about estrogen, you don't usually think about your liver. But some doctors now link estrogen-related disorders, like fibrocystic changes, to liver function. To keep your liver healthy, you need B vitamins. In fact, fibrocystic-change symptoms improved in one study where test subjects received supplements of this group of vitamins. To eat foods high in the B-complex vitamins, choose whole grains, beans, peas, and liver. They help your body turn carbohydrates, fats, and protein into energy, and they just might turn the tide against fibrocystic changes.

Consider vitamin E. There is some evidence that daily doses of vitamin E, between 100 and 1,200 international units (IU), can reduce the number of cysts you develop and even how large they become. If you're thinking about taking supplements, check with your doctor first. Vitamin E supplements can raise blood pressure in some people. Green and leafy vegetables, wheat germ, whole-grain products, nuts, and seeds are good, safe ways to add vitamin E to your diet.

Get more magnesium. Some experts think a supplement of magnesium is helpful in treating breast cysts. Eat nuts, legumes, whole grains, dark green vegetables, and seafood for magnesium the natural way.

Don't ignore iodine. The mineral iodine may protect you from breast lumps and cysts. Studies show that if you don't have enough iodine in your diet, you could be at a higher risk of developing fibro-cystic changes. The recommended dietary allowance (RDA) for iodine is 150 micrograms (mcg). One cup of milk or a little less than a half teaspoon of iodized salt, or an iodized salt substitute, supplies close to the RDA. Other dietary sources are vegetables; seafood, especially halibut and cod liver; fish liver oils; eggs; and bread. The antiseptic iodine, which is used on cuts and scrapes, is not the same thing and should not be taken internally.

Fight back with omega-3. One of the most annoying symptoms of fibrocystic change is painful breasts. You can control this discomfort by adding more omega-3 fatty acids to your diet. Fish oil is a wonderful source of these important nutrients. You can supplement with fish oil capsules, but a better solution is to get it naturally by eating cold-water fish. Try albacore tuna, lake trout, sturgeon, salmon, and anchovies.

Low-fat way to fewer lumps

Studies show that women with various forms of breast disorders eat more high-calorie, high-fat foods, especially the saturated fat found in meat and dairy products, than women who do not suffer from benign breast disorders. It may be that saturated fats and excess calories cause a higher production of female hormones. These, in turn, cause lumps and cysts to form in your breasts.

A good rule of thumb is to make dietary fats only 30 percent of your daily calories. It's also important that you lower your percentage of body fat by maintaining your ideal weight. If you take care of the rest of your body, your breasts will benefit as well.

Cut caffeine to cut pain

Caffeine is everywhere — in the coffee and tea you drink, the soda you swizzle, and the chocolate you let melt in your mouth — and it may be linked to fibrocystic changes.

If you suffer from painful breast lumps, experts suggest you cut caffeine completely out of your diet for about three to four months. This doesn't mean dropping back to only one cup of coffee a day, or drinking a couple of sodas only on the weekend. It means the end of caffeine. Substitute decaffeinated coffee or grain-based products, caffeine-free sodas, and carob for your usual fare. Also, check the labels on any pain medication you're taking. Some pain relievers contain hidden caffeine.

If you can quit "cold turkey," that's good. But if you're really used to a regular intake of caffeine, wean yourself off of it gradually. After four months of complete abstinence, see how you feel. For some women, there will be no difference. Others will notice fewer or smaller breast lumps and less pain.

Get rid of excess fluid to soothe breast pain

Just before you get your period, your body signals your kidneys to retain fluid. This extra fluid makes you feel bloated, and it can cause discomfort in your breasts.

Certain foods act like diuretics, which means they help your body eliminate fluid. Adding some natural diuretics to your diet, especially just before your period, may provide short-term relief from the pain and heaviness of breast cysts.

Foods that are considered natural diuretics are grapefruit juice, cranberry juice, lemon water, and watermelon. In addition, limit your salt and drink six to eight glasses of water each day to flush out excess sodium.

Herbs and herbal teas that have a mild diuretic action are rose hips, parsley, lovage root, horsetail, ginger, dandelion, chicory, buchu, and borage.

GALLBLADDER DISEASE

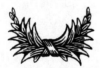

Quick weight loss can spell trouble

You've got to fit into that special dress or suit next month. In a panic, you turn to those alluring ads for quick weight loss. Be careful. Fad or crash diets that cause you to lose weight too fast can increase your risk of developing gallstones.

Some scientists believe that irregular, low-calorie meals (800 calories a day or less) cause too much cholesterol to stay in the gallbladder, where it settles into clumps that later form gallstones. So first of all, don't skip meals, especially breakfast. It's the most important meal of the day if you want to avoid this painful problem. Your gallbladder needs to empty regularly, and it only does this when your digestive system is working.

Be sure to eat lots of fresh fruits and vegetables. Balance this with lean meat for protein and a moderate amount of low-sugar carbohydrates to round up the calories. A slow but steady weight loss plan is safest.

The worst foods for gallbladder woes

Since gallstones are made from excess cholesterol, it only makes sense to keep your cholesterol levels low. So how do you know what foods to eat? Just remember that cholesterol is only found in animal products, especially the fatty part of any meat.

These probably include some of your favorites, like bacon, hot dogs and sausage, but unfortunately, they are the worst offenders. Others to worry about are egg yolks, shellfish, and dairy products. In fact, eggs are the number one problem food for people with gallstones.

Dried beans and peas, skinless chicken or turkey, and skim-milk dairy products are all healthy, low-cholesterol choices.

You might want to consider switching to a vegetarian diet. Studies have shown that this eliminates a lot of the troublesome foods, while leaving all the healthy natural alternatives.

Gallbladder good guys

Forever fiber. Does a spread of corn-on-the-cob, baked beans, and fresh raspberries sound like the perfect summer meal? This menu would not only appeal to your taste buds, but your intestines as well, since these foods are full of natural fiber. Eating 25 to 40 grams of fiber each day will lower your risk of developing all kinds of intestinal disorders, including gallstones.

Next time you're at the store, pick up more whole grain products, fresh fruits and vegetables, and dried beans. If you need help making out that high-fiber shopping list, start with spinach, dates, and bran cereals.

Hit a high C. The common orange, along with other foods high in vitamin C, may help lower your risk of developing painful stones. One study suggests that if you're deficient in vitamin C, you're more likely to get gallstones. Try adding more citrus foods to your diet, as well as brussels sprouts, strawberries, broccoli, collard greens, cantaloupe, tomato juice, and cabbage.

More E is easy. Want a simple way to lower your chances of developing gallstones? Eat more "E." That is, vitamin E. Start cooking with safflower or sunflower oil. Sprinkle some wheat germ on your peaches for a double dose of E. Make your salad with spinach, and take advantage of asparagus season. All these foods will give you at least 10 mg of vitamin E — the daily recommended dietary allowance. If you are vitamin E deficient, your doctor can prescribe a supplement.

Beef and cherry pie? It's an odd combination, but it seems to work. Researchers have tested various foods on people suffering from gallstones and have put together a combination of nine foods that cause no pain or other symptoms. See how many dishes you can come up with using only beef, rye, soy, rice, cherries, peaches, apricots, beets, and spinach.

Surrender the fat

If you have gallstones, you will soon learn that fat is your gallbladder's worst enemy. Eating fat causes your gallbladder to contract and empty bile into your intestines, a routine process, except when you have gallstones. These contractions cause the gallstones to rub and irritate the inside of your gallbladder, sending it into painful spasms.

To cut the fat in dairy products, choose skim, 1/2-percent, or 1-percent milk, buttermilk or yogurt; part-skim cheese products; and low-fat or fat-free ice cream, frozen yogurt, and sour cream.

When cruising the meat department, stroll past the sausage, bacon, frankfurters, and lunch meats, especially bologna and salami. It's all right to linger in the poultry section, just remember to remove that skin before cooking. Water-packed tuna and salmon are good low-fat fish choices. With all meats, think about reducing your serving size to three ounces.

For a happier gallbladder, season your food with herbs, lemon, or vinegar; not cream sauces, butter, gravies, mayonnaise, or salad dressings. If you cut the fat, be sure to add more carbohydrates and protein into your diet.

GAS

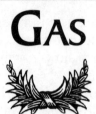

The incredible bean

Beans are good for you. Don't avoid them because of the intestinal discomfort they can cause. To get all the nourishing benefits without any gassy side effects, follow these tips:

- Soak the dried beans for about four or five hours, then drain.
- Cover with fresh water and boil for 10 minutes. Simmer for 30 minutes.
- Drain and cover with more water. Simmer until the beans are tender, about one to two hours.

Give up these gas-producers

The bad news is you can't cut out all gas-producing foods without seriously endangering your health. The good news is not all foods react the same way in everybody. You may have to experiment to see what foods give you that bloated, about-to-explode feeling.

A very general rule is carbohydrates can cause gas, while foods high in fats and proteins produce less. More specifically, these gas-producers are likely to make you uncomfortable:

- **Lactose.** This natural sugar is in milk, cheese, ice cream, and other milk products; bread; cereal; and salad dressing.
- **Fructose.** A fruit sugar found in pears, honey, onions, artichokes, and wheat.
- **Raffinose.** A complex sugar found in beans, cabbage, brussels sprouts, broccoli, and asparagus.
- **Sorbitol.** As a natural sweetener, you can find it in apples, pears, peaches, and prunes. It is also used as an artificial sweetener in sugarfree products and dietetic foods.
- **Starches.** Wheat, corn, noodles, and potatoes contain these gas-causing carbohydrates.
- **Soluble fiber.** This type of fiber, found in fruit, peas, beans, seeds, rye, rice bran, and oat bran, is not digested in the

small intestine. Bacteria break it down in the large intestine, releasing gas at the same time.

- **Carbonated liquids.** Beverages such as soda and beer fill your digestive system with carbon dioxide bubbles. If you can't go without your bubbly beverage, at least "de-fizz" it first by pouring it into a glass.

Humble herbs relieve gas

Even though many herbal remedies are based on superstition and folklore, the oils or seeds from some herbs are better at relieving gas than many commercial products.

Anise. Cakes flavored with anise were popular in Roman times to prevent indigestion after a particularly rich meal, such as a wedding feast. This is where the tradition of a wedding cake came from. Today, you can mix anise with caraway and fennel and drink it hot to relieve gas pain.

Chamomile. Tea made from chamomile is an old and familiar prescription for calming and healing the digestive system.

Peppermint. Peppermint leaves, either chewed or steeped in hot water, will relieve gas and indigestion.

Fennel. This herb was once used as a guard against witches, fleas, and bad spirits — quite a burden of responsibility for such a delicate looking herb. Crushed fennel seeds, mixed with anise and caraway, make a soothing tea.

Caraway. The seeds of the caraway plant add flavor and reduce the gassy side effects of foods like cabbage.

There are two ways gas gets into your digestive system: when you swallow air, usually caused by eating or drinking fast; chewing gum; smoking; or wearing loose dentures; and through bacteria breaking down certain foods in the large intestine.

Foods made up of insoluble fiber, the kind that won't dissolve in water, produce no gas at all. This fiber passes through the digestive system without being broken down. You can find insoluble fiber in whole grains, wheat bran, vegetables, seeds, and brown rice.

GASTRITIS

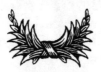

Soothing a stomach that says 'ouch'

You know you should say "no" to nachos and beer and bypass the bottomless cup of coffee. You should, but sometimes you just have to give in to those cravings — even if your stomach ends up paying for it later. And the price could be a painful bout of gastritis. This is an inflammation of the lining of your stomach, caused by infection, diet, or certain medications like aspirin or ibuprofen. Symptoms include loss of appetite, indigestion, cramping, nausea, and vomiting. If your doctor says you have gastritis, try these suggestions to help keep your tummy tranquil.

Eat small meals. Eating small meals throughout the day reduces the amount of digestive juices your stomach produces at any one time. This is gentler on your digestive system.

Drink water. One folk remedy that may just wash away your stomach pain is as pure and simple as summer rain. It's water. Drink 16 ounces of lukewarm water very slowly, without stopping. Since water can rid your body of many toxins, this is a healthy tip no matter what your trouble.

Enjoy fruits and veggies. Fruits and vegetables don't have the fat and cholesterol that meats and processed foods have, which means healthier, more natural digestion. Studies show that foods high in vitamin C reduce the risk of developing gastritis and stomach cancer. Citrus fruits, broccoli, cantaloupe, brussels sprouts, and sweet peppers are good sources of vitamin C.

Avoid caffeine, alcohol, and spicy dishes. These things eat through the barrier that protects your stomach lining, exposing it to harsh digestive acids which can cause sores and inflammation.

Stay away from milk. The real surprise for most people is that milk is no longer considered soothing to the stomach. Experts now know that dairy proteins cause the stomach to produce more acid. This can irritate the delicate tissues of your stomach and lead to pain, cramping, and indigestion.

GLAUCOMA

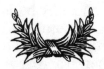

Grab hold of glutathione

A vital amino acid, glutathione does everything from fighting aging to building protein. This stellar substance also boosts your immunity, fights damage from disease and pollution, and protects your eyes. But when your body's supplies are low, it can cause problems.

In your eyes, glutathione plays a valuable role helping to fight off free-radical damage. Levels of glutathione in your eyes should normally be very high. In a recent study, researchers checked glutathione levels in the eyes of people with eye disease. They found those with glaucoma had a significantly lower level of glutathione in their eyes. Without adequate glutathione, antioxidants can't protect the eyes, making them more prone to disease.

Building up the natural supply of glutathione in your body is a good way to help protect your eyes from the ravages of free radicals. Here are four good ways to build up your supply:

- **Keep it fresh.** Eat fresh fruits and vegetables for the richest supply of glutathione. Foods that are canned, smoked, or otherwise processed contain much less glutathione than the same foods when they are fresh.
- **Get more C.** Studies show that consuming vitamin C raises your glutathione levels. So, if you eat lots of citrus fruits, you're giving your body a double boost of glutathione.
- **Lose the fat.** The more fat you eat, the more free radicals you have in your body. Glutathione works overtime to fight free radicals, which causes your glutathione level to drop. Cutting way back on your fat intake allows your body to build up its supply of glutathione.
- **Go for glutamine.** If you want to add even more to your glutathione stores, you can take supplements. But taking glutathione directly isn't as helpful as taking glutamine, another amino acid that converts to glutathione in your body. This food supplement can be found in health food stores.

Herbal help for glaucoma

As many as two out of every 100 people over the age of 35 are affected by glaucoma, the unhealthy buildup of pressure in the eyes. Laser surgery is effective for some people, but natural remedies may have a place in preventing and treating glaucoma, too.

According to herbal expert Varro Tyler, preliminary studies are being done using bilberries, a type of European dried blueberry, as a possible treatment for glaucoma and other eye diseases. Bilberry extract is sold as medicine in Europe and as a food supplement in the United States.

The pasque flower is an herb used to treat glaucoma and other eye problems. Like many herbs, it was used in "the good old days" before surgery was common. The herb can be made into a tea or infusion by steeping the whole dried pasque flower in hot water.

HAIR LOSS

The root of temporary hair loss

You've gone on a crash diet, and you're very pleased about all the pounds you've lost. However, excess weight isn't the only thing that has disappeared. You seem to be filling the shower drain with hair, and you're beginning to think you're going bald.

People normally lose 100 to 125 hairs per day. Fortunately, those hairs grow right back. However, if you suddenly begin losing more hair than usual, your diet could be the hair-robbing culprit. Extremely low-calorie diets can cause temporary hair loss, and a vitamin supplement could make things worse if it contains a lot of vitamin A. Excessive doses of vitamin A can cause you to lose hair.

To save your hair, try a more sensible diet, and get your nutrients from foods. Remember that slow and steady wins the race, so take your time and lose the weight, but keep your hair.

Hair-raising concerns

Trying to pick through the slew of products claiming to restore hair is enough to make you pull your hair out. Your options range from natural to surgical and permanent to temporary. No one treatment is right for everyone. With millions of men looking for hair loss cures, you're bound to have people trying to take advantage of you. To protect your health, wallet, and self esteem, carefully check out the pros and cons, and consult experts before you buy.

Although most oral and topical hair loss treatments have not proved effective, you may find an herbal mixture that works for you. Royal jelly, nettle, and jojoba oil all claim to stimulate hair growth. A mixture of lavender oil, calamus oil, gentian tincture, and rosemary spirit rubbed on your scalp is said to put hair on your head.

Serious causes to consider

If hair loss is a problem, have your thyroid and iron levels checked to be sure they're normal. Anemia (iron deficiency), a low blood count or thyroid problems could be responsible. You may need a simple blood test to determine if you have normal hormone and nutrient levels.

HEADACHE

Diet decisions can head off headaches

People will do almost anything to get rid of a headache. Some cavemen may even have drilled holes in their heads to relieve their pain. If you have frequent headaches, you probably don't want to wait until one strikes to decide what to do about it. There are ways to head them off without drilling a hole in your head or even reaching for the pill bottle.

Eat regular meals. Skipping meals or going a long time between meals can bring on headaches caused by low blood sugar. By eating at regular times and including some protein food at least three times a day, you may be able to avoid some of the pain.

Keep a food diary. Many foods seem to trigger headaches, but the same ones don't affect everybody the same. To help find out which foods bring on your headaches, make notes about what you eat and drink each day.

A headache usually occurs three to 12 hours after eating a trigger food, but it can take even longer. Look back as far as 24 hours before the headache occurred to see what may have caused it. Some foods may be a problem when combined with other foods, but are okay when eaten alone. Therefore, it may be helpful to list ingredients on a pizza or in a casserole.

You may also want to make notes about your moods and activities. Some people find that the troublesome foods may not cause headaches except when they are under stress, fatigued, or at a particular time of their menstrual cycle. Alcohol, especially red wine, is one of the triggers most often reported in connection with other factors, like stress or fatigue.

Avoid allergens. Although headaches usually result from a chemical in the food, sometimes an allergy is the cause. A 17-year-old girl in Italy suffered severe headaches off and on for more than 10 years. She had taken medication, but the headaches, which were not migraines, continued to get worse.

She realized that a severe headache started every time she went into a kitchen where eggs were being fried. Tests showed she was allergic to eggs and milk. Since taking those out of her diet, she has been relatively headache-free.

If you have headaches you can't explain, an allergy may be the problem. Your food diary can be the key to tracking them down.

Lick the ice cream headache

A dish of ice cream on a hot summer day can look inviting. But after a few quick bites, a sudden sharp pain may strike in the middle of your forehead. Ouch! The attack of an ice cream headache.

Ice cream is the most common cause of head pain, according to a report in the *British Medical Journal*. Eating or drinking this or other very cold foods and beverages can cause a stabbing pain that usually peaks in 30 to 60 seconds. It usually fades quickly, but in some people can last up to five minutes.

There's no need to give up ice cream to avoid an ice cream headache. Just eat slowly and try not to let the frozen treat touch the back of the roof of your mouth. If you find this hard to do, just wait for winter. One researcher experimented by pressing crushed ice to his palette. He found that in hot weather this produced pain within 20 to 30 seconds, but in cold weather he had no pain at all.

Savor scents-ible solutions

Some foods don't have to be eaten to soothe headaches. Try these unusual remedies for your pain.

An apple a day — or just a walk though the orchard — might be enough to keep the doctor away. If you like the smell of green apples, you may be able to reduce the pain of migraine headaches. A study of 50 "migraineurs" found that those who like the smell of green apples reported less severe headaches when they sniffed this scent. They aren't sure why. If pleasant smells distract and relax you, they can lift your mood. Maybe you feel happier, so it's easier to handle the pain.

Ease pain with herbal oils. Researchers in Germany found that peppermint oil was as effective as acetaminophen, the pain-reducing ingredient in Tylenol and Datril, in reducing headache pain. A mixture of 10 percent peppermint oil in ordinary alcohol brought pain relief within 15 minutes. The peppermint oil solution was not swallowed. It was rubbed over the temples and foreheads of people suffering from tension-type headaches. There were no complaints of side effects.

Rosemary, lavender, and chamomile are other essential oils that may also help ease your headache. For quick comfort, gently rub one drop of oil on the place where it hurts the most. The essence of the herb is very concentrated, so even though it seems like such a little bit, one drop should really be enough. You can buy essential oils in natural food stores.

Hot-foot it to relief. Believe it or not, an herbal footbath can soothe your headache. Mix one teaspoon of powdered mustard or ginger with water as hot as you can stand in a plastic basin big enough for both feet. Settle into a comfortable chair and ease your feet gently into the water. Drape a thick towel across the top to hold in the heat. Lean back, close you eyes, breathe deeply, and relax for about 15 minutes. By the time the water cools, your headache may be completely forgotten.

Think about ginkgo

It's hard to think about anything when you have a headache. But the herb gingko helps clear headaches and confusion by increasing the flow of blood to the brain. One study found ginkgo increased blood flow by 70 percent in persons between 50 and 70 years of age. People from 30 to 50 years old saw a 20 percent improvement.

Ginkgo usually comes in 40-mg tablets. The recommended dosage is three tablets a day with meals. It seems that the longer you take it, the more it helps. Ginkgo has no known serious side effects with extended use, but very large doses may cause some restlessness, diarrhea, nausea or vomiting.

Manage migraines naturally

Migraine misery has a long history. Hippocrates, the "Father of Medicine," was one of the first to describe it more than 2,000 years ago. If you're a migraineur, you deal with pounding pain and nausea, or what's known as a "sick headache." Although some people find that nothing gives them relief, others have discovered natural ways to help keep migraines away or at least lessen the pain.

Feverfew is often seen in English gardens but is known for more than just its pretty flowers. For more than 2,000 years, it has been used in the treatment of headaches. Recent research has found that its leaves contain chemicals that reduce the inflammation and muscle spasms associated with migraine headaches.

You can buy feverfew preparations at a health or nutrition store. Check the label to be sure the preparation you buy contains at least 0.2 percent parthenolide. That's the main ingredient that reduces pain and causes the migraines to come less often.

It was recently found that tanetin, a flavonol in feverfew, may also fight migraines by reducing inflammation. In the future, you may want to watch for it on the label as well.

The recommended dosage is 125 mg/day of the dried feverfew leaves. You can get the same amount by chewing one or two fresh leaves each day. Try masking the somewhat bitter taste by eating the leaves with other foods. If you are particularly sensitive to the fresh leaves, you can get mouth ulcers. In that case the dried leaves may be more suitable.

Magnesium deficiency can cause migraines. Studies show that taking magnesium can help reduce the number and intensity of headaches. In one study, 3,000 women were given 200 mg of magnesium a day. About 80 percent reported migraine relief.

Too much magnesium can interfere with your calcium absorption, and it could be dangerous to take more than 500 mg/day in supplement form. It's easy to get magnesium from your diet, but this nutrient can be washed or peeled away or lost in other processes. The closer foods are to the natural state, the more magnesium you'll retain.

Good food sources include brown rice, popcorn, oatmeal, corn-meal, broccoli, green peas, acorn squash, potatoes, sweet potatoes, shrimp, clams, and skim milk.

Calcium and vitamin D can help relieve migraines in people with low blood levels of vitamin D. When a group of women with premenstrual syndrome (PMS) were found to have low levels of vit-amin D, they were given a combination of calcium and vitamin D. They found that not only did the symptoms of PMS improve, their premenstrual migraines got better as well.

Two post-menopausal women who also had low levels of vitamin D found dramatic improvement with calcium and vitamin D supplements. Their headaches came less frequently and lasted a shorter time.

Scientists aren't sure exactly why calcium and vitamin D improve migraine headaches. It is clear, however, that the body needs vitamin D in order to absorb calcium. You can get both these nutrients naturally by drinking milk.

Riboflavin eases migraine pain as effectively as aspirin. In a study of 49 people who had migraine headaches, each one took 400 mg/day of riboflavin for three months. Half of them also took 75 mg of aspirin. Results showed that 68 percent had less severe headaches after taking riboflavin with no difference between those who took aspirin and those who did not. Riboflavin is found in foods such as milk, eggs, meat, poultry, fish, and green leafy vegetables.

Omega-3 fish oil can reduce the number of migraines as well as their intensity. Sixty percent of the people in a study at the University of Cincinnati reported improvement after taking fish oil capsules for six weeks.

There is some danger of getting too much omega-3 in supple-ments because the oil is more concentrated than it is in the fish. Your best natural source is fatty, cold-water fish like tuna, cod, and salmon. You can also get omega-3 oil from oat germ, flaxseed, soy bean products, and walnuts.

Ginger may be the root of relief for some migraine sufferers. A 42-year-old woman in Denmark suffered with severe migraine headaches for 16 years. Researchers at Odense University gave her 500 to 600 mg of powdered ginger mixed with water at the first sign of a headache. She felt better within 30 minutes after taking the ginger.

After a few days of using the ginger four times a day with no side effects, she began to include fresh uncooked ginger in her daily diet. She found she had fewer, less severe migraines.

Herbalists generally recommend 2 to 4 grams of ginger a day. For migraines, you might need more. At first, ginger may cause a burning sensation in your mouth or stomach, so add ginger to your diet gradually. Another alternative is to buy ginger in gelatin capsules.

You won't get much ginger from commercial ginger ale, but you can make ginger tea by simmering a couple of slices of fresh ginger root in a cup of water for about 15 minutes. Ginger root can usually be found in the produce section of the supermarket.

Avoid migraine triggers

Watch out for the three C's. Cheese, chocolate, and citrus are the three most common foods reported as headache triggers. They contain substances that may affect the brain in ways that bring on migraines. In the case of chocolate, however, it isn't clear whether it causes the headache or comes right before it. People often have food cravings before a migraine begins. That means the headache may already be on its way when they decide they can't live without that chocolate bar.

Avoid foods with amines. Two in particular, tyramine and histamine, make blood vessels in the brain expand, causing headache pain. Foods that contain these substances include red wine, bananas, avocados, aged cheese, chicken livers, sardines, sour cream, nuts, beer, sauerkraut, and pickled herring. You should also avoid the pods of broad beans like lima, lentils, snow peas, fava beans, and soy beans.

Caffeine — cause or cure of morning headaches? A cup of coffee may seem to relieve your morning headache. In fact, caffeine could be the cause of your pain. This probably sounds confusing, but remember that caffeine is a drug. If your body has come to count on it, missing that drink of cola, tea, or coffee can give you a headache. The headache then goes away when you drink the caffeinated beverage.

Caffeine withdrawal may cause what is sometimes called the "weekend headache." People who drink coffee to get going on work days may find they wake with a headache when they sleep late on weekends. Cutting back on caffeinated drinks during the week should help.

The National Headache Foundation recommends limiting caffeine intake to eight ounces a day. If you drink more than that now, it's best to cut back gradually to avoid headaches.

On the positive side, some of the most effective headache medications contain caffeine as an ingredient. And some migraine sufferers swear by a cup or two of strong tea or coffee at the onset of a headache to prevent or ease the pain

Alcohol attracts migraines. Red wines like Sherry, Chianti, and Burgundy as well as beer, ale, and other fermented drinks are especially likely to bring on the pain. The alcohol itself may not be the only cause of these headaches. Chemical substances called congeners, which give the distinctive taste and smell to fermented drinks, may also share the blame.

Food additives can add pain. Substances are often added to processed foods to preserve them and add flavor, but you may find these additives subtract from your comfort.

- **Aspartame** is an artificial sweetener found in low-calorie foods and diet drinks. Nutrasweet and Equal are two of the brand names. They come in powdered and liquid forms for sweetening foods and drinks. Some studies link aspartame with migraine headaches, and others do not. You might want to avoid this additive, or if you do use it, note how it affects you.

- **Monosodium glutamate (MSG)** is a flavor enhancer often reported by migraine sufferers as a headache trigger. Although once it was associated mainly with Chinese food, it is also used in Accent, meat tenderizers, canned meat and fish, and packaged and prepared foods. There was a time when MSG could be listed on labels as "natural flavor," or "hydrolyzed vegetable protein (HVP)," but new FDA requirements make it easier to identify as an ingredient.

- **Sodium nitrite**, apreservative used in processed meats like hot dogs, turkey, ham, and sausage, can cause migraines in some people.

A salty solution

A warm salt pack can relieve headache pain. Place the salt in a dry pan and heat until it's very warm but not hot. Wrap the salt in a thin dishtowel. If the headache is in front, press the pack to the back of your head and rub. The dry heat will draw the pain away from where it's hurting.

Give hangover headaches a holiday

The best way to avoid a hangover is to drink nonalcoholic beverages. But if you have too much of the spirits in your celebrating, these tips might help you avoid the morning-after blues.

Skip the champagne. You are more apt to get a hangover headache from fermented drinks like red wine, bourbon, and champagne. They contain congeners, substances that add flavor and aroma but can also cause headaches. With non-fermented drinks, there's less taste and smell, but you may feel more comfortable in the morning.

Liquids can lessen the misery. Alcohol can cause dehydration. If you overdo it, drink lots of water or other fluids. Drinking coffee may not sober you up, but it can relieve your headache by tightening the blood vessels that the alcohol has enlarged.

Fructose is a friend. A cup of honey-sweetened tea or a glass of orange juice before bedtime may help you avoid the morning-after blues. Too much alcohol can bring on a headache by lowering blood sugar. Fructose, found naturally in honey and fruits, can raise your blood sugar and help your body metabolize the alcohol.

Headaches may signal heart disease

If your headaches begin during exercise then go away when you rest, it may be a sign of heart disease. Researchers recently found that to be the case with seven patients who did not suffer other signs of heart problems.

It's not clear how exercise causes these headaches. It's possible that undetected chest pain travels along nerves from the heart to the head where it's more noticeable. Or, the diseased heart causes more pressure in the head because of poor circulation.

This type of cardiac headache may occur in people whose headaches begin after age 50 and who are at risk for heart disease because of high blood pressure, diabetes, smoking, or family history.

Hearing loss

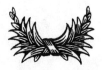

Protect your hearing with vitamin A

You already know that too much noise can cause hearing loss, but did you know that vitamin A can protect your hearing?

A deficiency of vitamin A can contribute to hearing loss indirectly by making your ears more sensitive to noise. This increased sensitivity makes you more likely to suffer hearing loss as a result of exposure to noise.

Add some vitamin A to your diet by eating tuna, salmon, butter, and liver. You can also get beta carotene, which is converted into vitamin A in your body, by eating green leafy vegetables, like spinach, or bright orange fruits and vegetables like sweet potatoes, carrots, cantaloupes, apricots, and pumpkins.

Heart attack

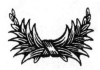

Fiber's amazing benefits

Up until the 1950s, people called it roughage. Today it's called fiber. Whatever you call it, call on it frequently to reduce your risk of a heart attack. A high-intake of fiber helps lower "bad" LDL cholesterol.

A study of 21,000 men in Finland found that the men who ate an average of 35 grams of fiber a day had 25 percent fewer heart attacks than men who averaged just 16 grams of fiber a day.

Fiber may sound like something you'd get from chewing on a rope, but it can be much tastier than that. In one study, American men with the healthiest hearts said cold breakfast cereal was their most regular source of fiber.

By studying those men, researchers determined that you can cut your risk of a heart attack by a third just by adding 10 grams of fiber to your diet every day. Check your favorite cereal box to see how much fiber it contains. Several popular brands have about 10 grams per cup. Some have even more.

You might want to chop up an apple or some almonds to throw in with your cereal. Fiber is abundant in fresh fruits and nuts, as well as in vegetables, seeds, and unprocessed grains.

If you aren't in the habit of eating much fiber, you may want to add it to your diet gradually. Sudden increases can cause gas and intestinal cramps. By drinking extra liquids, you may be able to avoid any digestive upsets.

A nutty way to avoid a heart attack

Don't squirrel away nuts for an occasional treat. This tasty, nutritious snack can save your life. Researchers who studied the diets of 30,000 men and women made a remarkable discovery. By eating nuts five times a week, you can cut your risk of dying from a heart attack in half, compared with people who eat nuts less than once a week.

A study of 40,000 postmenopausal women also found a lower risk of heart disease among frequent nut eaters. That's good news for women because their risk of heart disease increases after menopause.

Nuts are rich in vitamin E, folic acid, vitamin B6, and niacin, as well as the minerals magnesium, zinc, copper, and potassium.

Nuts are also high in fiber and a good source of protein. If you eat nuts, you can cut back on the amount of meat in your diet. Although meat provides a lot of protein, it's also high in saturated fat and cholesterol. Nuts are high in fat, too, but they have more heart-healthy monounsaturated fat. Of the 13 to 20 grams of fat in one ounce of nuts, only 1 to 2.5 grams are from saturated fat. And nuts are cholesterol free.

But remember, don't go too heavy on the nuts if you want to maintain a heart-healthy weight. One ounce has 160 to 200 calories.

The next time you reach for a snack, pass by the chips and grab a handful of nuts. You'll be doing your heart a big favor.

Heal your heart with fish

To protect your heart, eat fish — especially cold-water fish like salmon, tuna, sardines, herring, and mackerel. Fish are rich in omega-3 fatty acids. Omega-3 helps keep your blood from becoming too sticky and forming clots, which can cause heart attack and stroke. Studies show that eating one 3-ounce serving of fatty fish per week can cut your risk of heart attack in half. If you never eat fish, but start including even a moderate amount in your diet, you can lower your risk of heart disease by 50 to 70 percent.

Fish oil also lowers your bad cholesterol and triglyceride levels, and it helps protect against irregular heartbeats. If your high blood pressure is caused by hardening of the arteries, heart disease, or high cholesterol, fish oil may help lower it. The higher your cholesterol levels and the worse your heart disease, the better fish oil works to lower your blood pressure.

If you really want to live right, consider moving to Greenland. The Eskimos there are well-known for their low death rates from heart attack. Studies have shown their diet of seal, walrus, and mackerel puts them in fish oil heaven.

Antioxidants safeguard your heart

There is strong evidence that antioxidants help your body fight disease. Of all the antioxidants, vitamin E offers the most convincing evidence of its disease-fighting capabilities.

According to a two-year study in Great Britain, vitamin E protects people with atherosclerosis, or hardening of the arteries, from heart attacks. In the study, the participants took vitamin E or a fake pill. The people in the vitamin E group took either 400 or 800 international units (IU) of vitamin E daily. After 200 days, the risk of nonfatal heart attacks dropped 77 percent for the people taking vitamin E.

Not only does vitamin E prevent the build-up of plaque that clogs arteries, it helps break up existing plaque and prevents blood clots from forming. That's good news because both plaque and blood clots can cause a heart attack.

For some people, diet alone may provide enough vitamin E. One study found that women who ate foods high in vitamin E were 62 percent less likely to die of a heart attack than those with a low vitamin E intake. Some of the best food sources are sunflower seeds, wheat germ oil, and almonds.

To get enough vitamin E to stop the build-up in arteries already clogged with plaque, you would have to take supplements. Talk it over with your doctor and follow his advice.

Vitamin C, another powerful antioxidant, helps lower your cholesterol and blood pressure and strengthens your capillaries. It also lowers your risk of angina. In one study, researchers showed that taking an extra 60 milligrams (mg) of vitamin C a day — about one orange — lowered heart disease risk.

If you already have coronary artery disease, your blood vessels will sing the praises of vitamin C. It helps open those clogged vessels when your heart needs more blood during work or exercise.

Beta carotene is another antioxidant that helps prevent heart attacks by keeping arteries clear of plaque. In one study, women who got more than 15 to 20 milligrams (mg) of beta carotene a day had a 22 percent lower risk of heart attack than those who got less than 6 mg. Studies of men have shown similar results.

You can add beta carotene to your diet by eating lots of vegetables like carrots, sweet potatoes, butternut squash, and spinach. Beef liver is also a good source of beta carotene.

For more information, see the *Atherosclerosis* chapter.

Flavonoids fend off plaque

For your heart's sake, drink some tea and eat lots of fresh fruits and vegetables. According to a study of 693 Dutch men, these foods will provide you with a healthy dose of flavonoids. Flavonoids work like antioxidants and protect your heart by preventing the build-up of plaque in your arteries. This allows blood to flow freely, taking oxygen and nutrients to your heart to keep it healthy.

In the study, those who had the most flavonoid-rich foods in their diets had less than one-third the risk of a fatal heart attack than those who ate fewer of these foods. The main sources of flavonoids in the study were tea, apples, and onions. Other rich sources are kale, broccoli, endive, celery, and cranberries.

Magnesium vital for a healthy heart

Magnesium is a very important mineral for your heart. Low levels of magnesium can cause a number of problems, including interfering with normal sodium and potassium levels, which help maintain the electrical function of your heart.

In addition, a 10-year ongoing study of 2,182 men ages 45 to 59 suggests that dietary magnesium may provide long-term heart protection, according to Dr. Peter Elwood of the Medical Research Council Epidemiology Unit in South Wales. A good supply of magnesium can also protect your heart from the ravages of high cholesterol, which increases your risk of heart disease.

Magnesium seems particularly effective at protecting your heart from artery spasms. The lower your body is in magnesium, the less able your heart is to stop the spasms, which can lead to death.

Magnesium can be especially helpful for heart rhythm irregularities that occur after a heart attack has damaged the heart muscle.

A study led by Dr. Jerry L. Nadler at the City of Hope Medical Center in Duarte, Calif., suggests that magnesium can help prevent blood clots, which can block arteries and lead to heart attacks. Magnesium does this by slowing the release of thromboxane, a substance that makes blood platelets more sticky and more likely to clot.

It's easy to add magnesium to your diet, especially if you eat unprocessed foods. Good sources of magnesium include beans, brown rice, grains, popcorn, nuts, spinach, soybeans, broccoli, green peas, corn, acorn squash, potatoes, sweet potatoes, molasses, oatmeal, cornmeal, shrimp, clams, oysters, crab, and skim milk.

A 'grape' way to prevent a heart attack

Drinking a tall glass of purple grape juice can do more than give you a purple mustache. It can lower your chances of a heart attack by reducing your blood's ability to form harmful clots.

One study found that by drinking 10 to 12 ounces of purple grape juice each day for a week, harmful clotting was reduced by 39 percent. Grapefruit and orange juice were also tested, and while they helped some, purple grape juice was by far the most effective.

'Happy half-hour' for your heart

The relationship between alcohol and prevention of heart disease is one of those good news/bad news stories. What it seems to boil down to is this: If you drink alcohol in moderation, you may be able to cut your risk of a heart attack or angina in half. But if you have more than two drinks a day, your risk of high blood pressure, stroke, cancer, and many other serious health problems increases dramatically.

Moderate drinking means one to two drinks a day. If you drink more than this amount, the benefits are lost. With three or more drinks a day, the risk of death increases with each additional drink. One drink equals a 12-ounce bottle of beer, a 4-ounce glass of wine, or a 1 1/2-ounce shot of 80-proof spirits. They all contain the same amount of alcohol, one-half ounce.

Researchers think alcohol helps the heart by increasing HDL, the "good" cholesterol. HDLs remove the "bad" LDL cholesterol from the walls of the arteries and carry it back to the liver. Other research suggests it also keeps blood clots from forming and may even break up blood clots as they form.

Many researchers have focused on red wine and dark beer, thinking it may be antioxidants in wine and beer and not alcohol that protects the heart. Although the evidence is not conclusive, one type of alcoholic beverage doesn't seem to be better for your heart than another.

Clearly, there is both good and bad to be said for alcohol use. That's why the American Heart Association has developed the following guidelines:

- Talk to your doctor about your personal risks and benefits. If you have a family history of alcoholism, high triglyceride level, inflammation of the pancreas, liver disease, certain blood disorders, heart failure, or uncontrolled high blood pressure, drinking alcohol could be dangerous. Pregnant women and people on medication that interacts with alcohol should avoid drinking alcohol.
- If none of the above conditions exist, one or two drinks a day can be considered safe.
- Never operate machinery or motor vehicles when using alcohol.
- Go over the risks and benefits from time to time as part of your regular medical care. If you are having problems as a result of your drinking or you are drinking heavily, ask your doctor for guidance.
- Adolescents and young adults should be counseled about the risks and benefits before they develop any drinking habits.

Everyone is different, but if you follow this advice, you may reap the heart-healthy benefits from a glass of your favorite wine.

HEARTBURN AND INDIGESTION

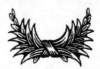

Relief for an upset stomach

If you suffer from gas, bloating, heartburn, and indigestion, and you're tired of chewing antacids, try these helpful hints:

Feast on fruits, veggies, and grains. Switch to a diet high in fiber and complex carbohydrates, like vegetables, fruits, and grains. These foods will speed up digestion and empty your stomach faster.

Eat small meals. Instead of eating two or three large meals a day, eat several small meals. Chew your food slowly and carefully.

Avoid problem foods. Fried, spicy, or fatty foods can send your stomach acid into overtime. Other popular offenders are lemonade; citrus fruits, especially grapefruit; alcoholic beverages, including wine; milk; and most tomato products. Some foods produce more gas when they are being digested than others. Beware of beans, cucumbers, cabbage, turnips, and onions.

Chew a stick of gum. Ever thought you could chew your way out of an attack of indigestion? Well, some researchers think if you chew gum after dinner you might be able to do just that. The chewing action produces saliva which counteracts your stomach acid. The result is no more acid indigestion. If you are going to give gum a try, just make sure it's sugarless.

Brush-off heartburn with toothpaste. Dr. Basil Rodansky of Lincoln Park, Mich., offers this simple home remedy for easing heartburn in adults: take one to two teaspoons of mentholated toothpaste followed by warm water or tea. But don't use the kind with baking soda or hydrogen peroxide. They can actually increase the acid level in your stomach.

Soothe your stomach with nature's remedies

When treating indigestion or heartburn, herbs may gently do all the things synthetic drugs claim to do. Plants and herbs gave man the first antibiotic, the first antacid, and the first adhesive bandage.

While most people take stomach-soothing herbs as teas, they are more effective as a concentrated extract known as an essential oil.

Peppermint, chamomile, anise, caraway, coriander, fennel, and turmeric are all essential oils that may improve your digestion. At the same time, they may rid you of the uncomfortable symptoms of heartburn and other stomach problems.

Not all of them work the same for everyone. Some evidence suggests that mint can actually cause heartburn in some people by relaxing the valve between the stomach and the esophagus, allowing stomach acid to back up. Try different types of mint to see how your body reacts.

Animals know to eat bitter plants when their digestion is suffering because bitter foods and herbs help get the digestive juices flowing. Watercress, endive, dandelion and collard greens, green leaf lettuce, artichokes, and orange peel are bitter foods that might soothe your digestion problems.

Some bitter herbs traditionally used as tonics for digestion are gentian root, wormwood leaves, goldenseal root, rue leaves, yarrow flowers and leaves, yellow dock root, angelica root, quassia bark, barberry root, elecampane root, and horehound leaves.

If you decide to try an herb, some herbal experts recommend taking it as a tonic, which is an alcohol or vinegar solution, rather than in a capsule. Either place it directly on your tongue or dilute it in a cup of hot water. It is your body's physical reaction to the bitter taste that seems to help your digestion the most.

No comfort from comfrey

Comfrey tea to ease digestion sounds harmless, and comforting, but don't be fooled. It contains enough toxins to permanently damage your liver and even cause death. It could also put you at risk for liver cancer.

While some herbalists still recommend comfrey tea for heartburn, why risk it when there are other natural alternatives? The Henry Doubleday Research Association says that unless future research shows comfrey is safe and effective, "no human being or animal should eat, drink, or take comfrey in any form." For now, consider the herb poisonous.

Herbs that may cause serious side effects

- **Comfrey.** Speeds healing and prevents bruises and swelling from injuries when used in a paste. Don't take it by mouth because it contains alkaloids that might cause cancer.
- **Chaparral.** Used as a cure for acne and for stopping the aging process, this supplement can cause liver disease.
- **Mistletoe.** Although a pharmaceutical version of mistletoe has been patented, home use is not recommended. The berries are poisonous, and the leaves may cause dangerous blood pressure problems.
- **Ephedrine.** Raises blood pressure and heart rate.
- **Germander.** Germander is used to fight obesity, but it may cause hepatitis, an inflammation of the liver.
- **Licorice.** Licorice candy may be dandy, but too much of it can raise your blood pressure to dangerous heights.

- **Pokeroot.** Extremely toxic.
- **Sassafras.** Contains safrole, which has been proven to cause cancer.

HEMORRHOIDS

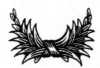

The bottom line on prevention

The number one way to prevent and treat hemorrhoids is to prevent constipation. And the number one way to prevent constipation is by adding fiber to your diet. Some fiber-rich foods are potatoes, beans, whole-grain breads, bran, and fresh fruits. To really get things moving, eat more vegetables like cabbage, corn, parsnips, brussels sprouts, cauliflower, peas, asparagus, carrots, and kale.

Drinking six to eight glasses of water or juice each day will keep your digestive system from becoming impacted, another cause of constipation. By softening and bulking up your stool, you will find that you don't have to push or strain during a bowel movement.

Foods low in fiber will only slow up the process and make your stools harder to pass. Avoid ice cream, soft drinks, cheese, white bread, and meat. Remember that alcohol is dehydrating, which means that it draws water from your body. This only contributes to constipation.

In addition, some people find that certain foods, like coffee, nuts, or spicy foods, make their hemorrhoid symptoms worse. For more information, see the *Constipation* chapter.

Age-old cures may do the trick

- **Butcher's broom** is an herb that will reduce the inflammation of hemorrhoids and work to shrink the veins.
- **Witch hazel** helps form a layer of protection over your skin which allows it to heal. This is important in preventing hemorrhoids from recurring. In addition, this astringent relieves itching and inflammation.
- **Myrrh** can be used as an antiseptic on external hemorrhoids.

- **Plaintain or psyllium** seeds are used as a bulk laxative. This means that if you take them with lots of water, they swell up and move through your digestive system quickly. This process softens your stool, reduces the straining of constipation, and relieves bleeding and pain during bowel movements. Some people have even found that other hemorrhoidal symptoms improved.

HIGH BLOOD PRESSURE

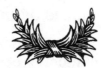

Try bulbs for better blood

Your garden may provide some helpful ingredients to regulate your blood pressure. Both garlic and onions contain certain chemicals that may help lower pressure by relaxing and opening up the blood vessels.

Be careful about taking garlic if you are on anti-clotting medications, however. Garlic could intensify the effects of some drugs, such as aspirin or warfarin. It's best to ask your doctor about adding garlic to your diet on a regular basis.

Most people with high blood pressure need to watch their salt intake. The spicy flavors of garlic and onions make them good substitutes. Try grating, juicing, or drying them for easy use in recipes.

You may want to take a tip from the ancient Greeks and nibble on rose petals to get rid of your garlic and onion breath. Or go the herbal route and chew on raw parsley, dill, or fennel seed. Either way, you'll enjoy sweeter breath while reaping the benefits of these bountiful bulbs.

Fatty fish fight blood pressure battles

If you go fishing to relax, it just might help lower your blood pressure. But whether you catch your own or buy it, eating fish two or three times a week is a good way to battle high blood pressure. It's the omega-3 oil in salmon, mackerel, sardines and other cold-water, fatty fish that makes it so beneficial.

Omega-3 helps keep your blood from becoming too sticky and forming clots that can cause heart attack and stroke. It also lowers your bad cholesterol and triglyceride levels.

Eating fish is more likely to help you if your high blood pressure is caused by heart disease, high cholesterol, or atherosclerosis. Apparently, the worse shape you're in, the better fish oil works to lower your pressure. If it's normal to begin with, fish oil doesn't seem to have any effect.

Fish oil cautions

It's easy to overdose on fish oil supplements because the oil in a pill is more concentrated than in the fish itself. And if you take too much, you can change your blood fat levels and worsen Type II diabetes. It can also harm your immune system, which makes it easier for you to develop infections or even cancer.

Fish oil supplements are made from fish skins and livers, which may contain toxic pesticides and other contaminants. Fish oil contains high levels of vitamins A and D, which can also be toxic if you take too much.

You're also risking free radical damage. Since omega-3 fatty acids are unsaturated, they're open to attacks by free-radical oxygen. This starts a chain reaction that can easily damage your cell membranes and may lead to cancer and heart disease. If you get too much omega-3 fat, you could be letting yourself in for more than you bargained.

Any benefits you'd get from fish oil supplements are probably outweighed by the dangers. Your best bet is to go straight to the source — eat fish.

Minerals: natural pressure relievers

The right nutrients and a healthy weight are natural ways to lower blood pressure. They also reduce your risk of heart attack, stroke, atherosclerosis, and kidney damage. Eating fruits, vegetables, and low-fat or nonfat milk products gives you minerals that work together to lower blood pressure. In addition, foods high in these minerals give you the added benefit of fiber, another helper in lowering blood pressure.

Potassium is a peach when it comes to preventing and lowering hypertension. Although you won't find this critical mineral in peaches, you will find it in bananas, cantaloupe, acorn squash, spinach, kidney beans, avocados, and baked potatoes with skins.

In one study, a potassium-rich diet led to a 36 percent reduction in the use of high blood pressure medications. Apparently, it works by stimulating the body to get rid of excess salt and release helpful hormones and chemicals into the bloodstream.

Potassium can be lost in cooking, so it's best to eat your fruits and vegetables raw. Or choose foods that are cooked in their skins, such as potatoes, which don't lose as much potassium.

This mineral can have serious side effects if you get too much, especially if you have kidney problems or are taking medications called ACE inhibitors. If you're thinking about taking potassium supplements, talk to your doctor first.

Calcium does more than just give you strong bones and teeth. Studies have shown that this mineral also helps lower high blood pressure, particularly in blacks and white women. For some reason, it doesn't seem to have as much effect on white males.

Calcium is especially helpful to those who are salt sensitive, so if you find salt raises your blood pressure, be sure to get plenty of calcium in your diet. Dairy products, sardines, kale, soybeans, and almonds are good sources.

Calcium from supplements does not seem to work as well on lowering blood pressure. But it's easy to get the recommended daily intake of 800 to 1200 milligrams (mg) from your diet. A cup of skim milk will provide 350 mg; a cup of nonfat yogurt has 450 mg; and four ounces of sardines provide 433 mg of calcium.

Magnesium, found in oysters, baked potatoes, spinach, and black-eyed peas, seems to relax blood vessels and allow them to open wider. This gives blood more room to flow freely, reducing blood pressure. Magnesium also may help neutralize stress hormones that raise blood pressure.

'C' your way to lower blood pressure

A glass of orange juice, a bowl of strawberries, or a serving of broccoli could help lower your blood pressure. Studies show that people with high amounts of vitamin C in their blood have lower pressure than people with low amounts. It may be that vitamin C strengthens and supports blood vessel walls, making them more resistant to high blood pressure.

The recommended dietary allowance for vitamin C is 60 mg per day. You can easily get that by eating five servings of fruits and vegetables each day. If you think you might benefit from a supplement, check with your doctor. Even though vitamin C is considered one of the safest vitamins, it does cause problems in some people, especially at high doses.

Can high blood pressure shrink your brain?

Unfortunately, the answer may be yes. A recent study from the National Institute on Aging concluded that older people with chronic high blood pressure are more likely to lose language and memory skills.

It seems that high blood pressure, combined with normal aging, promotes tissue loss in the cognitive areas of the brain. This occurs even in people whose blood pressure is controlled by medication.

The best way to help keep your mind sharp as you age is to exercise and eat right so you avoid the plague of high blood pressure altogether. If it's already too late, then make sure you don't delay in treating the problem. Earlier studies showed that regulating your blood pressure as soon as possible may lower your risk of cognitive impairment in old age.

5 food tips to lower risk

Eating nutritious foods that help bring your blood pressure down is a smart diet move. But it's only half the solution. You also need to take it easy on the things that send your blood pressure soaring.

Go slow on salt. You should limit your intake to less than one teaspoon a day if you are salt sensitive, which means your kidneys don't get rid of excess salt very effectively. That doesn't mean you should cut out salt completely. Your body must have about a quarter teaspoon a day to work properly.

Surprisingly, eating too little salt can cause your blood pressure to go up as well. It also puts you at risk of heart attack, high cholesterol, sleep disturbances, and loss of important nutrients.

If you're like most people, you get more salt than you need, especially if you eat a lot of fast foods or pre-packaged foods. They usually contain large amounts of salt that you might not even taste. Even worse, most of the minerals that help lower blood pressure are lost when fresh foods are processed.

Take corn, for example. A cup of cooked fresh corn has 226 mg of potassium and 8 mg of sodium, the main ingredient in salt. That's a healthy ratio in anyone's diet. But what if you ate a cup of corn flakes instead? After all the processing, the corn is left with only 20 mg of potassium and a whopping 228 mg of sodium. Obviously, you're better off with the fresh food.

You may be surprised to learn that some salty foods are actually better choices than foods that don't taste salty. Salted peanuts, for example, contain less sodium than instant chocolate pudding. But you notice the salt more because it directly touches your taste buds.

You may want to remember that when it comes to seasoning your food during cooking. A light sprinkling of salt at the table may be healthier and more satisfying than loading it on beforehand. You can also use salt substitutes. But if you have kidney problems, avoid those that are high in potassium.

Look before you lick. Black licorice, which is found in some candy and chewing tobacco, may contain glycyrrhizic acid. This can make your body retain salt and lose potassium, leading to higher blood pressure. That ingredient is usually removed from licorice-flavored foods and tobacco produced in this country, but watch for it on the label of imports.

Reduce fat. Societies that eat less meat usually have fewer problems with high blood pressure. Perhaps it's because they eat more high-fiber foods that contain other nutrients known to lower blood pressure. Or it may be that people who eat a lot of animal fat are more likely to have high cholesterol and atherosclerosis, conditions associated with high blood pressure.

Cutting fat is a good idea if you want to reduce your calories and maintain a healthy weight. Overweight adults have high blood pressure 50 percent more often than those of normal weight. Reducing fat is important to good health whether it affects blood pressure directly or indirectly.

Use caffeine with caution. A cup of coffee may raise blood pressure temporarily, but the effect usually doesn't last very long. So why should you worry about caffeine? Because it also causes your body to lose calcium, which could lead to higher blood pressure.

Restrict alcohol. Relaxing with a bottle of wine may seem like a good way to end a stressful day. That should be good for your blood pressure, right? Not necessarily. Having three or more drinks a day may be the sole cause of over 10 percent of all cases of high blood pressure. If you use alcohol, limit your daily intake to the recommended amounts of 24 ounces of beer, 8 ounces of wine, or 2 ounces of liquor.

Using good judgment about what you eat will go a long way toward controlling your blood pressure. Checking labels for hidden ingredients, and avoiding those you know are harmful, are steps in the right direction.

Race may affect your risk

If you are black, you should be particularly concerned about high blood pressure. It occurs in black people almost twice as often as it does in white people. It starts at an earlier age and grows more severe if not treated.

Why does this occur? It seems that salt sensitivity is especially high in blacks. This means your kidneys have trouble getting rid of excess salt, which leads to high blood pressure.

Blacks also have a higher rate of potassium deficiency. Since this mineral helps the body get rid of salt, it is very important in the diet. In cases of a deficiency, your doctor may recommend potassium supplements.

If you don't know what you blood pressure is, have it tested and continue to do so regularly. High blood pressure has no symptoms, so people often have it and don't know it until it has caused a serious problem like stroke, heart attack, or kidney problems.

DASH high blood pressure

If you want to lower your blood pressure without taking medication, a new diet might be the key. It's called DASH (Dietary Approaches to Stop Hypertension), and it more than doubles the amounts of fruits, vegetables, and low-fat dairy products Americans normally eat.

The diet includes daily servings of four to five vegetables, four to five fruits, seven to eight grains, two to three low-fat or nonfat dairy products, two meats or less, and a half serving of nuts, seeds, or beans.

Doctors say following this plan could reduce blood pressure-related heart disease by as much as 15 percent and stroke by about 27 percent nationwide.

The DASH diet is most useful in preventing and lowering high blood pressure if you follow a healthy lifestyle. That includes maintaining a healthy weight, exercising, eating foods low in salt and fat, and using alcohol moderately, if at all.

Of course, you shouldn't stop taking any hypertension medications without consulting your doctor.

Research on the DASH diet is continuing at five medical centers in different locations around the U.S. You can get more information, including menus, recipes, and tips for using the diet, at the DASH website at http://dash.bwh.harvard.edu/.

Spicy no-salt seasonings

Mix up a blend of your favorite dried herbs and spices to shake on foods instead of salt. Some possibilities include basil, bay leaf, chili powder, cinnamon, cumin, curry powder, dry mustard, garlic powder, onion powder, oregano, paprika, parsley, pepper, and thyme.

For a spicy treat, try some of this mixture on meat, chicken, or fish before cooking:

1/4 cup paprika	1 teaspoon black pepper
2 tablespoons oregano	1/2 teaspoon red pepper
2 teaspoons chili powder	1/2 teaspoon dry mustard
1 teaspoon garlic powder	

HIGH CHOLESTEROL

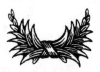

Everything you need to know about fats

A simple way to lower your risk of heart attack, stroke, gallstones, even vision loss, is to eat less fat.

Fat, especially saturated fat, combines with cholesterol in your bloodstream. There it can cling to artery walls and harden into plaque. This narrows the passageways, slows blood flow, and endangers the heart and other organs.

Since some fats are healthier than others, you need to choose carefully. Here are some tips for healthy adults from the American Heart Association.

- Limit your total fat intake to no more than 30 percent of your total calories. If you eat a high-fat meal, don't give up. Just balance it out over a few days with meals that are lower in fat.

- Saturated fat should make up no more than 8 to 10 percent of your calories. This kind of fat is usually solid at room temperature. It comes mainly from meat, especially fatty cuts of red meat, hamburger, and sausage, and full-fat dairy products like cheese, butter, and milk. These foods also contain dietary cholesterol, which raises blood cholesterol.

- Polyunsaturated fat should not exceed 10 percent of your calories. These fatty acids are found in corn, soy, sunflower, and safflower oils. They remain liquid at room temperature and in the refrigerator. They help lower LDL "bad" cholesterol, but they may also lower HDL "good" cholesterol.

- Monounsaturated fats can make up to 15 percent of your total calories. Olive oil and canola oil are examples of monounsaturated fats. They are liquid at room temperature but turn cloudy and begin to harden when chilled. They lower LDL cholesterol but not HDL cholesterol.

Remember, these guidelines are for healthy adults. If you already have high cholesterol or one of the related diseases, your doctor is likely to recommend lower amounts of fat.

Top cholesterol-cutting food choices

Toss up a salad. Choose dark leafy greens, juicy red tomato wedges, and some green peppers. Add some carrots, onions, and cucumber slices for a healthy garden salad. Or make it a fruit salad with apples, bananas, pears, and nuts. These salads do more than look pretty and taste good. They can save you from a heart attack or stroke.

Fruits and vegetables are full of vitamin C, vitamin E, beta carotene, and selenium. These antioxidant vitamins and minerals not only help lower cholesterol, they protect your body from damaging free radicals. As your body processes oxygen, it creates chemicals called free radicals that damage cells. When free radicals come in contact with LDL cholesterol, they cause even more harm to arteries already damaged by plaque. Antioxidants neutralize free radicals to help prevent that damage.

Chromium, another antioxidant, helps lower LDL cholesterol and raise HDL cholesterol. You can get this mineral by eating apples with skins, Brewer's yeast, fish and other seafood, mushrooms, liver, prunes, nuts, and asparagus. Don't expect to get this mineral from highly processed or refined foods like sugar or white flour. They are not good sources and can even cause you to lose chromium.

And the list of antioxidants goes on. The herbs ginger, ginkgo, and ginseng are included, as are black and green teas, red wine, and chocolate.

It's best to get antioxidant vitamins and minerals from your diet. Raw or lightly cooked foods have the most nutrients. Be careful about taking supplements. One study showed that vitamin E and beta carotene supplements actually increased the risk of fatal heart attacks in smokers who had previously had a heart attack. If this describes you, talk with your doctor before taking supplements.

For more information about cholesterol, see the *Atherosclerosis, Heart attack, Stroke,* and *High blood pressure* chapters.

Boost protein, lower cholesterol with soy

If you want to lower your cholesterol naturally, try replacing some high-fat meat and dairy products with foods made from soybeans. You'll get plenty of protein and help keep your arteries clear at the same time.

Research shows that the higher your cholesterol level, the more you will benefit from soy. In one study, those who had the highest cholesterol levels lowered them almost 20 percent by eating an average of 47 grams of soy a day.

Not long ago, soy foods like tofu and miso were hard to find. Now they are so popular you can find them easily in your grocery store.

For more information about soy, see the *Super foods* section.

Margarine vs. butter — Which one is healthier?

Margarine is usually made from liquid vegetable oil and hardened by a process called hydrogenation. During this process, trans fatty acids are formed. Research shows that trans fatty acids can raise your cholesterol level. But before you reach for the butter dish, don't forget that butter can also raise your cholesterol level. So what should you use, margarine or butter?

According to the American Heart Association, margarine is preferable to butter. That's because butter is high in both cholesterol and saturated fat. Margarine, because it's made from vegetable oil and not animal fat, has no cholesterol.

Look for margarine in tubs or liquid form. Soft margarine has fewer trans fatty acids. Read the label. Make sure the first ingredient is liquid vegetable oil. Check the fat grams. It shouldn't contain more than 2 grams of saturated fat per tablespoon.

If you limit your total intake of fat to the recommended five to eight teaspoons a day, trans fatty acids shouldn't be a problem for you.

How to eat eggs and still save your heart

Although the "incredible edible egg" commercials might lead you to think differently, egg yolks are not good for your heart. One large egg has an incredible 213 to 220 milligrams (mg) of cholesterol. The American Heart Association says a healthy adult shouldn't get more than 300 mg total cholesterol per day.

The AHA recommends that you have no more than three to four egg yolks per week. That includes eggs served as a main dish or as an ingredient in foods, like baked goods.

What matters most is the amount of cholesterol, not where it comes from. If you choose to eat more eggs, eat less meat and dairy products.

You can find commercial cholesterol-free egg substitutes at your supermarket. And remember, it's just the yolk that contains cholesterol. Some recipes work just as well with egg whites only.

No need to scrimp on shrimp

Although shrimp is low in fat, it's high in cholesterol, but that doesn't mean you shouldn't eat it. According to researchers, shrimp can be part of a heart-healthy diet. Shrimp raises the level of good cholesterol, which helps the body get rid of harmful cholesterol.

So go ahead ... enjoy some grilled shrimp or a refreshing shrimp cocktail. Your heart will thank you for it.

Garlic and fish oil pair up for heart protection

Garlic has been known as a healing food for a long time, and now tests can prove its benefits. In one study, men with moderately high cholesterol levels took supplements of aged garlic extract. Within 10 to 40 days, the garlic not only lowered their cholesterol levels, it also helped lower their blood pressures.

Fish oil, or omega-3, from fatty fish like salmon, tuna, and sardines is also good for your heart, but garlic and fish oil together pack a powerful punch. Not only do they reduce LDL cholesterol, they raise HDL cholesterol as well. A tasty salmon fillet and a tossed salad with garlic vinaigrette might be just what the doctor ordered.

The connection between alcohol and cholesterol

According to a recent study, one to two alcoholic drinks a day may be good for your heart. Alcohol not only increases HDL cholesterol, it may slow the formation of blood clots and even break up clots after they form. But moderation is the key. With more than two drinks, you increase your risk of serious health problems.

For more information about alcohol and your heart, see the *Heart attack* chapter.

Fabulous flax fights disease

If something seems fishy about flax, it's because they both contain healthy omega-3 fatty acids that reduce cholesterol. Flax may seem like a strange food to you, but it's easier to add to your diet than you think. Flax flour can be used for baking or in sauces. Stir in a few spoonfuls of flaxseed to add crunch and nutty flavor to cookies, breads, and muffins. Sprinkle flaxseeds in cereals, salads, and soups.

The fiber in flax is another plus for your heart, but it can cause gas if your body is not used to it. Add flax to your diet gradually, up to about three teaspoons a day.

This tiny seed does more than lower cholesterol and protect your heart. It also helps fight cancers of the breast, prostate, and colon. And if you are diabetic, flax may help you control your blood sugar.

If you have any health problems, talk with your doctor before adding flax to your diet.

Moove over skim milk

If you've switched to skim milk because it's better for your heart but miss the rich, creamy taste of whole milk, here's good news. Supermarkets will soon be selling a new type of low-fat milk that has whole milk's taste, look, and mouth-feel.

It's made from cow's milk, but the fat has been removed and Oatrim, a fat substitute, has been added. Oatrim is made from oat flour, so it's also high in fiber.

The new low-fat milk is being produced by Golden Jersey Products of Vero Beach, Fla. It's not clear yet what the brand name will be or when it will be available. Look for the name of the fat substitute, Replace or TrimChoice, somewhere on the label.

Another low-fat substitute, called Z-Trim, is being developed by the U.S. Department of Agriculture. Z-Trim is made from agricultural by-products like hulls of oats, soybeans, peas, and rice, or bran from corn or wheat. It has zero calories and can be used to make low-fat cheese products, lean ground beef patties, and baked goods. Brownies made with Z-trim got the seal of approval from a panel of testers when compared with regular brownies.

While products made with Z-Trim aren't in your supermarket yet, you could be seeing them in the not-too-distant future.

Lower cholesterol with high-fiber foods

Most Americans don't eat enough fiber, but those who do are enjoying the healthy benefits. Fiber, found in grains, fruits, and vegetables, helps lower LDL cholesterol, and it may even raise HDL cholesterol. There are two kinds of fiber, soluble and insoluble. Soluble fiber dissolves in water and insoluble fiber won't.

Soluble fiber softens and forms gels that bind cholesterol and carry it out of the body. It also seems to slow down the liver's production of cholesterol. Pectin, from apples and citrus fruits, is a soluble fiber. Oat bran is another good source.

Insoluble fiber helps with digestion and elimination. It passes quickly through your digestive system, taking toxins with it. Cellulose, found in the strings of celery and the outer skins of corn kernels, is an example of insoluble fiber.

Psyllium, which contains both soluble and insoluble fibers, also helps lower cholesterol. You can find it added to some cereals and in Metamucil.

Another good thing about fiber is it really fills you up, leaving less room for meats, eggs, and dairy products that are high in cholesterol and fats. It's easy to get soluble and insoluble fibers from a well-balanced diet because most plants contain both.

Since fiber and nutrients are lost in food processing, especially in refining grains, make sure you add plenty of whole grains and fresh fruits and vegetables to your diet.

Ask your doctor about niacin therapy

Some doctors prescribe niacin supplements to lower cholesterol, while others avoid recommending it. When niacin, a B vitamin, is used to lower cholesterol, it is considered a drug. High doses of niacin can cause side effects like itching, flushing, rash, and stomach pain, as well as more serious side effects like ulcers, liver damage, and symptoms of diabetes.

If your cholesterol level is high, ask your doctor if the benefits of niacin therapy outweigh the risks.

HIVES

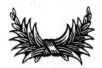

How to give hives the heave-ho

Hives pop up suddenly — and they can leave just as suddenly, or hang around for up to 24 hours. Hives usually just cause temporary swelling and red, itchy patches on your skin. They sometimes appear in clusters.

Finding the cause of your hives is the key to prevention. Sunlight, drugs, exercise, or exposure to heat or cold can all trigger hives, but food is the most common trigger. The worst offenders are nuts, berries, shellfish, bananas, grapes, tomatoes, eggs, and cheese. If these foods cause you to break out in hives, ban them from your diet.

IMPOTENCE

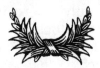

Eating right may save your sex life

Impotence may not be life-threatening, but it can be one of the most frustrating problems a man ever encounters. Although some cases of impotence involve mental or emotional factors, about 85 percent are due to physical causes.

Because your erection depends on blood flow to your penis, anything that interferes with proper blood flow can cause impotence. People with diabetes, heart disease, or atherosclerosis (hardening of the arteries) are more likely to have the problem. Although your chances of having impotence rise as you get older, it is not an unavoidable consequence of aging. Eating a proper diet now can help you avoid impotence in the future.

Limit your fat. Too much fat in your diet can contribute to high blood pressure or heart disease. These conditions can lead to impotence. Heart disease may interfere with proper blood flow, making impotence more likely. High blood pressure may not cause impotence directly, but many of the medications prescribed for high blood pressure can.

Vitamins provide antioxidant protection. Antioxidants combat free radicals, unstable particles in your body that attack your cells. Some particularly effective antioxidants are vitamin E, vitamin C, and vitamin A. These vitamins interact with free radicals and make them harmless, protecting your precious cells from damage. This includes the cells involved in having an erection, so make sure you get at least the recommended dietary allowance of these important vitamins.

Watch your weight. Excess weight could affect your sex life beyond just having unattractive "love handles." Too much weight can contribute to diabetes and high blood pressure, two major causes of impotence. Forty percent of men who have impotence problems are diabetics.

Put a lid on alcohol. Drinking too much alcohol in one night can cause even a young, healthy man to experience temporary impotence. However, too much alcohol over several years can cause nerve and liver damage. That can lead to impotence that may be irreversible.

Following a sensible diet can help prevent impotence in your future. If you already have a problem with impotence, don't be embarrassed to see your doctor. Successful treatment is possible in 95 percent of the cases, yet only 5 percent of men seek treatment.

You should also see your doctor because impotence may be caused by another medical problem that requires treatment. For example, impotence often occurs just weeks before a man suffers a heart attack or stroke.

Serious side effects from 'sexy' herb

Many men who have a problem with impotence are reluctant to see their doctor about it. Some of those men may be making a trip to the herb store instead. While many herbs provide safe, natural alternatives to prescription drugs, that may not be the case with supposed impotence cures.

If you see your doctor for impotence, he may prescribe yohimbine, a prescription-only drug that is made from the bark of an African tree. However, your local herb store may offer a similar herbal solution containing yohimbe. Yohimbe has a long-standing reputation as an aphrodisiac, and comes from the same source as yohimbine.

However, according to herbal experts, yohimbe can cause dangerous side effects including high blood pressure, irregular heartbeat, nausea, and vomiting. An overdose could even lead to paralysis or death. Although prescription yohimbine can help some men with impotence, it can also have potentially serious side effects and should never be used without a doctor's supervision.

Control cholesterol for a sexier you

Men with total cholesterol higher than 240 mg/dl are twice as likely to have trouble achieving or maintaining an erection than men whose cholesterol levels are below 180 mg/dl. Men who have low levels of HDL, the good cholesterol, are also twice as likely to suffer from impotence. Limit cholesterol you eat to less than 300 mg per day. An easy way to cut cholesterol is to limit your intake of butter, cheese, eggs, and meats, especially red meat.

Eat more garlic. Eating as little as a half of clove of garlic a day reduces cholesterol an average of 9 percent, according to researchers at New York's Medical College. It also lowers blood pressure and prevents the bad LDL cholesterol from being oxidized, which damages arteries. Since lower cholesterol means lower risk of fat buildup on your artery walls, a little garlic every day could do your body good.

Fill up on fiber. Fiber helps bind up cholesterol in your intestines, preventing it from being absorbed and clogging your arteries. You need at least 30 grams of fiber a day. Grains, fruits, and vegetables are all good sources.

Dr. Mary Dan Eades, author of *The Doctor's Complete Guide to Vitamins and Minerals,* recommends 50 or more grams a day. She suggests supplementing your diet with a vegetable fiber bulking powder such as Metamucil or Citrucel. Add more fiber to your diet gradually or you're likely to suffer from bloating, cramping, and gas.

Ginseng for sexual healing?

For centuries, ginseng has been one of the world's most popular herbs, consumed by people from hundreds of different generations for thousands of years. Today, millions of people around the world still take ginseng.

Because ginseng supposedly strengthens all the body's organs and makes them more resistant to disease, it has been given credit for curing almost every illness under the sun, from cancer to impotence. While you have the testimony of millions of people who've trusted ginseng with their health for several thousand years, scientists still have trouble nailing down exactly what, if anything, ginseng does.

Researchers believe that ginseng's healing powers come from its ginsenosides, steroid-like compounds found in the bark, or outer layer, of the root. In addition, ginseng also contains vitamins B1 and B2, manganese, phosphorus, iron, copper, cobalt, sulfur, and germanium, which probably contribute to the root's body-balancing effects.

Generally, the more ginsenosides a root contains, the more valuable it is. Because ginsenoside content of the root increases with age, normally only plants six years or older have roots with therapeutic value.

In Eastern medicine, ginseng is considered an adaptogen. This means it works to keep the body in balance in all circumstances, bad or good. An adaptogen also increases the body's resistance to unhealthy influences. It works only when needed or when the body has a deficiency. Since ginseng does contain antioxidants, it may be those compounds that give ginseng its body-balancing abilities. Researchers also suspect it's the antioxidant activities that help protect your heart, liver, and lungs.

Recently, United States Department of Agriculture scientists discovered that the mineral chromium works in a way similar to an adaptogen by raising and lowering blood sugar as needed. It's possible a number of foods and nutrients work this way, giving 20th-century credibility to the ancient health claims made for ginseng.

Ginseng's most famous claim to fame is its reputed ability to help men overcome impotence. Thus far, there's been little scientific support for the super sex claims made for ginseng.

Recently, however, Dr. Tony Lee, professor of pharmacology at Southern Illinois School of Medicine, uncovered information that gives some credibility to this age-old claim. According to Dr. Lee, ginseng contains compounds that stimulate nerve cells in the penis, which may help men maintain an erection.

If you use the raw ginseng root, herbal expert Varro Tyler recommends using 1/2 teaspoonful of the root to make a cup of tea, which can be taken one or two times a day.

For people who prefer supplements, look for one that is standardized to 4 to 7 percent ginsenosides. Seven European studies of ginseng extracts with this amount of ginsenosides found those supplements significantly improved the reaction time, alertness, and concentration powers of study participants.

Most studies report few, if any, side effects from taking ginseng. Generally, the most common problems are nervousness and excitability. These usually go away after a few days of use. Other reported side effects include insomnia, skin rashes, diarrhea, nausea, and vomiting. If you have high blood pressure or diabetes, you should consult your doctor if you want to take ginseng.

INFLAMMATORY BOWEL DISEASE

Change your menu to find relief

More than 2 million Americans suffer from Crohn's disease or ulcerative colitis, the two major types of inflammatory bowel disease (IBD). If you are one of them, you can manage most of the unpleasant symptoms simply by changing a few eating habits.

Forget the fiber. You probably never thought you would hear those words but that big bowl of popcorn or your favorite snack of sunflower seeds and nuts can make your colon cringe. Fiber has gotten so much attention lately as part of a healthy diet that most people still think "the more, the merrier." This is not true if you suffer from ulcerative colitis or Crohn's disease. Your colon is already narrowed and inflamed and doesn't need any more roughage tearing through it. High-fiber foods will only give you cramps, diarrhea, and grumpy intestines.

To avoid tummy troubles, stay away from beans; corn; raisins; raw vegetables; whole grains; and raw fruits, especially coconut and pineapple.

Eat less more often. Try eating five, or even six, small meals each day, instead of three large ones. Many IBD sufferers find that eating small meals more often reduces their symptoms.

Bone up on vitamin D. If you have Crohn's disease, you may be vitamin D deficient. Food producers make it easy to get vitamin D by fortifying milk and cereals. It just takes reading a label or two. Liver, eggs, and dark green leafy vegetables are also good sources of vitamin D. Don't take supplements without checking with your doctor. Too much vitamin D can be toxic.

Go easy on the spices. If salsa sends you screaming and curry causes conniptions, lay off the spicy foods. Even if your taste buds love that extra punch, it's your digestive system that pays the price. Experiment with leaving different foods, like hot peppers, off the menu until you find out what foods cause problems.

Learn to love low fat. Maybe you're already on a low-fat diet, but can you go that extra mile and cut out even more fat? Foods high in fat can cause miserable cramping and diarrhea in IBD sufferers. With Crohn's disease, the small intestine is often so damaged that it can't properly absorb fats; vitamins A, D, E, and K; calcium; and magnesium.

Low-fat foods can be very tasty. Try eating lean meat, fish, or poultry that has been baked, boiled, or broiled; fat-free or low-fat dairy products; fat-free broth and bouillon; breads, cereals, pasta, and rice; and fruits and vegetables.

Ditch the dairy. Does that gooey mozzarella stringing from your pizza cause you to spend the rest of the evening doubled over in pain? If so, you may be lactose intolerant, like many people with IBD. This means you don't have enough of the enzyme lactase that breaks down the sugar in dairy products. If you absolutely must have a bowl of ice cream, try taking a lactase enzyme caplet first. It will break down the dairy sugar for you.

Even if you are lactose intolerant, you can probably eat butter, hard cheeses, and small amounts of yogurt without any nasty side effects. Soy products and milk-free tofu can be tasty substitutions for milk and cheese, while still giving you plenty of protein. Don't forget your body needs calcium for strong bones and teeth. There are lots of nondairy foods high in calcium, like sardines, cooked greens, dried beans, and peanuts.

Cast off Crohn's with fish

Maybe you've heard of using fish oil to treat arthritis, diabetes, heart disease, headaches, and even cancer. Researchers now think it can even help people with Crohn's disease.

A recent study of Crohn's disease sufferers shows that the anti-inflammatory properties of fish oil can reduce the number of relapses. The people in the study who took specially coated, low-dose fish oil capsules for one year had fewer relapses than the people who took an inactive pill.

If you want to try fish oil supplements, check with your doctor first. To add fish oil to your diet naturally, eat salmon, tuna, mackerel, sardines, anchovies, and herring.

Maximize your minerals

When you have a bowel disease, your intestines aren't working as they should. They allow important nutrients to drift on by without being absorbed into your bloodstream.

Having the correct balance of minerals is extremely important, but loading up on mineral supplements "just to be safe" is dangerous. It's too easy to overload your system with toxic amounts.

Combine iron-rich food. Iron supplements can cause bowel irritation and cramping, and they can be dangerous if you take too much. If you're anemic, like many IBD sufferers, it's much better to get the iron you need from food. For instance, a meal of chicken, baked potato, and lima beans is just loaded with iron.

For an even healthier meal, make a citrus sauce for your chicken and top your potato with broccoli. This gives you a whopping dose of vitamin C, which helps your body absorb iron.

Zero in on zinc. This marvelous mineral helps wounds to heal. Beef, oysters, crab, chicken liver, dark meat turkey, cheddar cheese, lima beans, lean pork, and lobster are good sources of zinc.

The dangers of dehydration

If you have a digestive disorder, you could be losing fluid through a damaged or inflamed intestinal tract. This means dehydration — a serious problem.

To fight dehydration, you need at least four 8 ounce glasses of water each day. Active people need more, about six to eight glasses a day. If you're not used to drinking that much, it may take some time to get into the habit. Try adding a few lemon slices to a jug of water in the refrigerator for a thirst-quenching drink.

If you are having a difficult bout of vomiting or diarrhea, try sips of this concoction:

- 3/4 teaspoon table salt
- 1 teaspoon baking powder
- 4 tablespoons sugar
- 1 cup orange juice
- 4 cups water

Some drugs increase nutritional needs

Certain drugs used to treat Crohn's disease and ulcerative colitis can drain vitamins and minerals from your body. If this is the case, you need to take in more of these nutrients through the foods you eat or by taking a supplement. Check with your doctor and follow his advice.

If you take:	Increase your:
• Sulfasalazine	folic acid
• Corticosteroids	calcium
	phosphorous
	vitamin C
	potassium
	zinc
	nitrogen
• Cholestyramine	vitamins A, B12, D, E, and K
	folic acid
	calcium
	iron

INSOMNIA

Melatonin: sweet dreams or the stuff of nightmares?

How does a banana milkshake sound as a nightcap? Or a nice warm cup of tomato soup? Maybe rice pudding or hot oatmeal is more to your liking. These may not be your traditional bedtime snacks, but they may be just what you need for a deep, restful night's sleep.

What these foods have in common is a high dose of melatonin, a hormone made by the pineal gland in the middle of your brain. You may have heard a lot about melatonin in the news lately. It's one of the strongest antioxidants known to man and is said to cure everything from the flu to cancer.

Researchers do know that natural melatonin somehow controls your sleep cycle, and that you produce less of it as you age. This comes as no surprise to anyone over the age of 50 who finds their nights suddenly plagued by frustrating hours of wakefulness.

For those people whose bodies don't produce enough natural melatonin, a supplement could act as a sleeping pill. Scientists hesitate to recommend it, though, since melatonin supplements are still very much experimental. Synthetic melatonin has not been tested over the long-term and may cause a host of nasty side effects, including headaches, fatigue, nightmares, and insomnia, the very condition it is supposed to treat.

What may help is boosting your body's level of melatonin through foods, like sweet corn, ginger, barley, bananas, and Japanese radishes. To get the most benefit, experiment with these melatonin-rich foods about an hour before bedtime. It may be enough to send you happily off to dreamland.

Amazing amino acid helps you sleep like a baby

The amino acid L-tryptophan tells your body to produce more melatonin, which helps you sleep better. Eating foods high in this amino acid is the best way to regulate your natural melatonin levels.

Foods especially high in tryptophan are cheddar cheese, cottage cheese, fish, beef, pork, chicken, turkey, beans, eggs, figs, dates, soybean flour, and oatmeal. If you eat tryptophan-rich foods about an hour before bedtime, your melatonin levels may go up and your sleep might be sweeter.

Why did your grandmother always give you a cup of warm milk before bed? Was it just an old wives' tale that it would help you sleep better? Scientists wondered the same thing and examined all the elements found in milk. They discovered that it contains only small amounts of tryptophan, not enough to make much difference. However, it also contains a group of compounds called beta-casomorphins, which has a soothing effect on your nervous system.

So heat up a steaming mug of milk and snuggle in for a good night's sleep.

Herbs to sleep by

Herbal sleep remedies are almost as old as the herbs themselves, and modern science cannot come up with anything safer or more natural to send you nodding. Chamomile, valerian, and St.

John's wort are examples of herbs that brew up delicious teas to doze by. Sprinkle a little lavender oil on a pillow or in steaming bath water for some heavenly slumber.

The scent of a tropical breeze, the sun warm on your face, and the sound of waves rolling onto the sand. Feeling sleepy? If you're lying on a beach in the South Pacific, you might just be dozing off for an afternoon siesta. Or you might be feeling the effects of a ceremonial drink used for thousands of years by the people of Polynesia, Melanesia, and Micronesia.

Kava is made from the root of a certain pepper plant found only on these islands and is sweeping the international health food market like a Pacific typhoon.

Kava products have the same effects as mild tranquilizers — they relax muscles and remove sleep barriers. Because of this, they are useful for those suffering from sleep disorders like insomnia. Researchers have found no side effects except a type of scaly rash in heavy users. Talk to your doctor before taking kava and follow label directions carefully.

Vitamin deficiencies spell nighttime trouble

Several vitamins and minerals are necessary for your pineal gland to produce proper amounts of melatonin. Vitamins B-3 and B-6 are especially important.

To obtain more B-3 (niacinamide), eat dried apricots, barley, peanuts, pork, salmon, sunflower seeds, tuna, turkey, and wheat bran. Vitamin B-6 can be found in avocados, bananas, carrots, rice, shrimp, wheat germ, and whole wheat flour.

Calcium and magnesium are two minerals that are vital to melatonin production. Besides eating dairy products, you can get whopping doses of calcium in sardines, broccoli, almonds, and cheddar cheese. Foods high in magnesium include oysters, potatoes, spinach, and black-eyed peas.

If you and your doctor decide you need supplements, take about 1,000 milligrams (mg) of calcium and 500 mg of magnesium each day.

Don't lose sleep over the wrong foods

You know it's important to eat the right foods for a good night's sleep. But it's also important to avoid foods that will keep you tossing and turning.

The most common nighttime no-no's include coffee, tea, chocolate, and sodas — in fact, anything with caffeine. Alcohol and tobacco both will disturb your slumber, and large or spicy meals can bring on heartburn.

Drinking lots of liquids will keep you running to the bathroom, which can make getting back to sleep even more difficult. And if your blood sugar is too high from a sweet snack, it will interrupt normal sleep patterns. So plan your dinners wisely and choose late-night snacks for their sleep-appeal.

IRRITABLE BOWEL SYNDROME

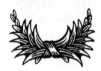

Distress-free diet

If you are one of the 15 percent of adults suffering from Irritable Bowel Syndrome (IBS), you may want to grab a pencil and paper. Writing down everything you eat could be the key to figuring out what's causing your intestinal distress. Experts recommend keeping a food diary so you can track exactly what triggers the painful spasms in your colon, or the gas, constipation, and diarrhea that are the symptoms of IBS.

Certain foods can give you a bumpy ride if your intestines are the least bit sensitive. Those to look out for are chocolate, peppermint, wheat, tomatoes, corn, citrus fruits, and caffeine — especially in tea and coffee. Also, avoid alcohol and fatty, fried, or spicy foods.

Foods like beans, cabbage, bananas, nuts, raisins, and some fruits and fruit juices can cause excess gas and bloating. So can dairy products if you are lactose intolerant. This means you have trouble digesting lactose, a natural sugar found in milk. If you must limit your intake of dairy products, make sure you get enough calcium by eating nondairy foods high in calcium, like sardines, cooked greens, cooked dried beans, and peanuts.

Eating fat stimulates the intestines. If you suffer from irritable bowel syndrome, avoid foods high in fat. Poultry skin, vegetable oil, margarine, shortening, avocados, whole milk, cream, cheese, butter, and whipped toppings are high-fat foods.

Try keeping track of what you eat for a week or two. You may be able to help your doctor figure out what's causing your distress.

Fill up with fiber

Abdominal pain and constipation are major problems for people with IBS. Increasing your dietary fiber by 15 to 20 grams per day will help move things along. Eat more wheat bran, oatmeal, oat bran, rye cereals, and fresh fruits and vegetables. Spend time in the produce section of your grocery store, and you'll discover some wonderful sources of fiber. Don't forget that figs, dried apricots, and prunes make chewy, fiber-filled snacks.

If you decide on a fiber supplement, eight to 10 teaspoons of unprocessed wheat bran once a day or one teaspoon of psyllium twice a day will do the trick. Just be sure to drink lots of liquids with these supplements. At least eight glasses of water a day will help the fiber move through your system.

Healing herbs soothe digestive woes

Herbs not only add zip to your cooking, they may offer relief from the painful symptoms of irritable bowel syndrome.

Peppermint oil. This fragrant oil relaxes your intestinal muscles and soothes your cramps. If you take it as an enteric-coated capsule, it will dissolve in the intestines, not in the stomach where it can irritate your stomach lining. Many IBS sufferers find relief by taking one to two 0.2 milliliter (ml) capsules three times a day, between meals.

Chamomile. To relieve cramps and intestinal irritation, you can steep the dried flowers and drink it as a tea, or mix an alcohol-based tincture of chamomile with hot water. Some herbal experts recommend drinking either brew three or four times a day, between meals.

Artificial sweetener causes diarrhea

Sorbitol is an artificial sweetener used in many sugar-free products like gum and candy. Even though you may think you're helping your body by reducing calories, you're actually sending a laxative through your intestines. Since your body can't digest sorbitol, it rockets through your bowel, irritating its already-sensitive lining and giving you diarrhea.

Recently, a flight attendant sought medical help for a severe case of diarrhea, only to discover the culprit was her sugar-free gum, which contained sorbitol. Before you swear off sugar-free gum, keep in mind that this woman chewed up to 60 sticks every day.

Our daily bread

Originally, all bread was brown or black, made only from unrefined flour. It was not until grinding and milling techniques were improved that millers began removing the outer husks of the grain, thus "refining" the flour. The resulting soft, white bread was considered a luxury since only the rich could afford it. Now, nutritionists tell us that the peasants actually had the healthier diet, and whole grain bread is once again the loaf of choice.

KIDNEY STONES

Calcium KO's kidney stones

If you have kidney stones, enjoying a cold, frothy glass of milk may seem out of the question. For years, doctors have told their patients who are "stone formers" to keep their calcium intake low to prevent kidney stones. But new research shows a glass of milk or a cup of yogurt may be just what your kidneys need.

Foods such as spinach, tomatoes, rhubarb, peanuts, coffee, tea, and chocolate contain oxalate, a substance suspected of causing kidney stones. When you eat high-calcium foods with high-oxalate foods, the calcium keeps your body from absorbing the oxalate. This makes you less likely to form kidney stones.

On the other hand, the study shows that taking calcium supplements may increase your risk of forming kidney stones. If you're a woman who needs extra calcium to prevent osteoporosis, what should you do?

The answer is to increase your intake of calcium naturally by eating plenty of low-fat dairy products. Have milk with your brownies, cottage cheese with your sliced tomatoes, and cream (or low-fat evaporated milk) with your coffee. By including delicious dairy foods, you can eat the high-oxalate food you love and still avoid kidney stones.

Shake the salt habit

According to new research, calcium is a friend, not a foe, of people with kidney stones. But shaking on the salt makes your body excrete calcium before it can do you any good. A recent study found a clear relationship between salt and kidney stones in people who are "stone formers." The more salt the people in the study ate, the more calcium was excreted from their bodies.

Calcium in your diet seems to protect your body from absorbing too much oxalate, a substance in kidney stones. So losing calcium from your body may encourage stones to form.

To be sure your body absorbs the calcium you take in, cut back on the amount of salt in your diet. Experts believe a salt intake between 500 and 1,000 milligrams (mg) of sodium per day is a healthy range for most people. You would get this amount of sodium in 1/4 teaspoon of salt.

To reduce the salt in your diet, you can do more than just avoid the salt shaker. Eat fewer fast foods and processed foods and more fresh fruits and vegetables. A quarter-pound cheeseburger contains around 1225 mg of sodium; a slice of bread, 200 mg; a bowl of cornflakes, more than 300 mg; and a bagel, around 245 mg. A bowl of canned soup can contain more than 1,000 mg of sodium, and a small can of tomato juice has 660 mg.

However, a fresh tomato has only 10 mg of sodium, and other vegetables and fruits are also naturally low in salt. By eating more fresh, healthy food, you can keep down the salt in your diet, hold on to your calcium, and keep your kidneys healthier.

Drink up for healthier kidneys

Water is essential to good health; it's involved in making every body system work. Without enough water, your urinary tract is especially open to problems. A kidney stone can be one of them.

Drinking water helps flush out harmful substances before they can bind together and form kidney stones. A five-year study showed that those who drank enough water to produce 2.5 liters of urine a day developed significantly fewer kidney stones. This occurred without any changes in their diets.

You need to drink a minimum of eight to 10 cups of water a day for healthy kidneys. In hot summer months, you may need as many as 12 to 16 cups a day.

If you want healthy kidneys but you're tired of plain water, what other liquids should you drink? A recent study shows that all drinks are not created equal as far as your kidneys are concerned. If you want to lower your risk of developing stones, you can drink regular or decaffeinated coffee and tea, even though they contain some oxalates. Beer and wine also seem to work. Low-fat milk is an especially good choice, since it provides both the fluid and the calcium you need to fight kidney stones.

Steer clear of apple juice and grapefruit juice, however. They seem to increase the risk of stones. Soft drinks are a bad beverage choice, possibly because of the phosphorus and sugar they contain. Another study found that fewer kidney stones formed in people who gave up soft drinks.

End kidney stones in 4 easy steps

You already know from past experience that you're a "stone former." And you'll do just about anything to avoid the awful, stabbing pain of kidney stones. So exactly what should you eat to keep that kidney-kicking pain away for good? Recent research has some answers for you.

- **Skimp on protein.** A diet high in protein, especially animal protein, encourages kidney stone formation. You need enough protein for good health, but no more. For an average-size woman, that translates to 50 grams of protein per day, and for a man, about 63 grams. You can get this amount of protein by having one serving of meat, two cups of milk, and one cup of yogurt. Try substituting high-protein beans for the meat serving to get even more protection from kidney stones.
- **Fill up with fiber**. You've probably heard that fiber is a wonder nutrient that helps digestion, lowers cholesterol, and protects your heart. Now you can add kidney stone prevention to the list. Researchers aren't sure exactly how it works, but studies have shown that kidney stone sufferers who eat 10 to 15 grams of bran fiber per day have fewer stones. To get that amount of fiber, you could eat a serving of bran cereal plus two cups of popcorn. Or try a sandwich with two slices of whole wheat bread and six whole-grain crackers.

- **Flee from fat.** Studies have shown a link between fat and kidney stones, but results have not always agreed. Since fat has a negative impact on other aspects of your health as well, it's safer to keep your dietary fat as low as you can.
- **Pump up your potassium.** If you are deficient in potassium, your risk of forming kidney stones may be higher. To supplement your potassium naturally, eat more fresh fruits such as cantaloupes, oranges, bananas, and avocados. Dried apricots, figs, and peaches are especially high in potassium.

Your diet is the strongest factor in determining whether you suffer from kidney stones. Take control of it, and you'll see a healthier, pain-free life.

LEG PAIN

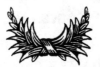

Ironing out restless legs

Do you twist your bedcovers into knots with your legs at night? If so, you may have restless legs syndrome. This syndrome causes creeping, aching, or writhing sensations deep in your legs. The unpleasant sensation only occurs when you're resting and goes away when you move your legs.

If you have this syndrome, you may have difficulty sleeping. As you lie still, trying to fall asleep, the sensation strikes and the urge to move is irresistible. This syndrome doesn't cause your body any real harm, and it may go away on its own. However, it is annoying, especially when it keeps you from sleeping.

Restless legs syndrome is often associated with iron deficiency anemia, so have your doctor check your iron levels. Eating iron-rich foods like red meat, nuts, and beans may help, but because too much iron can be harmful, never take supplements without a doctor's advice.

Kick leg pain goodbye with this herb

Traditional Chinese doctors have been unlocking the mysteries of the ginkgo in the Orient for more than a millennium. The Chinese use ginkgo to relieve chilblains — the swelling of hands and feet after exposure to moist, cold weather. They also use ginkgo as a digestive aid and infection-fighter. But it's only been in the past 20 years that Western studies have proven what the Chinese have known all along — ginkgo offers significant health benefits.

For instance, do you ever have leg pain or constant cramping in your calf muscles after even a short walk? As many people get older, their legs don't get an adequate blood supply because of hardened or blocked blood vessels. This painful condition is called intermittent claudication. Fifteen clinical studies show that ginkgo extract relieves the symptoms of intermittent claudication by improving circulation.

In the health studies on ginkgo, researchers most often used 40 mg three times a day. You will probably have to take the supplements for four to six weeks before you notice any difference in your health.

Lupus

Alfalfa alert

Researchers stumbled onto some fascinating information while testing alfalfa sprouts for cholesterol-lowering benefits. They found that an amino acid in alfalfa sprouts seems to trigger lupus in some people. Alfalfa is found in more than sprouts today. It's a concentrated ingredient in a number of health food pills and potions. People with lupus who unknowingly take these pills might find their lupus getting worse.

A few alfalfa sprouts on a sandwich probably won't hurt you once in a while, but you don't want to make them part of your daily diet. Check any "natural" supplements you take to be sure you're not getting a little alfalfa every day.

Counteract the effects of cortisone

Cortisone can be a godsend for controlling some symptoms of lupus. However, some of cortisone's side effects are problems in their own right. A plan of "defensive eating" can help soften its effects and keep you healthier and feeling better.

- **Fight your appetite.** Taking cortisone can give you an appetite that won't quit. The drug suppresses hormones that regulate your appetite, so you feel hungry all the time. The best strategy is to map out a meal plan that will give you all the nutrients you need without extra calories. You might want to consider a visit to a dietitian for help with your diet plan. The cost is moderate, and you could reap the benefits for a long time.

- **Pump up your protein.** Your need for protein is greater than normal when you take cortisone. Cortisone binds with proteins in your body so they can't be used for other functions. This could be a problem if you have a poor appetite or don't eat much protein. If you are on a low-protein diet because of kidney problems, check with your doctor before adding more to your diet.

- **Control your carbohydrates.** Cortisone also can interfere with the way your body processes carbohydrates. Higher doses of medicine cause more problems; some people can even become diabetic from the cortisone. So managing your intake of starches and sugars is vitally important. Weight gain can nudge you toward diabetes, so try to maintain a healthy weight. To defend yourself from diabetes, eat a balanced diet that includes plenty of complex carbohydrates such as whole grains, fruits, and vegetables. Stay away from simple sugars.

- **Frown on fat.** High doses of cortisone can cause fat buildup in your blood, which puts you at higher risk for clogged arteries. Limit the amount of fat you eat so you can keep this problem to a minimum.

- **Slow down on salt.** Cortisone makes swelling problems even worse because it interferes with hormones that balance the fluids in your body. That causes side effects of puffiness and weight gain. Try to avoid fast foods, canned and other highly processed foods, lunch meats, and salty snacks such as chips and pretzels.

- **Pick up your potassium.** Steroid drugs such as cortisone tend to use up the potassium in your body. Replace it by eating potassium-rich foods such as dried peaches, dried figs, dried apricots, and fresh avocados. Check with your doctor before filling up on these foods, however. The right balance is important.

- **Concentrate on calcium.** Over the long run, cortisone can make your body short on calcium. It cuts down on your ability to absorb this mineral and makes you excrete much more than normal. It also interferes with the way your body uses vitamin D, which works with calcium to build strong bones. All this puts you at higher risk of developing osteoporosis, or brittle bones. You may need calcium and vitamin D supplements, but check with your doctor first. To add more of these nutrients to your diet naturally, drink lots of vitamin D-fortified skim milk.

Fight lupus with fish oil

Living with lupus may feel a little like you're swimming upstream all the time. Having the energy and ability to perform everyday tasks can be challenging. A recent study shows that a gift from the sea may be just the remedy you need. Fish oil contains omega-3 fatty acids, already shown to be helpful in treating or preventing heart disease, arthritis, diabetes, and Crohn's disease. Now researchers have documented fish oil's effectiveness against lupus.

A joint British and American study tested the results of fish-oil supplements and a low-fat diet on people with lupus. Researchers found that lupus symptoms improved for those who took the fish oil and followed the diet; but for those taking the placebo, the disease either stayed the same or got worse.

It probably isn't practical to take such a large amount of fish oil every day. Because of the impurities and contaminants sometimes found in concentrated fish-oil supplements, it probably isn't even safe. To get the disease-fighting benefits of fish oil, it's best to get it from the source. Fill your diet with tuna, salmon, sardines, trout, sturgeon, mackerel, herring, mullet, whitefish, bluefish, and anchovies. Develop a lasting appetite for cold-water, fatty fish, and it may help you stay ahead of the pack where lupus is concerned.

Your best attack plan

The jury is still out on how much influence diet has on the progression of lupus. There's no doubt, however, that a healthy diet can strengthen your body and help keep you from other diet-related diseases. You also need to take into consideration some of the special demands that lupus puts on your body.

A good balance of nutrients will give your diet a solid base to combat this disease. Eat 50 to 60 percent of your calories as complex carbohydrates, 20 to 30 percent as proteins, and 20 to 30 percent as fats. For carbohydrates, choose plenty of fresh vegetables and fruits as well as whole grains. Pick lean protein from low-fat dairy products, legumes (beans or peas), lean meat, and egg whites.

One ingredient you should avoid is salt. Lupus often causes swelling in the arms and legs. Eating lots of salt can make you retain water and have even more problems. High blood pressure is also a problem for some people with lupus. If you happen to be salt-sensitive, taking in more salt can push your blood pressure even higher. Staying away from obvious sources of salt and going light on processed and fast foods will help you control this problem.

You should also limit your cholesterol intake to no more than 300 milligrams a day.

Evidence increasingly supports the idea of a link between diet and disease. A carefully chosen food plan, such as that recommended by the American Heart Association or American Diabetes Association, is a good place for lupus sufferers to start.

MACULAR DEGENERATION

Limit fat for better eyesight

Medical research in the past several years has shown that Jack Sprat, of nursery rhyme fame, was ahead of his time with his "eat no fat" policy. Of course, you do need a little fat in your diet to keep your body functioning. But for most people the problem isn't getting enough fat — it's getting too much. A high-fat diet is linked to a rise in your blood cholesterol and the risk of atherosclerosis, the buildup of plaque in your arteries. Narrowed arteries cut down on blood flow to your heart, your brain, your legs, and even your eyes.

Two recent medical studies, one in The Netherlands and one in the United States, show a link between atherosclerosis and macular degeneration, the eye disease that affects so many elderly people. In the American study, researchers found people who ate diets high in saturated fat and cholesterol were much more likely to develop macular degeneration. In the Dutch study, researchers found people with a buildup of plaque in their arteries were more than twice as likely to develop the condition. So how can you avoid the problem?

To keep your arteries healthy and lower your risk of macular degeneration, concentrate on controlling the fat in your diet. Instead of fatty meat, choose only the leanest cuts. For your protein servings, rely more on chicken and fish, legumes (beans and peas), and tofu (soybean curd). Give up frying your food and bake, broil, roast, or microwave instead. Use only low-fat or fat-free dairy products. Eat more fresh fruits and vegetables, whole-grain breads, cereal, and pasta. And watch out for hidden fat in prepared foods and baked goods. Limit the fat factors in your life, and your eyes will thank you for it.

Zinc may stem macular degeneration

Zinc plays various roles in your body, from helping your stomach digest protein to helping your liver take the toxins out of alcohol. Zinc is found in your eyes, especially in the tissues of the retina, where it's important in chemical reactions. So, it seems logical that when you're deficient in zinc, your eyes would suffer.

That's what researchers reasoned in a medical study in the 1980s, when they used zinc supplements to treat people with macular degeneration. For the people who took the supplements, the disease seemed to stop progressing. But the researchers were reluctant to recommend zinc supplements based on the study. They felt the supplements would be dangerous if people took too much. Unfortunately, further research in this area has had mixed results.

A 1996 study showed zinc to have a protective effect against macular degeneration, but the effect seemed to be a weak one. Doctors still disagree about the usefulness of taking zinc supplements for macular degeneration. So you'll have to make your own decision.

If you choose to take supplements, don't take more than 50 milligrams (mg) daily. The recommended dietary allowance (RDA) is 15 mg for men and 12 mg for women. If you choose to get your zinc from food, think "lean red meat." This is a safe and available source of dietary zinc, and your body can easily absorb it. Other good sources of zinc are oysters, turkey, chicken liver, black beans, and lean pork.

'Just say no' to Olestra

Cutting fat from your diet is a good way to protect your vision and lose weight. But if you miss that rich, buttery texture in foods, don't go in for fat substitutes. It seems that Olestra, the fat substitute recently approved by the FDA, is still a little rough around the edges. Because of concerns about its safety, the manufacturer of a snack chip containing Olestra set up a hotline for consumers who were bothered by ill effects when they ate the chips. Many of the callers complained of stomach cramps and diarrhea. In another survey, one-fifth of people who ate the chips had digestive problems. Understandably, most people ate the chips only once.

An even bigger problem with the fake fat is that it may prevent your body from absorbing fat-soluble carotenoids, vitamins that help protect your body from such illnesses as cancer, heart disease, and macular degeneration. A consumer interest group has asked the FDA to take Olestra off the market, but the government is still investigating. Watch for more news on Olestra in the future, but for now, try to limit your fats to healthier, natural ones. Monounsaturated fats such as olive or canola oil are good choices.

Grape seeds provide antioxidant protection

You know that bitter little crunch you experience when you find out the grapes you're eating aren't seedless? Well, that hard, round grape seed packs a powerful wallop in the world of antioxidants. It contains a substance called PCO, sometimes sold under the brand name Pycnogenol, which works along with vitamin C and vitamin E to fight free radicals in your body. Free radicals are thought to be part of the process that damages your eyes and causes the central blindness of macular degeneration. PCO also helps keep the walls of your blood vessels, including those in your eyes, healthy and strong.

You can buy PCO in the form of grape seed extract or the more expensive pine bark extract. If you choose to take PCO supplements, experts recommend that you jump-start the antioxidants in your body by taking 100 to 150 milligrams (mg) a day for a week or two. Then you can scale back to a daily dosage of 50 mg. If you prefer, you can get your PCO from foods. A recent Australian study found PCO in the skin of red grapes. You can also find a good supply of this potent antioxidant in citrus peels, apples, onions, blueberries, cranberries, and peanuts.

Add greens to your diet for healthier eyes

If you think collard greens and spinach are icky, here's some news that should make them taste much better. Dark green, leafy vegetables are the healthiest things you can eat to protect your eyes from age-related macular degeneration. Vegetables and fruits contain carotenoids, the antioxidant pigments that help give them their color. Two carotenoids, lutein and zeaxanthin, are found mostly in green, leafy vegetables. A recent medical study showed them to be protective agents against macular degeneration.

The study was designed to test whether eating more foods that contain carotenoids and vitamins A, C, and E might help ward off the eye disease. The results were dramatic in one area. It turned out that people who ate the most spinach and collard greens had about half the macular degeneration risk of those who ate the least.

Some other studies have shown beneficial effects on macular degeneration from antioxidant vitamins and minerals such as vitamins C and E and selenium. Lycopene, another carotenoid found in abundance in tomato sauce, also had positive results in studies.

If you put the emphasis in your diet on leafy greens and other vegetables, fresh fruits, and whole grains, you'll be getting a good supply of all these protective nutrients. When you shop for groceries, put these items on your list and set your sights on the benefits of a healthy diet.

MEMORY LOSS

Sugar may provide sweet memories

As you get older, your brain's ability to retain new information slows down. So, you may have a hard time remembering the sermon you just heard or the article you read yesterday. But help may be as close as your kitchen in a surprising form — ordinary sugar.

A recent study examined the effects of glucose, or sugar, on elderly people's memory. The test was done early in the morning before anyone had eaten breakfast. One group drank lemonade with sugar before taking the test, and another drank lemonade with saccharin. Researchers found that those who drank the sugar-sweetened drink performed better on memory tests a short time later.

In a related study, people who ate sugar just after reading something remembered it better a day later than those taking saccharin. Researchers aren't sure exactly how sugar works in the brain to enhance memory but hope to find out more in the future.

This doesn't mean you can eat all the sugar you want. Too much is still harmful. The important thing is to keep your blood sugar on an even keel. Don't skip meals or wait too long between meals to eat. If you're tired and cranky and have trouble remembering things, your blood sugar is probably low. Try the sweet approach in the form of fresh fruit, a glass of orange juice or lemonade, or even a piece of hard candy. You might find the sweet success of remembering everything you want to.

Ginkgo may improve the following symptoms of cerebral insufficiency:

- difficulty concentrating
- absentmindedness
- confusion
- lack of energy
- tiredness
- decreased physical performance
- sadness or depression
- anxiety
- dizziness
- tinnitus (ringing in the ears)
- headaches

Gear up your memory with ginkgo

Ginkgo is a popular herb in Europe and China, where it has been used for centuries to treat elderly people for problems of memory and thinking. Now, medical researchers in the United States are beginning to sing the praises of ginkgo to treat cerebral insufficiency, also known as dementia.

Confusion, absentmindedness, difficulty concentrating, and memory loss are some of the symptoms of this condition. It stems from a lack of blood flow to your brain. Medical studies show that ginkgo helps open up your blood vessels and get more blood flowing to your brain. As you age, that's the kind of help your brain needs to work better. And there seem to be few, if any, side effects.

To give your brain a steady supply of ginkgo, experts recommend dividing your doses throughout the day. A dosage of 40 milligrams three times daily is a standard amount. Make sure to look for pure ginkgo biloba extract, also called GBE or GBX, instead of a formula with just a little ginkgo in it. Don't get discouraged if you don't see improvement in your memory power right away. It takes several weeks for the ginkgo to show its effects.

Nutrients to boost your brain power

It can be annoying and frustrating when you can't remember your best friend's phone number or your car's last oil change. But don't automatically assume a memory lapse is a sign of Alzheimer's disease. Depression or other illness, stress, or even certain medications can all affect your memory. Vitamin and mineral deficiencies can also cause memory problems.

If a vitamin deficiency is sabotaging your brain power, then simply getting more of the vitamin may solve the problem. Taking extra doses, however, probably won't give you a super-charged memory if you didn't have one before. These are some of the nutrients that will help boost your brain power and avoid memory problems:

Vitamin B12 and folic acid. If you don't have enough of these two B vitamins in your body, your mind probably isn't working at peak performance. A recent psychological study tested people between the ages of 75 and 96 for their ability to recall words. The people with the least vitamin B12 and folic acid in their blood had more trouble remembering than those with higher levels.

Another study showed that people with vitamin B12 deficiency may permanently lose brain power unless the deficiency is caught early. Those most vulnerable include people over age 65, alcoholics, vegetarians, people with digestive problems, or those who have recently had surgery or are under severe stress.

To make sure you get enough vitamin B12 in your diet, eat chicken liver or sardines, sirloin steak, tuna packed in water, and cottage cheese. The best sources of folic acid are raw spinach, broccoli, and romaine lettuce. You can also get folic acid from oranges, calves' liver, brewer's yeast, whole grains, and beans and peas.

Vitamin B1 (thiamin). A lack of thiamin can make you tired, irritable, and nauseated. It can also affect your appetite, sleep, concentration, and memory.

Most people get enough thiamin from a healthy diet; young children and the elderly are more likely to be deficient. You may need extra thiamin if you take antibiotics, birth-control pills, or sulfa drugs. This vitamin is also important if you are under unusual stress; have recently had surgery; or have kidney, liver, or thyroid disease. If you drink large amounts of alcohol, coffee, or tea or eat a diet high in carbohydrates or low in calories and nutrients, you should also make sure you get enough thiamin.

Brewer's yeast and wheat germ are excellent sources of natural thiamin. Other good food sources are whole grains, seeds and nuts, peas and beans, lean pork, and salmon. If you prefer supplements, a B-complex vitamin can meet your need for thiamin as well as B12, folic acid, and the other B vitamins.

Vitamin C. A 20-year British medical study showed that people over 65 who lost some mental ability had a higher risk of death, especially from stroke. They also turned out to be the ones with the lowest vitamin C intake.

Researchers speculated that the key was in the blood vessels of the brain. A high intake of vitamin C helps keep your blood vessels strong so your blood can circulate properly and nourish your brain. The result is healthier blood vessels, a lower incidence of stroke, and improved ability to think and remember.

To get more vitamin C naturally, you can eat more citrus fruits, broccoli, cantaloupe, strawberries, and sweet red peppers. If you want to take a supplement, a dose of 200 to 500 milligrams of vitamin C daily seems to be a safe amount.

Vitamin A (beta carotene). Beta carotene is a substance that is turned into vitamin A in your body. Along with vitamin C, it's an important antioxidant that affects your long-term mental ability.

A 22-year Swiss study measured the effect of certain nutrients on memory. Beta carotene proved to be a real asset in helping people retain their ability to think, reason, and remember.

It's safest to get your beta carotene from foods, rather than supplements, since it can be toxic if you take too much. Spinach, turnip greens, carrots, sweet potatoes, butternut squash, and cantaloupe are good natural sources.

MENOPAUSE

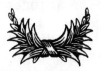

Protect your heart and bones

Menopause is sometimes referred to as the "change of life." Between the ages of 40 and 50, many women find that not only do their bodies change, but their personal and professional lives change as well. Even as you try to cope with all the different physical and emotional surprises, two potentially life-threatening conditions are waiting to ambush you.

Beware of weakened bones. Osteoporosis is a condition that possibly began when you were a teenager. During those adolescent years, you set yourself up for the quality of bone density you would have as a mature adult. Consider yourself fortunate if your mother made you drink lots of milk. That means stronger bones and a better chance of evading the crippling effects of osteoporosis.

However, even if you didn't grow up drinking a lot of milk, all is not lost. You can begin strengthening your bones today. The key word is calcium.

The National Research Council has determined that a healthy premenopausal woman needs 1,000 to 1,200 mg of calcium a day. If you're postmenopausal, you need up to 1,500 mg of this bone-strengthening mineral. That's a lot of calcium for anyone. Of course, it's best to get it from natural sources: dairy foods, seafood such as oysters and sardines, and vegetables like kale and beet greens. But if you don't feel you can eat that much calcium, you can turn to supplements.

Because of the decrease in estrogen during menopause, you are probably going to gain weight. It's a sad fact for most women but simply your body's reaction to the change in hormones. Being more physically active will help you avoid this problem. Be careful about dieting at this time though. At least one study has shown that weight loss in postmenopausal women significantly increases bone loss, and that means a higher risk of osteoporosis.

The heart of the matter. During and after menopause, you are more at risk of developing heart disease than at any other time in your life. But by adjusting your diet, you can say good-bye to this concern and really enjoy your golden years.

Heart-healthy eating is simple — low fat, high fiber. But one study has shown that this advice probably should be modified for postmenopausal women. It seems that a high-carbohydrate, low-fat diet increases risk factors for heart disease in these women. Replacing saturated fat with the monounsaturated and polyunsaturated kind found in olive, canola, vegetable, and soybean oils may actually work better than adding more carbohydrates to your diet.

Plants provide natural estrogen therapy

One term you may often hear in connection with menopause is phytoestrogen. It's a plant compound that acts like the estrogen in your body. That means there are certain foods you can eat that are healthy and a natural source of estrogen. By eating these, you may not have to rely completely on hormone or estrogen replacement therapy (HRT/ERT). While they have no specific recommended doses, it is just smart to make these foods part of your balanced diet.

Beat the heat with soy. Researchers around the world say soybean products reduce hot flashes and vaginal dryness in postmenopausal women. Just imagine, two of the most uncomfortable symptoms of menopause eased by a small, brown pea. Whether you bake with soy flour, drink soy milk, or explore the hundreds of ways to add tofu to your own recipes, you'll get a rich source of protein as you relieve the difficulties of menopause.

Fight "flashes" with food. If you suffer from hot flashes, try adding wheat, barley, oat, and rye flour to your shopping list. Or how about green beans, carrots, peas, and potatoes? Cherries, apples, rice, garlic, and alfalfa also sound like the ingredients in some deliciously healthy meals. But these foods also give you something extra — phytoestrogens, the plant compound that can ease your menopausal symptoms, especially hot flashes.

Researchers have even studied grains like red clover sprouts and linseeds and found they have effects similar to hormonal estrogen. Women who supplemented their diets with these grains for six weeks had significant changes in their estrogen levels.

So, don't be afraid to experiment with unusual ingredients such as soybeans and different varieties of grains. They'll not only spice up your recipes — they'll give you extra menopause protection as well.

Enjoy caffeine in moderation

All you poor coffee-holics who simply have to have your morning cup, but agonize over the health risks, can now relax. A little.

The old news from several studies was that drinking caffeine, especially more than two to three cups a day, caused bone loss in postmenopausal women if they took in less than 800 mg of calcium per day.

However, a new, more carefully controlled study did not find this to be true. Even those women who drank up to eight or more cups of coffee per day showed no changes in bone density. Of course, caffeine can affect you in other ways, so it's still best to limit your intake.

If you are a healthy, postmenopausal woman who likes her morning cup of coffee, go ahead and enjoy it. But be sure to take the recommended amount of calcium, and switch off the coffee pot after breakfast.

Learn the ABCs of menopause

The calcium-zinc connection. Your body is a complex machine where every nutrient you take in interacts with something else. Calcium is no different. If you take a calcium supplement with a meal, you could be decreasing your body's ability to absorb zinc by as much as 50 percent.

Most women within this age group don't get enough zinc anyway. (If you are over 50, you need 12 mg a day.) So, it may be wise to eat more zinc if you plan on taking a calcium supplement. You can get lots of this mineral by eating black beans, crab meat, steak, and oysters.

The calcium-magnesium connection. Like so many minerals, magnesium plays an important role in your body's delicate balance. If you don't have enough magnesium, your bones don't absorb calcium as efficiently. In fact, the calcium can end up deposited in the soft tissues of your body instead of your bones. Tests have shown that if you take in the proper amount of magnesium, calcium levels in your body rise, even if you don't take calcium supplements.

Eat tofu, raisins, beans, peas, grains, green leafy vegetables, avocados, and nuts and seeds for more magnesium. As a menopausal woman, you need 400 to 750 mg of magnesium each day. If you plan on taking a supplement, buy the buffered form, like magnesium gluconate or citrate, to protect your digestive system. To make life simpler, you can even buy calcium/magnesium combinations.

A dose of D. Watch your vitamin D, too, since it plays an important role in how much calcium your bones actually absorb. Eat eggs and shrimp, and drink fortified milk to get your calcium at the same time. Since sunshine helps activate your daily dose of D, remember that during the winter you are exposed to less sunshine and may experience more bone loss.

In addition, summertime sunscreens will block some of your body's absorption of this important vitamin. You don't need to sunbathe in January or give up your summer sunscreen — just make sure you take in 400 to 800 IU of vitamin D from other sources each day.

Enough E? You've heard it a million times — eat more fruits, vegetables, and grains. You know they're good for you and they really do taste delicious, but old habits are hard to break. If you aren't used to grabbing a handful of almonds instead of that candy bar for a snack, you may not be getting enough vitamin E.

Many of us fight this uphill battle by taking the easy way out — we buy a supplement. And in many cases, that's okay. But if you're a postmenopausal women, taking vitamin E pills will not protect you against heart disease as much as eating foods high in vitamin E. Researchers have found that supplements simply may not do the trick. So boil up some shrimp or bake a sweet potato. They're rich in vitamin E — the natural kind.

Herbal cures for menopause problems

Dr. Susan Lark, author of *The Estrogen Decision,* suggests that herbs, when used wisely, are a healthy addition to a nutritious diet. She has developed three special menopause formulas, which you can buy in an herb shop or make yourself at home by combining small amounts of the herbs listed for each formula.

Formula 1: This combination of herbs helps relieve hot flashes and vaginal dryness. Mix the following herbs together in equal amounts: black cohosh, dong quai, false unicorn root, fennel, anise, and blessed thistle.

Formula 2: This formula helps relieve tiredness and weakness. Mix together equal amounts of ginger, oat straw, ginkgo biloba, and Siberian ginseng.

Formula 3: These herbs help combat anxiety, insomnia, and irritability. Combine valerian root, catnip, chamomile, and hops in equal amounts for a little rest and relaxation.

Lark recommends that you add the herbs to tea or take them with meals. Do not take more than one to two herbal capsules or drink more than one to two cups of herbal tea daily. Although all of these herbs are considered safe, check first with your doctor, and stop using them if any symptoms make you uncomfortable.

Avoid nutritional pitfalls

You know that certain foods make your menopause symptoms worse. You can feel the hot flash coming on after that spicy enchilada or mug of hot drink. It's also been shown that alcohol will make every symptom you have stronger and more intense. Not just the hot flashes, but the mood swings, fatigue, depression, and insomnia.

Recently, a small study found that two alcoholic beverages, beer and bourbon, contain beneficial phytoestrogens, the plant compound that acts like estrogen. Beer gets its benefit from hops, and bourbon, from corn. The negative effects of these beverages probably outweigh the benefits, however.

Sugar also is a menopausal hazard. Too much sugar can upset your balance of B-complex vitamins, causing nervous tension, anxiety, and irritability. It may even affect how well your body metabolizes estrogen. Talk to your doctor about this side effect of too many sweets, and read your product labels. Most processed foods have hidden sugar.

Believe it or not, broccoli may be a no-no as well. Researchers recently discovered that this vegetable contains an anti-estrogenic substance, which means it could work against any diet or replacement therapy you are using. Try eliminating this vegetable for a while, and see if you notice a change in your symptoms.

On the positive nutritional side, fish high in omega-3 fatty acids, like Atlantic mackerel, lake trout, and bluefin tuna, can help your body cope naturally with menopause.

MOTION SICKNESS

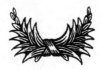

Anti-nausea nutrients ease motion sickness

If you've ever felt the dizzy, unconnected feeling of motion sickness, you know how easily it can ruin a trip. Whether you're traveling by car, boat, or plane, you probably don't care why you're feeling miserable, you just want to feel better.

Motion sickness starts in your ears. That's because they're your body's center of balance. Inside your ears are thousands of tiny nerve endings filled with fluid. The fluid supports tiny pebbles, one in each nerve ending, and when your body moves, the pebbles move with it. The motion of these pebbles sends messages to your brain, telling it what your body is doing, whether you are sitting, standing, or in motion. When this mechanism is not working right, your brain receives confused or incorrect messages from the nerve centers in your ears, and this confusion can cause nausea.

These mismatched signals can result from an ear infection; ear damage; or from drastic, unusual motion. Sometimes, if your eyes are focused on something moving, like a wave, and your body is moving differently or not at all, like on deck, your brain receives two sets of conflicting messages. Your eyes tell your brain the world is moving, but your ears tell your brain you are standing still.

While it is not known why some people suffer from motion sickness and others don't, it is clear that several factors, including nutritional deficiencies, can lead to ear damage, which can impair the balancing function of the ear.

The following vitamins and minerals can help keep your inner ear in top shape and help fight motion sickness.

Vitamin D and calcium are important to inner ear health. Not only is vitamin D important by itself, a lack of vitamin D can lead to a calcium deficiency. One of the best sources of vitamin D is fortified milk, and it's also a great source of calcium. Other good sources of vitamin D include eggs, green leafy vegetables, and fortified cereals. For a nondairy source of calcium, try some peanuts or broccoli.

Magnesium deficiency is linked to hearing loss. Squash, potatoes, skim milk, and oatmeal are all good ways to boost your intake of magnesium. Magnesium supplements are available at most drugstores, and they are often combined with calcium.

Zinc is another important nutrient that many older people don't seem to get enough of. Some studies suggest this may contribute to the ear damage and hearing loss that frequently occurs in older people. Zinc is abundant in meats, shellfish, and poultry. You can also get it from legumes, such as black beans, and whole grains. Don't take zinc supplements without checking with your doctor. Zinc supplements can cause serious side effects in high doses.

Common kitchen spice soothes stomach

Ginger has been used for thousands of years to treat everything from constipation to impotence. However, numerous recent studies prove that ginger is an effective remedy for the symptoms of motion sickness. When taken a half hour before traveling, ginger can prevent the nausea that comes from rocking boats or swerving cars.

In one test, powdered ginger was tested directly against Dramamine, an over-the-counter motion sickness drug. The people who took ginger lasted, on average, almost twice as long in a rotating chair as those who took the drug. In fact, half the people treated with ginger did not experience motion sickness at all.

Ginger doesn't affect your inner ear, and it doesn't work on your central nervous system. Rather, it works in your gastrointestinal tract to soothe the vomiting reflex and reduce the feeling of nausea.

You can buy ginger at any supermarket or health food store. You'll find it in its natural form or as a pill or a powder. A typical capsule, containing 500 mg of ginger, should usually be enough to head off your weak stomach. Some herbal experts recommend taking one or two tablets 30 minutes before your activity, then repeat as symptoms develop.

Candied ginger is a tasty way to enjoy ginger's benefits. This sugary treat can be found at many Oriental markets. A one-inch square of the crystallized snack equals the amount of ginger in one 500 mg tablet.

If you're still not sure about this natural remedy, try a variation that could very well be in your refrigerator right now. That's right ... ginger ale has been used for years to calm hostile stomachs and tame nausea.

Foods that fight the waves of nausea

What should you eat to help soothe a queasy stomach? Ask 10 motion sickness sufferers and you'll probably get 10 different answers. Although very little research has been done on home remedies for motion sickness, miracle foods and folk remedies abound. You never know what may work for you.

Pickled okra, anyone? Strange as it may seem, some people swear by pickled okra as a way to fight the motion of the ocean. Dill pickles, olives, and cheese are other pet remedies often used to prevent seasickness. Others suggest sucking on a wedge of lemon to reduce saliva in the mouth and reduce nausea. The most widely recommended food for dealing with the nausea of motion sickness is soda crackers. These plain, dry snacks help get rid of excess saliva and absorb stomach acid that can upset an empty stomach. Soda crackers seem to be the most tried-and-true of all folk remedies.

Keep your strength up. If you've already gotten sick, it's a good idea to eat something, if you can, to prevent weakness and increased discomfort. Nutrients and electrolytes that you lost during vomiting need to be replaced. Once again, soda crackers can come in handy, since they are bland and absorbent. If you can't eat, try drinking some ginger ale or a cola drink. As a last resort, sucking on some hard candy is better than nothing at all.

Although these remedies haven't been tested in the lab, they have been proven in the field. The best idea, however, is the same as for any allergy or sensitivity. Don't be afraid to experiment a little in order to find what works — and what doesn't work — for you.

Motion sickness aggravated by certain foods

While some foods can help ward off motion sickness, there are others you should definitely avoid. In one study, researchers measured motion sickness in pilots and found that the pilots who ate foods high in sodium, such as preserved meats and potato chips, had much higher rates of sickness. The same was true for high-protein foods, like cheeses and meats, as well as foods high in thiamin, such as pork, eggs, and fish. Foods high in calories also tended to increase the frequency of motion sickness.

In general, avoid strong-smelling, strong-tasting foods. These have a way of filling you up, and they are more likely to trigger a reaction in your sensitive gastrointestinal tract. Instead, try to eat light meals when you know you will be traveling. Reach for bland, low-fat, starchy foods that provide more substance than spice.

Caffeine is an irritant for many people who suffer from motion sickness, and it can bring on bouts of dizziness, especially in people who suffer from Meniere's disease. The same is true for salt. Reducing your intake of these might serve to lessen the uncomfortable effects of motion sickness.

Smoking cigarettes or using other tobacco products increases your risk of motion sickness. Another very common irritant is alcohol, which directly affects your sense of balance. There's no better way to ensure a bout of motion sickness than to start a trip with a drink or a hangover.

MULTIPLE SCLEROSIS

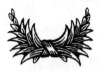

Low-fat diet may help MS

Treatments with steroid or interferon drugs can help control multiple sclerosis (MS), but they're not a cure. Until there is one, you want to do all you can to keep the disease at bay. Fortunately, there is something within your control that may make a huge difference in your life — your diet.

Dr. Roy Swank began his study of the effects of diet on multiple sclerosis in 1950. Many years later, the results are in. Over this long period of time, people who ate less than 20 grams of fat a day had a dramatically lower rate of disability and death than people who ate more than 20 grams of fat a day. People who began a low-fat diet early in the course of their disease fared better than those who started later.

The diet Dr. Swank recommends is one that is low in saturated fats and high in essential fatty acids. This means you should:

- **Make meals without meat.** Most meat is full of saturated fat. Eat only low-fat meats, and only occasionally.
- **Go light on dairy products.** Whole milk, butter, and sour cream are full of fat. Switch to skim milk and other dairy items that are low-fat or fat-free.
- **Eat fresh, not processed.** Avoid processed foods, since they often contain hidden fat. Read labels and avoid items containing coconut and palm oils.

Essential fatty acids, or EFAs, are nutrients your body needs but can't manufacture, so you have to get them from outside sources. EFAs are involved in building the membranes of cells and the myelin sheath which covers your nerves, and also in maintaining your central nervous system. Omega-6 fatty acids and omega-3 fatty acids are the two important types of EFAs you should eat. Here's what to look for:

- **Go to seed.** Omega-6 fatty acids are found in vegetable and seed oils. Choose safflower, sunflower, and soy oils; seeds; nuts; and whole grains.

- **Find some fish.** Omega-3 fatty acids are found mostly in oily, cold-water fish. To get the most benefits, choose salmon, sardines, trout, tuna, anchovies, bluefish, herring, mackerel, mullet, sturgeon, and whitefish. Try to eat fish at least three times a week.
- **Plant a healthy habit.** Omega-3 fatty acids also come from plant sources, although they aren't as good a source as the fish. Oat germ is the plant food richest in omega-3; dried beans, flaxseed, soybean products, walnuts, and wheat germ oil also contain it.
- **Keep your balance.** Experts say you should eat one serving of omega-3 foods for every four servings of omega-6 foods to get the proper balance of nutrients.

Dr. Swank's treatment for MS is controversial; some doctors feel his studies are not reliable. But there is no danger in following the healthy recommendations of his eating plan. It is essentially the same diet recommended by medical experts to help prevent or cure heart disease and stroke.

An interesting German study on the incidence of multiple sclerosis throughout the world backs up the basic idea of Dr. Swank's diet. Researchers found that MS occurs most frequently in colder climates where people eat more meat and dairy products and less fish.

The benefits of vitamin B12

Vitamin B12 works hard in your body, and one of its important jobs is to help maintain the myelin sheath that surrounds and protects your nerve cells. If the myelin sheath gets damaged, your nerves are open to injury. This situation can occur when you have a vitamin B12 deficiency. It also happens when you have multiple sclerosis.

Japanese researchers recently looked further into this relationship. They discovered that the people in their study with multiple sclerosis had a problem getting vitamin B12 into their cells. So they gave those people very large doses of vitamin B12 over a period of time. The results were promising.

Those who received the vitamin showed improvement in their sight and hearing, but not in other areas. Still the researchers were encouraged by the improvements. More research needs to be done to see how useful vitamin B12 may be in developing future treatments for MS.

Don't deny your D

If you are a woman with multiple sclerosis, you may not have thought much about osteoporosis, the bone disease that affects so many women. But a recent study shows you really should give it some thought. Vitamin D has an important role to play in fighting osteoporosis, and this study showed women with MS to be deficient in vitamin D.

The best way to get vitamin D naturally is to spend a little time in the sun each day. Your body uses sunlight to manufacture the vitamin D you need. You can also get it from vitamin-D-fortified skim milk and from supplements. Ask your doctor to check for a vitamin D deficiency, and discuss the options with her if you need more D. If you have MS, you certainly don't need the additional problems of osteoporosis to worry about. The solution could be as simple as a daily dose of vitamin D.

Nausea and Vomiting

Herbal remedy quiets a queasy stomach

Feeling a little queasy? Forget the pink stuff. Instead, why not try ginger. Folks the world over have been using this proven natural remedy for nausea and vomiting for more than 2,000 years.

Ginger, long known for its ability to lessen and prevent the symptoms of motion sickness, may also be effective in treating nausea and vomiting from other causes as well, including pregnancy and surgery.

Because ginger works directly in your gastrointestinal tract, it reduces both the symptoms and the causes of your nausea. In several studies, ginger outperformed commercial anti-nausea drugs. Newspapers and herbal magazines are filled with testimonials by people whose nausea was uncontrollable until they discovered the powers of ginger.

The most popular way to take ginger is in pill form. Capsules, usually from 250 to 500 mg in strength, are available at most health food stores. The German government's Commission E, similar to our FDA, recommends a dose of 2 to 4 grams per day to aid digestion and treat nausea.

A more tasty alternative is candied ginger. Candied ginger is a chewy, sugary treat, shown to be just as effective as other forms of the herb. Powdered, grated, and whole ginger are all widely available. One cup of boiling water poured over two teaspoons of powdered ginger and steeped for 10 minutes makes a soothing tea.

You can also get a smaller amount of ginger from ginger snaps and ginger ale. Ginger ale has been a home remedy for upset stomachs for generations.

If you use raw or dry ginger, don't swallow it by itself. Dry ginger is very spicy and can burn your throat.

Even though ginger has been used to successfully treat cases of severe, even life-threatening, vomiting, dosages in these cases can be pretty high. Check with your doctor before taking unusually large amounts of ginger, especially if you are pregnant. Ginger also shouldn't be used to treat nausea following chemotherapy if your platelet count is low because it interferes with blood clotting.

3 tips to relieve nausea

When you have that nauseous feeling, usually the last thing on your mind is eating, but sometimes that's the best thing you can do. When you vomit, you also lose large amounts of water, vitamins, and electrolytes. Failing to replace these can result in weakness, fatigue, and continued nausea. As if that's not bad enough, an empty stomach is usually very unstable, so it's a good idea to get something in there.

- **Drink clear liquids.** One of the most dangerous things about vomiting is the risk of dehydration. It is very important to put back the water you lose when you are sick. The best and easiest way to do this is with clear liquids. Broth, tea, and light soups are usually much kinder on your stomach than more solid foods. Carbonated drinks, especially ginger ale, can help settle an upset stomach. At the very least, drink some fruit juice or water.

- **Eat bland, starchy foods.** Although eating might be what caused your nausea in the first place, it can also help you recover. The key is to start small. Go slowly and don't overdo it, even if you are feeling a little better. Avoid strong-smelling and strong-tasting foods. These are more likely to irritate your stomach. Bland, starchy foods like dry toast and crackers are generally a safe bet. The best food for quieting queasiness might still be the soda crackers your mom gave you as a kid.

- **Try the BRAT diet.** One formula for getting yourself back on solids is called the BRAT diet. Designed to ease your digestive system back into eating after a bout of food poisoning, it works just as well for vomiting from other causes. Instead of moving right from water to normal eating, the BRAT method suggests a transitional diet of Bananas, Rice, Applesauce, and Toast. These foods are both nutritious and gentle on your digestive tract.

A spot of tea soothes stomach upsets

Drinking tea is a gentle way to soothe an upset stomach and replace lost liquids, but one particular tea seems to do a better job than others. In Europe, chamomile is almost as popular a remedy as ginseng is in America. Chamomile seems to fight spasms in the gastrointestinal tract that can result in vomiting.

Although the powerful extract of chamomile oil is not widely available in the United States, a very effective tea made from the plant's leaves is . To prepare chamomile tea, steep the leaves in hot water, covered, for at least 10 to 15 minutes.

Because chamomile solutions are prepared from a pollinated flower, it is possible to have an allergic reaction to chamomile tea. If you are very allergic to pollen, especially ragweed, asters, or chrysanthemums, check with your doctor before trying chamomile.

Skip the medicine, keep the vitamin

One of the most common, active ingredients in commercial anti-nausea medications is pyridoxine, otherwise known as vitamin B6. In clinical testing, vitamin B6 relieved the severe nausea and vomiting of early pregnancy, but it didn't work as well in women with only mild to moderate symptoms.

Since most anti-nausea medications have unpleasant side effects, such as drowsiness, taking B6 might be a better choice. Although you can get B6 from chicken, pork, dried beans, and whole grains, the amounts in these foods are probably not enough for the anti-nausea effect. If you're thinking of taking supplements, ask your doctor how much you can safely take.

Unproven folk remedies

Although ginger has proven itself to be a powerful remedy against nausea and vomiting, there are plenty of other folk remedies that are very dangerous or just don't work.

Don't jump for juniper. While juniper and juniper preparations might have some value as stomach remedies, there doesn't seem to be much reason to use them, since more effective and much safer options are available. Juniper in high concentrations can damage your kidneys and is dangerous for pregnant women. Under no circumstance should you take juniper if you are pregnant or have any history of kidney trouble.

Leave catnip for kitty. While it might drive felines wild, catnip doesn't do much for humans. Some people swear by catnip as a treatment for colds, indigestion, and upset stomachs, but studies can't back up any of these claims. Unlike juniper, however, side effects seem to be minor.

Lose the lemon balm. Like catnip, lemon balm is supposed to soothe an angry stomach and help quiet storms of vomiting. And, much like catnip, no scientific studies can support these claims. However, stirring a few teaspoons into hot water does make a delicious tea, and if you like the taste of lemon, it won't do you much harm. Just don't expect it to solve the problems in your stomach.

The potato chip question

When your stomach is upset, you want to feed it something bland and absorbent, like soda crackers, right? Well, at least one doctor isn't sure. She found that salty and tart foods, not bland, provided relief from nausea.

Dr. Miriam Erick didn't understand why many morning sickness sufferers were asking for foods like potato chips and lemonade until she studied what was in these foods. Potato chips, she learned, contain more vitamin C, folic acid, and potassium than soda crackers. These three are essential nutrients to replace if you have been vomiting. Also, the tartness of lemonade reduces the amount of saliva in your mouth that can lead to vomiting.

So, the choice is yours ... soda crackers or chips. Experiment a little and try to find out what works best for you.

OSTEOPOROSIS

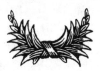

Avoid the breaks of osteoporosis

When you fell out of a tree and broke your arm when you were a kid, it was kind of cool to get extra attention and have a cast for all your friends to sign. However, when an older person falls and breaks a bone, the consequences can be much more serious. More than 250,000 people suffer a broken hip due to osteoporosis each year. Of these people, 12 to 20 percent will die within a year, and the ones who do survive may become unable to walk and many end up in nursing homes. The best way to avoid the life-threatening effects of osteoporosis is to avoid getting the disease in the first place.

- **Call on calcium.** When you were in school, cramming before a test was probably a common occurrence. Hopefully you were cramming calcium into your body at the same time. Your bones build in strength until you hit your 30s, when you reach your peak bone mass, and calcium is one of the building blocks of healthy bones. The amount of calcium you take in during these years is a strong predictor of whether or not you get osteoporosis later. However, if you didn't get enough calcium during those formative years, don't give up. You can still give your bones a boost by making sure you get plenty of calcium now. This is always important because if you don't have enough calcium in your diet, your body will draw it from your bones. Dairy products are the best source of calcium, but other good sources include green vegetables like turnip greens, beet greens, and kale, and fish like salmon and sardines (with bones). If you are lactose-intolerant or just don't like dairy products and have trouble getting enough calcium in your diet, supplements can help.

- **Keep up your vitamin D.** Just making sure you eat plenty of calcium-rich foods may not be enough to prevent osteoporosis. You need vitamin D to help absorb calcium so it can do its bone-building duty. Your body can manufacture vitamin D from sunlight, but if you are indoors a lot, you need to get your vitamin D from foods or supplements. About 400 IU of vitamin D daily will help you use your calcium supply to its fullest.

- **Get your fill of fluoride.** You know that fluoride can help you have healthier teeth. It can also help you have healthier bones. Though most people get fluoride through their water supply, if you drink well water or other water without fluoride, you may want to take fluoride supplements.
- **Team up with trace minerals.** Other minerals may help your body use calcium more effectively. One study found that postmenopausal women who were given supplements that included copper, manganese, and zinc lost less bone mass than those who received no supplements. However, too much of some of these minerals, particularly zinc, can actually decrease the amount of calcium you absorb. To get these minerals from food sources, eat plenty of seafood, potatoes, beans, and whole grains, but don't get more than the RDA, which is 15 mg for zinc. There is no RDA for copper and manganese, but the estimated safe and adequate daily intake is one and a half to three milligrams for copper, and two to five milligrams for manganese.

Calcium-sappers weaken bones

You've always loved milk and other dairy products, and you feel confident that you've given your body plenty of calcium to build strong, healthy bones that will carry you upright through your old age. Good for you! However, there's more to keeping those bones strong than just draining your milk carton. Other substances can cause all that calcium to go straight through your body and right down the drain, so go ahead and fill up on dairy products, but also watch out for calcium robbers like these.

- **Skip the sodium.** You sit down to eat a well-balanced meal full of calcium, but did you know that shaking too much salt on your potato could cancel out the calcium in your glass of milk? Sodium competes with calcium for absorption, so too much sodium can cause calcium to pass right through your body without being used.
- **Can the caffeine.** That cup of coffee may help get your bones moving in the morning, but it may keep them from moving when you're older. The caffeine in one cup of coffee can increase your need for calcium by 30 to 50 mg for the day.

- **Ax the alcohol and toss the cigarettes.** If you feel like you need a drink, your bones would prefer that you make it milk instead of liquor. Research finds that alcohol abuse is associated with a greater risk of bone loss and broken bones. However, studies haven't yet provided a clear answer as to whether an occasional drink can increase your risk of osteoporosis. One study of elderly male twins did find that bone loss increased by 10 percent among those who had an above-average intake of alcohol and cigarettes. Other studies have also found a connection between smoking and a higher risk of bone loss and fractures.
- **Drop the drug interactions.** Certain drugs can interfere with your calcium absorption. For example, antacids that contain aluminum hydroxide may cause calcium loss. Ask your doctor or pharmacist whether any medications you are taking might be stealing calcium right out from under your nose.

It's never too late for calcium

You passed on the cottage cheese and milk when you were younger, and now you're paying for it with your very bones. You have osteoporosis, but it's not too late to start taking calcium now. Even if your doctor has prescribed medicine for your osteoporosis, calcium can still help by making your medicine more effective. One study found that people with osteoporosis who increased their calcium to about 1,100 to 1,400 mg a day raised the bone-protecting ability of the drug calcitonin by 125 percent and more than tripled the effectiveness of estrogen. The National Osteoporosis Foundation recommends that women over the age of 50 take in about 1,500 mg of calcium daily. Although you can take supplements, getting that extra calcium in your diet isn't difficult. Just add a container of yogurt and a couple of glasses of milk to your usual diet. You may develop a taste for dairy, and your bones will thank you.

PMS

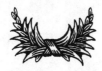

Balancing the scales of PMS

Just what is making you feel so lousy? Researchers know the root of the problem is your body's shifting play of hormones — everything from estrogen and progesterone to cortisol and insulin. All these enter your bloodstream in wildly different amounts, each capable of causing chaos in its own special way.

But how these various substances can make you irritable, crave sweets, or retain water is still somewhat of a medical mystery. Now, though, even modern scientists acknowledge that what you eat can tip your body's delicate balance of chemistry either toward turmoil or tranquillity.

Don't do it. You want it. You crave it. You've got to have it. Whether it's that chocolate bar, those cookies, or that can of soda, you want sugar. It might come over you like a flash or grow in the pit of your stomach like a gnawing ache, but it just won't go away. Be strong. It's quite normal to crave foods during PMS, but if you give into this particular craving, you may feel worse later, and it won't be from the guilt over the extra pounds.

Doctors have discovered that sugar, corn syrup, high-fructose corn syrup, and even molasses all cause water retention, mood swings, and other PMS symptoms. Stay away from refined foods and convenience foods which are full of these simple carbohydrates and sugars.

You may be dying for a few potato chips or peanuts too, but all that salt spells water retention and bloating. And you may think a quick cup of coffee is just the pick-me-up you need if you're feeling slow, or that a glass of wine or cocktail with dinner will ease some of your PMS anxieties. But you couldn't be more wrong. Caffeine is a stimulant, sure, but not only will it pick you up, it will put you back down, too, by increasing your irritability, tension, and insomnia. Alcohol will exaggerate emotions, so if you're feeling a bit weepy or cranky before that drink, just imagine what you'll feel like after.

So, what should you eat? Lots of protein, fiber, and complex carbohydrates like potatoes, whole grain breads, and crackers.

These will relieve your cravings and put you in a better frame of mind. Eat low-fat and pick up a piece of fruit when you long for some sugar.

Fish high in omega-3 oils may reduce symptoms of PMS by helping produce a group of fatty acids that reduce inflammation in the body. Your best source of omega-3 is seafood. Herring, mackerel, salmon, trout, tuna, and whitefish all contain about one gram of omega-3 in every three or four-ounce serving.

Try to eat fish at least twice a week to receive a good dose of this important nutrient. If you have trouble doing this, try buying some oat germ — it is the best plant source of omega-3.

Learn the ABCs of PMS

A-OK with A. Some of those foods you may have hated as a child could be your salvation if you suffer from PMS. We're talking about liver, spinach, broccoli, and sweet potatoes. They're all rich in beta carotene, which is converted to vitamin A in your body.

Of course, now that you're all grown up, you appreciate the delicious flavors and important nutrients in squash and carrots, apricots and cantaloupe. But you'll appreciate even more the way these foods can improve your PMS symptoms.

When you're shopping, pick out fruits and vegetables jam-packed with beta carotene by their dark, rich colors. They'll look beautiful on the plate and make you feel wonderful inside.

Better believe in B6. If you want to get rid of all those nasty PMS symptoms, that is. By helping to manufacture certain chemicals called neurotransmitters, vitamin B6 may improve fatigue, depression, breast pain, fluid retention, mood, sleep, and memory.

Too much of a good thing, though, isn't good, since high doses of B6 can be harmful. So check with your doctor before you take supplements. Eat green leafy vegetables, chicken, shellfish, and beans for natural doses of B6.

Calcium with a C. You should be loading up on calcium already. After all, osteoporosis is so easily avoided with a few dietary safeguards. And here is yet another reason to say yes to calcium: studies have shown that taking anywhere from 1,000 to 1,300 mg of calcium a day can reduce depression, bloating, back pain, irritability, and headaches associated with PMS. Talk to your doctor for a dose that's right for you.

Magnificent magnesium. Can you imagine relieving half a dozen symptoms of PMS with one little mineral? Well, you could say good-bye to nausea, headaches, dizziness, cravings, mood swings, and cramps, just by getting more magnesium.

The theory is that too little magnesium in your system lowers certain chemicals in your brain and causes emotions to run amuck. If you decide to take a supplement, take around 350 mg a day. To get more magnesium naturally, eat nuts, peas and beans, spinach, broccoli, and seafood.

Zinc is "ze end." According to a study at Baylor College of Medicine, women with PMS symptoms measured low but still acceptable levels of zinc and copper. This means that even if there is no evidence of a real deficiency, a minor drop in mineral levels may trigger certain PMS symptoms.

Researchers believe that a low level of zinc may affect the production of certain hormones. Eating more foods high in zinc is a reasonable, healthy way to ensure that you have enough of this important mineral in your body. Zinc-rich foods include black beans, crab meat, turkey (dark meat), lima beans, oysters, and steak.

Old herbs give new relief for PMS

All that was old is new again. Like so many other things, the popularity of herbal remedies is enjoying a rebirth. And today it's not just fashionable, it's smart. Several herbs offer safe, natural ways to deal with the distressing side effects of premenstrual syndrome.

Chaste tree is a plant that has been known as a cure for female problems for centuries. The name is a giveaway, isn't it? Recently a large German study showed that chaste tree liquid extract relieved PMS symptoms by bringing progesterone and estrogen back into balance. It's also available in capsule form.

Black cohosh is an herb native to North America, where it was once called squaw root, perhaps because it is helpful in treating a variety of female problems. Scientists have determined that it contains ingredients similar to estrogen. An alcoholic extract of this herb can be very helpful in treating the pain, discomfort, and tensions of PMS.

Ginkgo, one of the wonder herbs of the decade, can also improve PMS symptoms, particularly breast pain.

The next time you're out to dinner and you see that sprig of parsley on the side of your plate, go ahead and take a bite. It has a distinctly sharp flavor but is loaded with vitamin C. In addition, researchers say it will relieve menstrual pain.

The sweet smell of success

Aromatherapy is the use of highly scented oils from herbs and flowers to treat various health problems. Many professionals claim that certain aromatic oils can relieve period pain, tension headaches, stress, and anxiety.

For these PMS symptoms, they recommend lavender, as a hot compress or massage; chamomile, in your bath or as a massage; and rose geranium.

What a soothing, fragrant recipe for pain relief!

PROSTATE ENLARGEMENT

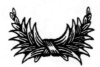

3 herbs to lower prostate pressure

As many men get older, their lives begin to revolve around the bathroom, and not because they spend more time fixing their hair. A frequent urge to urinate can turn your bathroom into the most visited room in your house. An enlarged prostate gland could be the cause of those frequent visits.

When most men hit middle age, their prostate begins to grow. This might not be a problem, except for its location. Your prostate surrounds your urethra, the tube that carries urine and semen out of your body. Since your prostate's main job is to manufacture most of the fluid that makes up semen, it makes sense that it would be located right where the action is. However, when it begins to grow, it can cause pressure on your urethra and your bladder and lead to urinary problems like frequent urination, difficulty urinating, or dribbling. This enlargement of the prostate is called benign prostatic hyperplasia (BPH), and it affects almost half of all men over forty and 75 percent of men over sixty. The treatments for BPH include drugs like finasteride or surgical removal of the prostate. If you want a more natural alternative, however, some herbal remedies have proven to be very effective.

- **Saw palmetto.** A small palm tree that grows in the southeastern United States could help reduce your BPH. A concentrated extract of saw palmetto berries has been shown in several studies to be at least as effective as finasteride in treating BPH. One study found that men with BPH who took saw palmetto for three months reported that their urine flow was more than twice as good as that of men who took finasteride for a year. About five percent of the men taking saw palmetto report side effects, most commonly gastrointestinal symptoms like nausea, constipation, and diarrhea. About five percent of men taking finasteride also report side effects. However, the side effects of finasteride include impotence, incontinence, and decreased sexual drive. Most men would probably rather have the diarrhea.

- **Pygeum.** Another type of tree may also supply you with prostate help. The bark of the *pygeum africanum* tree (which grows in Africa) is used to make an extract for treatment of BPH and prostatitis (inflammation of the prostate.) It may be a little less effective than saw palmetto for treatment of BPH symptoms. However, according to one study, it may improve sexual performance in some men with prostate disorders.
- **Nettles.** The stinging nettle might be able to put the sting to BPH symptoms. The root of this plant has been used to treat urinary difficulties caused by BPH. The suggested dosage is 4 to 6 grams daily. The leaves of the same plant may also increase urinary flow. The usual way to consume nettle is in a tea made with 3 to 4 teaspoonfuls of nettle leaves. Drink a cup of this tea 3 to 4 times daily. Be sure to drink plenty of water, too, and get your urine flowing smoothly again.

PROSTATITIS

Your best infection fighters

If you get a respiratory infection, you probably accept it as pretty routine. However, if you have a prostate infection, you might be a little more concerned. Your prostate can become infected just like any other part of your body, but sometimes men think that it signals a much larger problem. If you have the symptoms of a prostate infection, known as prostatitis, you should see your doctor. He can test you to make sure that is your problem and prescribe antibiotics to clear your infection up. To avoid this painful problem, you can follow a few simple diet guidelines.

- **Water, water, everywhere.** Supplying your body with plenty of refreshing water can help wash out bacteria and prevent prostatitis. Drink at least six to eight glasses of water daily. If you do get prostatitis, water can also help give you some relief. Try sitting in a tub of warm water or a whirlpool three times a day.
- **Pick a peck of pumpkin seeds.** You might like to snack on sunflower seeds, but did you know that pumpkin and squash seeds are rich in zinc and magnesium, two important nutrients for prostate health? Zinc helps guard your prostate from infection. Other good sources of zinc include oysters and black beans.
- **Go for low fat.** Too much fat and cholesterol in your diet can be particularly tough on your prostate.
- **Skip the spicy food.** Spicy foods may irritate your prostate, so if you have an inflammation, maybe you should cut down on the jalapeño peppers.
- **Choose drinks wisely.** Drinking lots of water may be good for your prostate, but drinking lots of alcohol isn't. Too much caffeine can also add to your prostate problems, so consider cutting down on your coffee intake.

Symptoms of prostatitis

- Bloody or cloudy urine
- Fever, chills
- Impotence (sometimes)
- Low back pain
- Difficulty urinating
- Frequent urination with burning sensation
- Pain between scrotum and rectum

RAYNAUD'S DISEASE

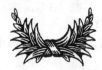

Improve circulation with these nutrients

Raynaud's is a disorder of the circulatory system involving your body's reaction to cold, whether it's the snow on your car windshield or the ice cubes from your freezer. So, if you suffer from this condition, winter can be a time of agony, and unfortunately, even household tasks can leave you in pain.

Recent studies suggest that if you have Raynaud's, you may need more vitamin C and selenium, a mineral found in unprocessed foods. Without these two important nutrients, you are more apt to suffer irreversible tissue damage.

In order to protect your fingers and toes, eat lots of citrus, cantaloupe, strawberries, peppers, papayas, mangos, vegetables, grains, and organ meats like liver. A multivitamin containing an antioxidant formula would be a good idea, too.

In addition, the herb ginkgo will help dilate your blood vessels, which can improve circulation. It helps move your blood to the tips of your fingers, which relieves pain and restores the normal color of your skin. Be sure to follow label directions carefully.

ROSACEA

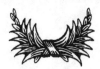

Flush the foods that cause flare-ups

Rosacea (rose-AY-see-uh) sounds like the name of a flower, and it may begin like the soft blush of a rose on your nose and cheeks. But when the bloom deepens and spreads over your face, breaking out in bumps and pimples that look like a teenager's acne, the flower image fades quickly.

This skin disease usually occurs on the faces of adults over 30 years old. Though it may resemble acne, it doesn't involve blackheads and whiteheads. Women get it most often, but men tend to have the most severe cases. The symptoms may come and go, but without treatment it grows progressively worse. It can become quite severe, even spreading to the eyes where it can cause vision problems.

Sometimes the nose becomes red and lumpy with a condition called rhinophyma. The swollen schnozzles of J.P. Morgan and President Bill Clinton have been immortalized by the cartoonist's pen. The bulbous nose of W.C. Fields may also come to mind. Because Fields frequently drank, this facial characteristic is wrongly linked with alcohol abuse. Alcohol can increase symptoms in some people, but it can be just as serious in someone who doesn't drink alcohol at all.

No one knows what causes rosacea, and there is no cure. It can be controlled, however. Here are some ways to limit the flare-ups:

- **Keep your cool.** Anything that makes you flush — whether food, drink, sun and wind, exercise, or the onset of menopause — can trigger an attack of rosacea. Other culprits include emotional stress, smoking or being in a smoky room, taking a sauna or hot shower, and even using hair spray. Cool your body temperature by sucking on ice cubes or drinking cool beverages in hot weather.

- **Lower the heat.** The "hot" in spices and the temperature of hot drinks and solid foods are among the biggest triggers of the symptoms of rosacea. To prevent heat from rushing to your face, avoid foods with black and white pepper, paprika, red pepper, and cayenne. It's the heat, not the caffeine or any other substance, in hot coffee or tea that causes problems. You should be able to continue to enjoy these if you reduce the temperature. Letting hot foods cool to room temperature before eating can help prevent a flare-up as well.

- **Watch out for these high-histamine foods.** Tomatoes, eggplant, spinach, cheese, chocolate, chicken livers, citrus fruits, bananas, raisins, red plums, figs, avocados, yogurt, and sour cream are foods that are high in histamines or release histamines into the body. They cause flushing because that's part of the job histamines normally do. When a burn on your skin turns red, for example, histamine is the reason. When your face turns red from flushing, it increases the skin irritations of rosacea. Try taking an antihistamine about two hours before a meal that includes these high-histamine foods.

- **Hold the pickled, smoked, marinated, and fermented foods.** Problem-causing ingredients like vinegar, soy sauce, and vanilla in foods prepared in these ways are likely to cause symptoms of rosacea to return. Alcoholic beverages, especially red wine, beer, bourbon, gin, vodka, and champagne can also stir up an outbreak.

- **Say no to niacin and ban the beans.** Flare-ups are sometimes caused by foods containing niacin, like liver and yeast. Breads made with yeast, however, seem to be okay for most folks. The pods of broad-leaf beans such as limas, navy beans, and peas sometimes stir up the flushes that bring on the roughness and redness of rosacea. Try taking an aspirin before eating foods that contain niacin.

Not everybody is affected by the same foods and beverages. It's a good idea to keep a diary of what you eat and drink to help you decide which ones affect your condition. You'll learn which ones to avoid, and maybe you'll find that you can safely continue some of your favorites.

You can get a free rosacea diary checklist and a free newsletter, *Rosacea Review,* by writing to the National Rosacea Society at 800 S. Northwest Highway, Suite 200, Barrington, IL 60010.

Could treatment for ulcers cure rosacea?

In 1994 a 53-year-old woman in Slovakia was admitted to the hospital. She had suffered with rosacea for nine years and her condition had worsened. Doctors learned that off and on for a long time she had also suffered with stomach pain and diarrhea.

Stomach tests found *Helicobacter pylori,* a kind of bacteria believed to be a cause of ulcers. She was treated for the *H. pylori* infection. Within four weeks her stomach problems were cured and her rosacea cleared up as well. Two years later, without any additional treatment, she was still free of symptoms of rosacea.

Recently a small study confirmed that 81 percent of people with rosacea in the study had *H. pylori* in their stomachs. More research is needed to see if there is a connection that will lead to new and better ways to treat rosacea.

SKIN PROBLEMS

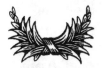

Vitamins for vibrant skin

Beauty is only skin deep. While true beauty lies on the inside, most people would also like to keep their outside beautiful and youthful. Taking care of your skin is a good start, and the right vitamins are essential.

Vitamin C for collagen. Among its many duties, vitamin C is responsible for helping make and maintain collagen. Collagen forms the basis of connective tissues in your body, including skin. It makes scar tissue to help heal wounds and burns, and supports tiny blood vessels to prevent bruises.

If you want your skin to look fresh and young instead of dry and saggy, get plenty of vitamin C in your diet. You can even buy vitamin C formula creams that claim to reduce wrinkling and prevent sun damage that can lead to skin cancer.

Niacin for nice skin. Niacin deficiency causes a disease called pellagra, meaning "rough skin." That should tell you how important this B vitamin is for healthy skin. Without it, you can develop the red rough skin that gives pellagra its name.

Your body converts tryptophan, which is found in almost all proteins, into niacin. Plenty of skin-saving niacin can be found in meats, including fish and chicken. Since most people get plenty of protein in their diet, niacin deficiency is uncommon today.

Be careful not to self-dose with niacin supplements, however. Too much of this vitamin can also be harmful to your skin and your health.

Vitamin A for added protection. Your skin is more than just pretty packaging. It also serves as a barrier to infections that would like to invade your body. Vitamin A helps maintain the cells that form this skin barricade.

If you don't have enough vitamin A, some of those cells are replaced by cells that secrete keratin. This is the substance that makes your hair and fingernails tough. It also makes your skin dry, hard, and cracked, which increases your chances of infection.

If you have a problem with acne or wrinkles, Vitamin A products like Retin-A may help. They are available in cream form to apply directly to the skin.

While you're eating healthful, vitamin-packed foods for better skin, wash them down with a tall glass of cold water. Water works its own moisturizing magic on your skin, and teams up with vitamins to help keep your skin soft and smooth.

Shade yourself from sun damage

Sunshine and fresh air go hand-in-hand with the image of good health, but that seemingly beneficial sunshine can sometimes cause health problems. For example, skin cancer kills almost 10,000 people a year, so sheltering your skin from damaging sun rays is a wise choice.

Although your grandmother may have chosen a bonnet and parasol to protect her skin, you probably slather yourself with sunscreen. Covering your skin may be your best protection, but studies find your diet may also help keep the sun's harmful rays at bay.

Trim the fat. Fat is the bad guy in many nutrition-related conditions. Now you can add skin cancer to that list. A study found that people with a history of non-melanoma skin cancer were more likely to get it again if they ate a high-fat diet. The people who cut their fat from 40 percent of their calories to 21 percent of their calories were five times less likely to develop more skin tumors.

Beta carotene beats harmful rays. The sun's rays may cause more than just skin cancer. Although sunscreens block ultraviolet-B (UV-B) rays, ultraviolet-A (UV-A) rays can still get through. UV-A rays can weaken your immune system, making you more susceptible to infections.

One study found that people exposed to artificial UV light were less able to fight off infections. However, people who took beta carotene supplements maintained the infection-fighting ability of their immune system. If you spend a lot of time in the sun, you may need more beta carotene than most people.

Stop psoriasis with diet

Silvery scales may be pretty on a fish, but you don't want them on your body. People with psoriasis have to deal with red, inflamed patches of skin covered with silvery-white scales.

When your body replaces skin cells too rapidly, the cells pile up and create these scales on the skin's surface. These rough patches are called "plaques," and they may itch, burn, or crack. They occur most often on your knees, elbows, scalp, face, lower back, soles of your feet, and palms.

Vitamin D does wonders. Sunshine or the "sunshine vitamin" may help clear up psoriasis. Some people with psoriasis improve after taking vitamin D supplements, and your doctor may prescribe a cream form of vitamin D that may help. Sitting in the sun for short periods also improves some peoples' conditions, but be careful not to get sunburned.

Zap it with zinc. People who have psoriasis lose more zinc through their skin than other people. Your body needs zinc to absorb linoleic acid, which is necessary for healthy skin. So, keeping up your zinc intake may be especially important if you have this condition.

Lay on the linoleic acid. If you don't get enough of this fatty acid, your skin will become dry, rough, and blotchy. Eat plenty of foods rich in linoleic acid, like nuts, wheat germ, and vegetable oil.

Fight it with fish oil. Some research indicates that a daily fish oil supplement might help control outbreaks of psoriasis. The fatty acids in fish oil help stop inflammation, which may prevent your skin from forming the red, inflamed patches of skin that psoriasis causes.

Eliminate the itching of eczema

Everyone has to deal with itchy skin sometime. A mosquito bite, a bout with chicken pox, or an allergic reaction to a wool sweater can set off an irritating episode of itching. However, people who have eczema, or chronic atopic dermatitis, must deal with red itchy skin for a long time, some for their entire lives.

Eczema tends to flare up, make you miserable for a while, then disappear. Just when you think you're safe from this itchy intruder, it can strike again, especially during periods of stress. However, you can exercise some control over this annoying problem.

Avoid food allergens. Eczema can be caused by allergies, either to environmental factors such as dust or pollen, or to certain foods. The foods most likely to set off an eczema episode include cheese, egg white, cow's milk, wheat, fish, and nuts. Taking suspected food triggers out of your diet may help, but be careful to eat a balanced diet.

Sunshine — friend or foe? Sunshine may either aggravate or relieve your eczema. Some people are sensitive to sunlight and should avoid exposure. Other people may find relief from their eczema if they get a reasonable amount of sun. Ultraviolet light therapy may be helpful, but only under professional supervision. Home sun lamps or tanning beds are not recommended because of the dangers of overexposure.

Oil it away. A recent study found that fish oil and corn oil can improve eczema symptoms. People who took fish oil for four months improved 30 percent, while those who took corn oil improved 24 percent.

Skip the salt. Salt may add flavor to your food, but if you have eczema, it might also make you itch. Doctors found that one girl with severe eczema who was put on low-salt, low-calcium water improved dramatically within two weeks. When they gave her water that was high in salt, her eczema symptoms returned. Since most people eat too much salt anyway, cutting down may be an easy, healthful way to help control your eczema.

Licking your wounds

When you cut your finger, do you immediately stick that finger in your mouth? Don't be embarrassed; it's a natural reaction. People have long known that dogs lick their wounds to help them heal. Some researchers believe that human saliva may also aid in the healing process.

One study found that the skin of people who had licked their hands contained higher amounts of nitric oxide, a substance that discourages infections. Researchers speculated that when saliva comes into contact with your skin, a chemical reaction occurs that creates this helpful substance.

Does this mean you should lick your cuts instead of putting antiseptic on them? Probably not, but the next time you prick your finger, you'll know why you impulsively want to lick your wound.

Win the war on warts

When you hear the word "warts," you may have a vision of frogs, witches, and burying something in the backyard under a full moon. People have been trying all sorts of methods to get rid of these pesky growths. Warts probably don't seem like a major health concern if you don't have them, but if you do, they are a major annoyance. Here are two examples of people who took wart treatment into their own hands and won.

An Ohio dentist had tried conventional wart treatment for eight months with no success. The warts had begun to interfere with his work. His dermatologist at the Medical College of Ohio suggested a bold course of treatment. He prescribed massive doses of beta carotene. The dentist took eight 15-milligram (mg) capsules of beta carotene daily. By the end of the second month, the warts were smaller, and by the end of the fourth month, they were gone.

The dermatologist treated several other people with the same good results. The negative side effect of this treatment is that your skin temporarily looks yellow from all the beta carotene. But the effect goes away after you stop taking the megadoses of vitamins.

An elderly Florida man successfully used an old family remedy to get rid of a wart on the sole of his foot. Every night, he would smooth the wart with a pumice stone and then cut a very thin slice of raw potato slightly larger than the wart. He would tape the potato over the wart for the night. After six weeks of this treatment, the plantar wart was gone. This method hasn't been clinically proven, but it's certainly an easy and inexpensive wart treatment.

STRESS

Stamp out stress with better nutrition

You've got to pick up your clothes at the cleaners, drop Fluffy at the vet, pack, and drive to your sister's by 9:00. Feeling a little stressed? You may not know it, but your pulse is faster, your blood pressure is higher, and your senses are sharper. You know you feel tense, irritable, emotional, and anxious. Probably the last thing on your mind is eating a healthy dinner, but it should be the first thing you think about. Studies show that if you haven't eaten well before a stressful situation kicks in, you're going to feel even hungrier during and after. And that's when you're going to grab something quick to eat, and it probably won't be healthy.

Experts agree that poor eating habits during times of stress can suppress your body's natural immune system. This makes you more susceptible to illness and disease and can even increase the effects of stress. It could also explain why you always seem to get a cold just when you've got an important deadline at work, relatives coming for the weekend, or a holiday party to prepare for.

By staying away from alcohol and eating nutritious foods, you will be giving your body the extra ammunition it needs to fight off the damaging effects of stress.

Protein. You always need protein, but even more so when you're under physical and emotional pressure. If your body doesn't get it from your diet, it will steal protein from your heart, lungs, and brain. Make sure you provide your body with a steady supply of nutritious foods. Lean meat, fish, low-fat milk, and egg whites will "beef" up your protein intake.

Carbohydrates. Complex carbohydrates like bagels, whole-grain muffins, cereals, and fruit will give you fast energy. They will also stick with you through the thick and thin of stress. Since they are quick and easy to digest, they won't place additional stress on your body.

Carbohydrates are packed with all kinds of nutrients, so you get plenty of fuel to take you through all those exhausting moments in your life. Many nutritionists believe that complex carbohydrates should make up 75 percent of your diet. Just be careful to stay away from the sugary carbohydrates like donuts, candy bars, and cookies.

Minerals. In a recent study, test subjects under physical and psychological stress experienced a dramatic fall in zinc, iron, and selenium levels. If you are stressed out, consider eating foods high in these minerals, such as beans, crab meat, yogurt, steak, clams, and oysters.

Vitamins. Stress very often goes hand-in-hand with digestion problems and malabsorption. This means your body can't take in and use all the nutrients you may be feeding it. If this happens, you could very well be vitamin deficient. The B-complex vitamins, in particular, are quickly used up during times of stress. Foods high in this group are peas, beans, lean meat, poultry, fish, whole-grain breads and cereals, bananas, and potatoes.

Stoke up on vitamin C during those hectic times, too, since your adrenal gland needs it to make stress hormones. Citrus fruits, strawberries, red and green peppers, broccoli, brussels sprouts, and cantaloupe are loaded with vitamin C.

If you decide to take a multi-vitamin, choose one high in vitamins C, B12, folic acid, and pantothenic acid (vitamin B5). Vitamin B5, sometimes called the "anti-stress" vitamin, is necessary to keep your adrenal glands healthy and functioning properly, which is critical during times of stress.

Herbs help you carry the weight of the world

Fight stress with ginseng. The Asians call it "man-root" because it has the rough shape of a person. In fact, the more closely the root resembles a human, the more expensive it is — sometimes costing thousands of dollars. Grown on special farms in the United States, Russia, China, Korea, and Japan, it takes at least three years to reach maturity. It is called ginseng and has been used as a natural medicine for more than 20 centuries.

Although it may treat illnesses in almost every part of the body, Western medicine has concentrated on ginseng's anti-stress qualities. Many experts now agree that ginseng contains a substance known as an adaptogen, which increases your body's vitality and helps fight off the effects of all kinds of stress. Ginseng can be taken as a tea or capsule. If you decide to try it, follow manufacturers' dosage recommendations carefully.

Relieve tension with valerian. The Pied Piper is said to have used valerian to entice the rats out of Hamelin. It may be attractive to rodents, but most people find the scent of this tall, perennial herb distinctly unpleasant. Don't let that put you off, though. Valerian is probably the most effective of all the herbs as a sedative or mild tranquilizer. It lowers your heart rate, blood pressure, and the amount of oxygen you take in.

It has been taken for hundreds of years to calm and relieve tension and was especially helpful during both World Wars. Soldiers and citizens alike used valerian to treat their stress reaction to battle and the anxiety of living under constant threat of air raids.

Unlike many synthetic sedatives, there are few, if any, side effects from valerian. You shouldn't wake up during the night, suffer from morning drowsiness, or experience reactions the next night. There is, however, some concern over long-term use. But if you are suffering from stress that lasts longer than a couple of weeks, you should see your doctor anyway.

You will need to take what may be considered fairly high doses of this herb to notice any effect. According to herbal experts, there is little danger of overdosing.

You can take valerian in three different forms. For a cup of tea, add two teaspoons of the dried root to a cup of hot water. To use valerian tincture, drop at least one teaspoon of the tincture into a glass of water or dissolve it on a sugar cube. Experts say you can take this dose every 15 to 30 minutes, up to three times a day. You can combine these two forms for an even stronger brew — add one teaspoon of prepared tincture to your cup of valerian tea.

Valerian extract is not as widely available and is more complicated to use. If you buy this form, follow label directions carefully.

Relax with kava. Even if you can't hop a plane to the nearest tropical island for a little rest and relaxation, you can use a surefire tropical remedy to relieve your tension.

The plant is called kava, and it has been used in South Pacific traditional ceremonies for thousands of years. Kava products act as mild tranquilizers — they will relax you and lessen nervousness and depression.

You may feel some sleepiness after using kava, so be careful if you must drive or operate machinery. Also, high doses may have an intoxicating effect.

Before using kava, ask your doctor for his advice. If you decide to give it a try, follow label directions exactly.

Quiet stress with chamomile, and melissa (lemon balm). These herbs make wonderful teas that act as gentle sedatives. According to a study out of Heidelberg University, the volatile oils in melissa protect your brain from outside stimulation. So brew a cup of natural healing and let an age-old remedy quiet your stress.

Try aromatherapy for stress relief

If you feel like pursuing the ancient practice of aromatherapy, there are several oils recommended for anxiety. These include bergamot, cedarwood, frankincense, geranium, hyssop, lavender, sandalwood, and ylang ylang. Dilute them in your bath or combine them with a massage oil. Some herbalists recommend taking essential oils internally, usually by placing drops on the tongue. Talk to your doctor before doing this, since many oils can be harmful if taken internally.

Break the caffeine cycle

Ever wonder why some people automatically refill their coffee cups when a deadline is approaching or the boss is on their backs? One study discovered that when people came under stress, about half of them increased the amount of coffee or soft drinks they consumed. Maybe they thought it would help them respond more quickly or get their work done faster.

There does seem to be a strange relationship between people under stress and caffeine. Another study out of Japan found that employees who worked the longest hours had the poorest sleeping habits, got the least amount of exercise, had irregular meal times, and were under the greatest amount of stress. They were also the ones who drank the most tea or coffee.

Unfortunately, this behavior doesn't help you cope with a fast-paced world. You drink more caffeine because you're under stress, and the caffeine makes you feel even more stressful, so you drink more caffeine, and so on ... the pattern continues.

To get off this unhealthy merry-go-round, go ahead and reach for your cup, but fill it with something decaffeinated instead. Try an herbal tea, spiced cider, or instant soup if you crave something hot. And substitute juice or water for those sodas. You can give into the habit of having a drink in your hand if you must — just make it a healthy one.

Is tea your bag?

The next time you feel the demands of your life closing in on you, take a few moments, grab a pillow, and settle down on the floor. No, not for an afternoon nap, but for a Japanese Tea Ceremony. A recent study reported on the calming effect such a ceremony had on those suffering from stress.

Even though traditional Japanese green tea contains caffeine, it has significantly less than coffee, black tea, or even oolong tea. The important thing seems to be the act of taking a normal, everyday chore and turning it into a ritual. This makes you focus more on the present moment. Thinking too much about past or future problems is the root of most tension.

So, if you must have a cup of something hot to drink, choose green tea, and take some time out to actually enjoy it. Sit down, close your eyes, and find a moment of peace.

STROKE

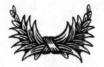

Stay away from salt

Older people may cut their risk of stroke by eating less salt, even if they don't have high blood pressure, a new British study says. Lowering your salt intake by 5 grams per day may lead to a drop in blood pressure, even if your pressure is usually normal. This, in turn, can reduce your chance of having a stroke.

Although high blood pressure puts people more at risk for stroke, those with pressure in the upper normal range, who are not trying to lower it, are more likely to suffer a stroke, researchers said.

If your favorable blood pressure has made you less concerned about your salt intake, you may want to reconsider. A good idea is to follow the American Heart Association's recommendation of no more than 2.4 grams of salt per day. That's a little more than a teaspoon, and it provides your body with all the sodium it needs.

Go easy on the salt shaker, and be sure to watch for hidden sodium in packaged and processed foods.

Milk works a stroke of magic

Kids are taught to drink milk for strong teeth and bones, but milk is important to older folks as well. A study that followed 3,150 middle-aged men for 22 years found that men who drank no milk had twice as many thromboembolic strokes, the most common kind of stroke, as the men who drank at least 16 ounces of milk a day.

Researchers aren't sure what it is about milk that makes the difference. Milk is rich in calcium, but calcium from other sources didn't have the same protective effect. Lifestyle could be a factor. The milk drinkers tended to be leaner and more active than those who drank no milk, and their diet was healthier in general.

Although most of the men in the study drank whole milk, drinking low-fat or nonfat milk is still a good idea to protect your arteries from clogging. Almost 50 percent of the calories in whole milk are from saturated fat, a contributor to high cholesterol that can lead to atherosclerosis, high blood pressure, and strokes. For more information on these problems, see the *Atherosclerosis* and *High blood pressure* chapters.

Vitamin C is the key to a healthier brain

Eating tomatoes and green leafy vegetables, and drinking lemonade or orange juice, may be the way to keep a sharply functioning brain.

In a study of men and women over 65, those who ate a lot of vitamin C had a lower risk of death from stroke. They scored higher on mental tests as well.

It's probably the antioxidant activity of vitamin C that protects the brain. Strokes are often caused by atherosclerosis, a kind of hardening of the arteries. The clots that form seem to be responsible for much of the brain's deterioration over the years. Fruits and vegetables that are rich in vitamin C and other antioxidants help combat this condition by keeping blood vessels clear.

Summer diet changes may cause problems

Do you eat the same kinds of food all year long? Probably not. A bowl of hot chili helps fight the chill of winter. But when the weather warms up, you may prefer cool, fresh salads.

If you are taking the anti-clotting drug Coumadin, a brand of warfarin, this could be a big mistake. Sudden major changes in your diet may throw off the balance of vitamin K and this medicine in your system, causing serious problems.

Vitamin K is found in green leafy vegetables, broccoli, canola and soybean oils, and some dietary supplement drinks. Its main job is to help your body form clots. Coumadin is prescribed to do the opposite — prevent blood clotting in people at risk for stroke or certain heart problems. If you suddenly eat lots of leafy vegetables, you may get too much vitamin K, which could seriously affect the way the drug works.

If you take Coumadin, talk it over with your doctor before making any major changes in your menu.

Vitamin E and aspirin — a winning combination?

Most strokes occur when a blood clot blocks an artery leading to the brain. Aspirin has long been thought to reduce stroke risk because it helps keep blood from clotting.

One study has found that vitamin E may help aspirin lessen your chances for a stroke because it also keeps your blood vessels clear. When 100 stroke sufferers took both vitamin E and aspirin for 18 months, they had significantly fewer attacks during that time than those who took just aspirin.

You can get vitamin E from whole grains, green leafy vegetables, avocados, seeds, nuts and vegetable oils. But it may be difficult to get the most helpful amount from diet alone, especially without adding fat and calories.

For most people, it's probably fine to take a supplement of 100 IU to 400 IU a day. Extremely high doses, however, could lead to hemorrhagic stroke, caused by bleeding in the brain. In fact, some researchers think that combining vitamin E with aspirin, or other clot-preventing medicines, may raise your risk for this type of stroke.

Talk to your doctor before taking vitamin E and aspirin together. He'll be able to determine if the combination is right for you.

Say nuts to stroke

Walnuts and vegetable oils, especially canola, olive, and soy, contain an ingredient called alpha-linolenic acid that may lower the risk of stroke. Researchers at the University of California, San Francisco, found that the risk of stroke dropped 37 percent for each 0.13 percent increase of alpha-linolenic acid in the blood.

Alpha-linolenic acid is a type of omega-3 fatty acid, the kind that helps thin your blood and reduce blood clots. Researchers think this may be the reason it's so helpful in lowering stroke risk.

Nuts are high in protein, so substituting some for meat protein in your diet may be a good idea. That way, you'll benefit on both counts.

Fish for a solution

A poached salmon steak, or sardines and crackers. Whether plain or fancy, fish can reduce your chances of having a stroke.

A four-year study found that white women and blacks of both sexes who ate fish more than once a week were half as likely to suffer a stroke as those who ate no fish at all. That's especially good news for women since stroke is the third leading cause of death in women.

For some reason, white men didn't fare so well in that study. But the news from other research is good for men, too. A 25-year study found those who didn't have strokes ate 50 percent more fish than those who did.

Fish helps thin the blood, reducing blood clots that can cause strokes. There is one drawback, however. Too much fish oil can cause bleeding in the brain and possibly a stroke. But if you limit your servings to two or three a week, you can get the benefits without doing any harm.

If you are taking vitamin E supplements, which also thin the blood, or any blood-clotting medications like aspirin or warfarin, you might want to talk to your doctor about how much fish to eat.

Stroke victims need extra 'D'

If a stroke has left you paralyzed on one side of the body, be sure to get plenty of vitamin D. Hip fractures are common in this situation, and a vitamin D deficiency seems to be partly responsible. Taking extra vitamin D reduces bone loss and the likelihood of broken bones, especially when it's combined with calcium.

Getting plenty of sunshine is the best way to increase your body's vitamin D. But if you can't get outdoors, you can rely on foods and supplements. The richest food sources are fortified milk and other dairy products. You can also get vitamin D from fortified cereals, egg yolks, liver, and fatty fish like salmon, tuna, and sardines.

Supplemental vitamin D may have some serious side effects, especially if you are over 55, so check with your doctor before taking supplements.

THYROID DISEASE

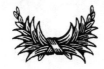

Reverse 'false senility' and regain youth

The symptoms of thyroid disease can mimic those of senility and even Alzheimer's disease. When the disease is corrected, many symptoms that were "chalked up to old age" are reversed.

Shaped like a butterfly and located just below your Adam's apple, the thyroid gland produces hormones that control your body's metabolism. Sometimes the thyroid produces too little hormone, which causes your body to use energy too slowly. This condition, known as hypothyroidism, can cause fatigue, poor memory, depression, and obesity — symptoms often associated with old age.

In hyperthyroidism, the thyroid produces too much hormone, causing your body to use energy too fast. Symptoms include a rapid heart rate, high blood pressure, insomnia, nervousness, increased perspiration, and weight loss.

Although thyroid trouble is often inherited, it can result from a poor diet. To reduce your risk, make sure you're getting all the vitamins and minerals your body needs.

- **Key nutrients for hormone production.** Your thyroid gland needs zinc, vitamin A, and vitamin E to function properly. Far and away, the best source of zinc is oysters. But if you find shellfish a little slimy, there is always lean meat, lima beans, and whole grain breads and cereals.

  The easiest way to get vitamin A is from liver. Eggs and dairy products are loaded with this important vitamin, but like liver, they are also loaded with fat and cholesterol. If fat-watching is a concern — and it should be — your best bet for vitamin A is fortified low-fat or nonfat milk.

  Vitamin E is found in vegetable oils, seeds, wheat germ, and some nuts. Wheat germ oil has the highest concentration of vitamin E, if you can find it. If not, sunflower oil is also very good.

- **Don't forget your B's and C's.** B vitamins are also very important for healthy thyroid function. Riboflavin (B2) can be found in dairy products, liver, and dark green vegetables. As a rule, Americans get about half of their riboflavin from milk, so be sure not to skimp. The best sources of niacin (B3) are high-protein foods, such as lean meat, peanut butter, and dried beans. These foods, as well as bananas, avocados, potatoes, and dried fruit, are also good sources of vitamin B6.

  It seems like vitamin C is good for everything, and your thyroid is no exception. This vitamin helps keep hormone production at the proper speed. So go ahead ... pour yourself a refreshing glass of orange juice.

- **Go fishing for vitamin D.** A deficiency of vitamin D can lead to hyperthyroidism. Vitamin D fortified dairy products are the most easily available source. If you are a seafood fan, you're also in luck. Many fish, especially salmon and sardines, are rich in vitamin D.

Keep a step ahead of thyroid disease

Exercise is a valuable weapon in the war against thyroid disease. You already know the positive effects of a regular exercise program on your overall health, but did you know exercise actually stimulates your thyroid gland and improves its ability to function?

Exercise helps eliminate obesity, lethargy, and fatigue, common symptoms of hypothyroidism, by raising your metabolism. It also increases your body's sensitivity to the thyroid hormones.

Avoiding a goiter

A goiter is an uncomfortable swelling in the neck that can be a symptom of just about any type of thyroid disease. When not working properly, your thyroid becomes inflamed and can expand to several times its normal size, causing this visible lump to form.

The number one cause of goiter throughout the world is iodine deficiency. Iodine is the most important element to the function of the thyroid. Without it, the thyroid can't produce hormones. In America, however, most brands of table salt are fortified with iodine. Most estimates put the typical American intake of iodine well within safe range. This is because we generally eat more than enough salt. If you follow healthy eating habits, there is rarely a need to supplement your iodine intake, but there are exceptions to the rule.

- **Think low salt and iodine rich.** Paying attention to a low-salt diet, as many older people do, can lead to an iodine deficiency. If you don't use table salt and avoid salty dishes, there are many foods that offer natural sources of iodine. Seafood is very rich in iodine, as well as dairy products and some breads. Foods such as sweet potatoes, carrots, spinach, and broccoli provide iodine and are good sources of vitamin A, an important vitamin in the absorption of iodine.
- **Watch the pine nuts and rutabagas.** Iodine may be your thyroid's most needed ingredient in the making of hormones, but getting the right amount of iodine might not be enough.

Some very healthy foods can get in the way of your body's ability to use iodine. These foods, which contain elements called goitrogens, do not reduce your level of iodine. They simply make it hard for your thyroid to convert the iodine into hormones. If you ate enough of these foods, you could actually develop hypothyroidism from iodine deficiency, without being iodine deficient.

Items to avoid include turnips, rutabaga, cabbage, soybeans, and millet. Other popular trouble foods are peanuts, pine nuts, and mustard. These foods do not have to be avoided entirely, but you should be aware of their effects if you are watching your iodine. On the plus side, cooking usually makes the goitrogens in these foods inactive.

Self-test for thyroid disease — basal body temperature

Since your body temperature is controlled by your metabolism, which in turn is controlled by your thyroid, unexplained changes in your body temperature could signal thyroid problems. Here's a simple test you can do at home using a special basal temperature thermometer available at most pharmacies.

- Before bed, shake your thermometer until it reads below 95 degrees.
- When you wake up, before moving around, place the thermometer under your armpit for 10 minutes. Remain very still with your eyes closed.
- When finished, record your temperature and the date.
- Do this for at least three days in a row.

Note: If you are menstruating, the test must be taken on the second, third, and fourth days of menstruation.

The acceptable range for body temperature is between 97.6 and 98.2 degrees. If your readings are lower, it is possible your metabolism is operating too slowly and you have hypothyroidism. If your temperature is above 98.2, your thyroid could be overactive, and you might have hyperthyroidism.

A word of caution. Because many different things can affect your metabolism, some experts believe that measuring your body temperature does not provide a reliable indication of thyroid function.

TINNITUS

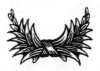

Give up certain foods to silence tinnitus

Eating certain foods may make your taste buds sing, but did you know that certain foods may make your ears ring? Millions of people have tinnitus, a condition that causes ringing, buzzing, or hissing sounds that no one else can hear.

Although the most common cause of tinnitus is exposure to excessively loud noises, some people find that food is at the root of their problem. Cheese, red wine, and salt are the most likely ring-starters. Alcohol, caffeine, and nicotine can also make tinnitus worse.

If you suspect a food allergy is causing your ears to ring, remove that food from your diet for at least a month. If your hearing improves, try adding the food back into your diet slowly to see if it causes a return or worsening of your tinnitus.

TOOTH AND GUM DISEASE

Put the bite on cavities and gum disease

To keep your pearly whites in good working order, you must keep plaque away. Plaque is a sticky film that builds up and hardens on your teeth if you don't care for them properly. Since it is filled with millions of germs, plaque can lead to tooth decay and gum disease.

If your gums bleed easily and look red and swollen, you might have a mild form of gum disease called gingivitis. This often leads to a more serious condition called periodontitis. Periodontitis causes your gums to pull away from your teeth, which opens the door for severe inflammation, infection, and tooth and bone loss.

What you bite into also plays a big role in keeping your chompers strong and healthy. In the fight against tooth and gum disease, a good diet is as important as brushing.

Eat less sugar and more fiber. Mom always said sugar would give you cavities, and she was right. It's a good idea to limit your intake of refined sugars. These sugars, which include most commercial sweeteners like corn syrup, tend to stick to your teeth and gums and allow plaque to build up.

Fiber, on the other hand, helps prevent this from happening. The fiber from foods such as apples, celery, and cereals works like a natural toothbrush, keeping your teeth clean while keeping your body healthy.

ACE your diet. Three of the most important nutrients for healthy teeth and gums are vitamins A, C, and E. You can get vitamin A from milk, dairy products, and fish. Good sources of vitamin E are fortified breakfast cereals, wheat germ, sweet potatoes, and greens. Besides the obvious citrus fruits, vitamin C can be found in papaya, bell peppers, kiwi, and cantaloupe.

Zinc, vitamin B12, and folic acid are also important for healthy teeth and gums. Low levels of these nutrients have been linked to unhealthy gums.

Rinse after meals. Rinsing out your mouth after meals helps get rid of lingering bits of food and stimulates the flow of saliva. Try rinsing with water. It's economical and works great.

Chew some sugarless gum. Chewing sugarless gum after meals also gets the saliva moving through your mouth. This helps to keep leftover food and plaque-causing debris from sticking to your teeth.

Easy way to check your brushing skill

You brush your teeth. You floss. You've been doing it for years, and you're pretty good at it by now, right? Maybe not.

A good way to check your technique is by using disclosing tablets. These small, chewable tablets will show you where plaque is hiding in your mouth by temporarily staining it red. You can buy disclosing tablets at most pharmacies and grocery stores.

For an even simpler way to check your skill as a brusher, look no further than your kitchen. With a cotton swab, rub green food coloring on your teeth, covering all surfaces. The green will appear darker on spots where plaque has built up.

Gum massage therapy relieves discomfort

Massage not only feels good on sore muscles, the gentle pressure applied in a slow, circular motion can stimulate circulation, soothe tenderness, and speed healing. It can also work wonders for your gums. A gum massage not only strengthens them, it eases pain and bleeding and prevents infection.

To massage your gums, use the soft part of your fingertips and rub along your gums gently, in a small, circular motion. The American Dental Association suggests 15 minutes of gum massage every day.

To improve the effectiveness of your gum massage, you might want to try some of the following suggestions.

Keep bacteria down by massaging your gums with some lemon juice. Combine the juice of half a lemon with one cup of water. The acid in the lemon juice will help kill off the bacteria that form in your mouth.

Fight infection in your gums by rubbing them down with goldenseal or echinacea tea. These solutions can lower your risk of infection in bleeding gums, and they are also good for preventing canker sores. To make echinacea tea, boil one or two tablespoons of echinacea root in one cup of water. After boiling, simmer for 10 minutes. Let cool and massage slowly into your gums and along the tooth line. Follow the same procedure for goldenseal tea, mixing two teaspoons with one cup of water. You can also make some chamomile and sage tea to use as a mouthwash.

Reduce inflammation with the use of myrrh. Add some myrrh to boiling water and make into a tea. You can apply it to your gums or simply drink.

If you are pregnant, don't use myrrh. Ask your doctor to recommend a safe treatment for you.

ULCERS

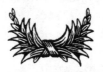

Take up the ulcer challenge

If you want some basic guidelines on a stomach-friendly diet, think of your heart. Experts say that heart-healthy foods are also what is best for your digestive system. This means eating low-cholesterol, low-fat foods, reducing the amount of salt, and piling on the complex carbohydrates, like grains, fresh fruits and vegetables. Sounds simple enough. These foods keep your arteries clear, your heart strong, and your intestines running smoothly.

- **Fiber proclaimed as ulcer foe.** The results are in. A recent study by Harvard University researchers states that eating lots of high-fiber fruits and vegetables means a lower risk of developing ulcers. Your digestive system will get the most benefit from insoluble fibers, the tough, indigestible parts of certain foods that will not dissolve in water. Foods high in this kind of fiber are wheat bran, whole wheat breads, brown rice, beans, fruits and vegetables.

- **Vitamin A gets an A+.** This same study gave vitamin A high marks for preventing ulcers. So, fill your pantry with the most colorful fruits and vegetables you can find; these will be highest in vitamin A. Whether you choose apricots, sweet potatoes, carrots or spinach, or take supplements or multi-vitamins, you'll be protecting your body from the pain of stomach ulcers.

- **The healing power of ... cabbage?** For many Irish households, corned beef and cabbage is the centerpiece of a traditional Easter dinner as well as a St. Patrick's Day feast. It has an aroma that either makes your mouth water or makes you wish Lent lasted another 40 days. Either way, you should commit to cabbage in your diet if you suffer from stomach ulcers. In addition to having generous amounts of vitamin A and insoluble fiber, it also contains glutamine, an amino acid that may help heal ulcers. So, the next time you're pondering the produce aisles, pick up a leafy head of cabbage. It can speed the healing of ulcers of any nationality.

Honey from Down Under works wonders

You knew it was sweet and gooey and delicious on hot biscuits, but did you know that honey can cure your ulcers? A 15-year study in New Zealand has discovered that one particular type of honey, "Active Manuka Honey," has antibacterial properties which get right to the source of stomach and intestinal ulcers. This special honey actually kills *Helicobacter pylori,* the bacteria thought to cause ulcers.

Since Active Manuka Honey is the only variety that fights *H. pylori,* you won't get the same results from your average local honey. The manuka bush is found only in certain wild areas of New Zealand. Active Manuka Honey is not a brand name but identifies this honey as the unique ulcer-fighting variety.

At this time, you can only purchase this product through mail order from the beekeepers in New Zealand. The honey is air mailed to you in about a week. The cost for a 500 g (11.6 oz) jar is about $22.00, which includes shipping and handling. You can pay by U.S. postal money order or by credit card. Write to:

William and Margaret Bennett
Richards Road
R.D. 8
Hamilton, New Zealand

Or you can fax them at 64-7-8297642.

Researchers recommend eating the honey one hour before meals, with no fluids, and again at bedtime. Spread about one tablespoon on a piece of bread. Putting it on the bread keeps the honey in your stomach longer, giving you maximum benefit. What could be more delicious?

The truth about ulcers

The milk myth. It's a remedy that's been around a long time: drink milk to cure an ulcer. The belief was that dairy foods soothed and coated the stomach lining, protecting the inflamed tissue and giving it a chance to heal. But experts now know this is wrong. In fact, they have learned that dairy can even slow down the healing process. Milk proteins cause the stomach to produce gastric acid, which only irritates the ulcers more. If you have ulcers, you still may be able to enjoy milk and other dairy products without problems, but keep the portions small.

Dull is just plain dull. If you've been diagnosed with an ulcer, you may think all you have to look forward to is a lifetime of bland food. No more spice, no more zest. Dull, dull, dull. But the truth is, it has now been proven that the bland diet will neither effectively treat nor prevent ulcers.

So don't throw out that salsa just yet. Instead, you can do trial-and-error elimination of the foods that cause your stomach pain. Some people can tolerate spicy, fatty, or acidic foods in spite of their ulcers. Make a list of your "hot" foods and discuss them with your doctor. You may be lucky enough to get the green light on your favorite chili.

Can you 'catch' an ulcer?

Since 1982, when the *H. pylori* bacterium was first discovered, scientists have tried to pinpoint exactly how this organism enters the stomach and is transmitted from one person to another. One theory is that houseflies pass it on when they land on your food. This should certainly remind you how important it is to keep your food covered whenever you're outdoors. Another group of researchers studied cultures which share common food portions and eating utensils, like the Chinese. Their tests supported the theory that the bacteria can be transmitted through saliva. Until more definite answers are found, keep the fly swatter handy and use your own chopsticks!

Ye old herb shoppe

Deglycyrrhizinated licorice is really a mouthful, in more ways than one. Its name means that the potentially dangerous part of the licorice root extract which can increase blood pressure, glycyrrhizinic acid, has been removed from the compound. It also means possible relief from stomach pain.

Don't think that those licorice candies will do the same job, though. Most are not even made with real licorice, but flavored with anise, which has a similar taste. You must take the genuine herb compound, glycyrrhizinic acid-reduced licorice, to get ulcer-healing benefits. Take 250 to 500 mg before you eat and before going to bed to protect your delicate digestive tissues from stomach acid. Some studies reported better results when the licorice was taken along with antacids.

Ginseng and ginger may have ulcer-healing properties, but there are no conclusive studies to support this. Taking recommended amounts of either of these two herbs for a trial period is certainly not dangerous, and you may just be one of the lucky ones to find ulcer relief in your health food store.

It has been suggested that peppermint oil may help stop the growth of *H. pylori* bacteria in your stomach and intestines. Talk with your doctor and follow label directions carefully.

Ulcer irritants

Alcohol, black tea, and coffee (even decaffeinated) are all known to irritate your digestive tract. While drinking these products may not give you an ulcer, they can certainly make the one you have feel worse and maybe even take longer to heal. It may be hard to give up your morning cup of java, but try substituting a hot drink that is milder on your stomach. Chinese green tea is okay; in fact it's a potent antioxidant, so it will help you in other ways. (For more information on the antioxidant powers of green tea, see the *Green tea* chapter.)

And while you are changing your dietary habits, you should cut out as much sugar and saturated fats as possible. This means reading labels and making choices. It may sound like a lot to sacrifice, but after all, it's your body and your pain.

For spaghetti, vampires, and . . . ulcers?

That deliciously versatile food, garlic, may just be the answer to your ulcer woes. A recent study tested garlic extract against *H. pylori* and garlic came out the winner. Although this was a laboratory test, scientists are hopeful that the results will be the same for the thousands of ulcer sufferers across the country.

In any event, you can't go wrong by pressing a clove or two into almost any dish you prepare. Garlic has so many benefits that you'll come out the winner, as well.

URINARY TRACT INFECTIONS

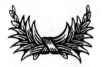

Natural help for painful infections

If you are one of the millions of people who get urinary tract infections (UTIs) every year, you're probably familiar with the painful, burning urination that usually accompanies a UTI. You'll probably also do whatever you can to avoid having another one.

Women are more likely to develop UTIs than men. And once you have one infection, you're 20 percent more likely to have another. However, it isn't just a women's problem. Men over 50 often get UTIs because of an enlarged prostate. Anything that interferes with urine flow can contribute to an infection. Because urine stays in the urinary tract longer, bacteria have more time to get a grip and multiply.

If you have a urinary tract infection, you'll probably need an antibiotic from your doctor to get well. However, some natural nutritional strategies may help heal a UTI or prevent you from getting one in the future.

Cranberries carry away infection. Cranberry juice may be a tart, delicious way to keep UTIs from cramping your style. For years, cranberries were believed to help prevent urinary problems, and modern research now supports those beliefs.

Some doctors think cranberries slow the growth of bacteria by making your urine more acidic. Other studies show that cranberries keep bacteria from clinging to your urinary tract. The bacteria just slip right through and out of your body.

However it works, if you're likely to get UTIs, you may want to add about three ounces of cranberry juice cocktail to your diet every day. One study found that the protective effects of cranberry juice appeared only after four to eight weeks, so for the most protection, drink cranberry juice regularly.

Wash it away with water. You can use water to clean almost anything, so it shouldn't surprise you that it may also cleanse your urinary tract. Most doctors agree that water can help wash bacteria out of your body. Drink at least six to eight glasses of water every day. If your urine is pale-colored, you're getting enough. A dark color means you need to visit the water fountain a little more often.

Take some vitamin C. Like cranberry juice, vitamin C supplements may make your urine more acidic, thus making it more difficult for bacteria to grow.

Help yourself to some herbs. Some natural herbs can increase your urine flow, making you less likely to get a urinary tract infection. Among these are goldenrod and parsley. You can find them at your local health food store, or look for fresh parsley in your grocery store.

The next time a restaurant puts some decorative parsley on your plate, don't just admire it and set it aside. Try eating it for an extra bit of urinary protection. However, beware of staying outdoors too long afterward. Parsley can increase your sensitivity to the sun.

Another herb, bearberry, has an antiseptic effect so it neutralizes bacteria before it can do its dirty work. Bearberry was used effectively for years to battle UTIs before sulfa drugs and antibiotics came along. This herb can be toxic, so if you try it, use it for a few days at most.

If you have a kidney disease, you should consult your doctor before trying any herb for urinary tract infections.

Vaginitis and Yeast Infections

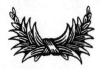

6 key nutrients battle bacteria

Not enough of this vitamin; not enough of that nutrient. Before you know it, you have an infection. It happens all the time. In fact, that's how you get vaginitis, an inflammation of the vagina. There are several key nutrients that fight off the specific bacteria that like to take up residence in a woman's genital area. Without them, the door is open to all kinds of nasty microorganisms.

Folic acid. This B vitamin not only protects you from vaginitis, it may decrease your risk of cervical cancer. According to researchers, low levels of folic acid may cause body tissue to become more vulnerable to cancer-causing substances.

To get folic acid naturally, eat cantaloupe; asparagus; beets; liver; and green, leafy vegetables like spinach and turnip greens. If possible, eat folic acid-rich fruits and vegetables raw, since the heat from cooking destroys up to half of this important vitamin. If you decide to take supplements, take folic acid as part of a complete B-vitamin complex, since they work best together.

Iron. Foods high in iron include shellfish, red meat, and dried fruit. For a winning combination, stir-fry some broccoli with your shrimp, or make a salad full of citrus fruits and dried apricots. Adding foods high in vitamin C will help your body absorb the iron better. Check with your doctor before taking iron supplements because it's easy to take too much in pill form.

Magnesium. Researchers discovered those suffering from one yeast infection after another tested low in magnesium. Nuts, whole grain foods, dark green vegetables like spinach and broccoli, and seafood are all rich in magnesium.

Zinc. Zinc fights yeast. Without it, you may develop yeast infections. Are you getting enough zinc? If you aren't eating seafood, red meat, poultry, legumes, and whole grains, you may not be.

Selenium. Scientists don't know how selenium fights vaginal infections, but they do know that women with chronic cases of vaginitis have low selenium levels. Don't bother taking selenium supplements. Just make sure you eat lots of unprocessed foods, like vegetables and grains grown in the United States. Our selenium-rich soil guarantees you enough of this important mineral.

Vitamin A. Your lungs, intestines, urinary tract, bladder, and vagina all have linings that act as protective barriers against bacteria — sort of a living armor. If cells die, bacteria can invade and cause infection. Vitamin A keeps the cells in this armor alive and well. Think of it as your first line of defense against vaginal infections. Some foods rich in vitamin A are liver, fortified dairy products, eggs, spinach, carrots, and papaya.

Vanquish vaginitis with the right foods

To give your body the best possible chance of fighting off vaginitis or yeast infections, you need to think about your total diet. In other words, what kinds of foods do you eat over the course of, say, a week, and in what proportions? Consider the following:

Avoid starchy vegetables. The two most important categories for you are lean proteins and low-starch vegetables. Examples of vegetables high in starch are corn, potatoes, dried beans, and peas. So stay away from those. Fill your plate with poultry, fiber-rich vegetables, and fruit.

Eat less sugar. The bacteria that cause vaginitis thrive in a high-sugar environment, so you need to eat less sugar. And it's not just the sodas, candy bars, and desserts you need to worry about. There is hidden sugar in lots of today's fast and processed foods. Read the labels on your cereal boxes, canned fruits, spaghetti sauces, and diet products. You may be unpleasantly surprised. Watch out for corn syrup, molasses, and honey, too.

If you are diabetic, you may suffer from more yeast infections than others because you have a higher concentration of glucose in your body. Talk to your doctor if this is the case. She may be able to recommend a more aggressive treatment for your infections.

Eliminate foods with yeast. Not all doctors agree, but some recommend eliminating yeast-containing foods if you are prone to yeast infections. Breads, aged cheese, vinegar, and beer are all high in yeast. If you are troubled by recurring infections, you might try this approach. You've nothing to lose.

Include some fatty acids. To reduce the inflammation that often accompanies vaginitis, eat more essential fatty acids. You've heard of omega-3 and omega-6? Well, that's what you need. If you eat fish two or three times a week and get small amounts of vegetable oils, like canola, safflower, sunflower, or olive oil, you will be getting a good balance of both omega-3 and omega-6 fatty acids. Seeds, nuts, poultry, and eggs contain fair amounts of fatty acids as well.

Enjoy garlic. Some experts believe garlic extract may be able to fight fungal infections. Even though the results are inconclusive, adding some heart-healthy garlic to your meals is probably a good idea.

Yeast infections may yield to yogurt

Lactobacillus acidophilus is a good kind of bacteria found in the vagina. Scientists believe this is what fights off the bad, infection-causing bacteria that result in various forms of vaginitis. So, it would make sense that increasing the amount of *L. acidophilus* in your system would help safeguard you from those irritating bouts of inflammation and itching. The problem is how, exactly, to introduce these good bacteria into your body.

In a number of studies, researchers had their subjects eat 8 ounces of yogurt, containing *L. acidophilus* cultures, every day for several months. The majority of women showed a decrease in the number of vaginal infections. Sounds like an easy and delicious way to fight those annoying infections.

Another proposed method of treatment is inserting yogurt directly into the vagina. A small study out of Japan found that over half of the women tested got either partial or complete relief.

Other studies have not had such positive results, however. This could point to biological differences in the women tested or differences in the yogurt products used. One study discovered that out of 16 nonprescription products advertised as containing *Lactobacillus,* (yogurt, milk, powder, tablet, and capsule), only four actually contained *Lactobacillus acidophilus* and 11 contained one or more contaminants. How manufacturers prepare yogurt can make a difference, too, on the amount of *L. acidophilus* that remains active in the product.

To be assured of the yogurt's quality, you can always make your own. Many cookbooks provide directions for making homemade yogurt.

A matter for men

Men can suffer from an embarrassing itch, too. It's called tinea cruris or, more commonly, jock itch. Although the symptoms and some of the treatments are the same, a different fungus causes this condition in men. Basically, your discomfort comes from organisms that like warm, moist areas and cause a fungal skin disease. The result is itching and a scaly rash around your genitals.

You are more likely to develop jock itch if you are overweight, which causes the skin in your groin area to rub and stay irritated. If you play sports, perspiring a lot and wearing tight clothing, such as a jock strap, can also increase your risk.

If you suffer from jock itch, don't share towels, clothing, or personal sportswear, since this condition can be contagious.

To treat this skin infection, keep your groin area as dry and cool as possible, and try the diet and nutrient recommendations for vaginitis.

Relief from Down Under

Early explorers to Australia used the leaves from a local tree to make an aromatic tea, so naming it "tea tree." They found out later that the oil from the leaves is also an effective germicide, and they began using this tea tree oil on bites, burns, and cuts. Today, as it gains popularity around the world, its uses are expanding. Several experts believe that applying tea tree oil to the vagina will treat infection, while others say not enough research has been done to recommend its use.

VARICOSE VEINS

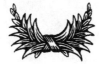

Bolster blood vessels with ginkgo

This ancient Chinese tree has been a source of beauty and healing for thousands of years, but only recently have scientists begun to explore the full potential of its therapeutic powers. When blood vessels lose strength, they allow pools of blood to form in the veins and in the surrounding tissue. This condition is called varicose veins.

We now know that the concentrated extract of ginkgo (GBE) protects the walls of blood vessels and strengthens the tiny capillaries that connect arteries to veins. This helps keep your fragile vascular system from becoming damaged through injury, stress, or age. Taking ginkgo will not heal existing varicose veins, but it may keep you from developing more.

High fiber and low fat — a sensible strategy?

What can you eat to improve or prevent varicose veins? Dr. Denis Burkitt, a British physician, believes he has the answer. He theorizes that constipation is directly related to varicose veins. He says if your diet is low in fiber you're more likely to strain during bowel movements. That, in turn, will increase the pressure on the veins that run down your leg, causing them to enlarge.

Although not proven, his theory suggests that eating high-fiber foods like whole-grain cereals and breads; fruit with skins, like apples, strawberries and cherries; and lots of vegetables and legumes will help prevent varicose veins.

On the other hand, some people are more likely to get varicose veins because of their weight. The more fat you have, the less muscle there is to support your veins and aid in circulation. In addition, extra weight around your middle and in your legs puts more pressure on the walls of your leg veins.

All this adds up to a greater likelihood that you will develop varicose veins. Keep your diet low in fat, salt, and sugar, and high in fiber, and you may avoid this painful and unsightly condition.

'C' is for collagen

Collagen has gotten a lot of press in the last few years with regards to cosmetic surgery. It is, of course, the natural protein that many people inject under their skin to reduce wrinkles.

Well, in the case of collagen, beauty is indeed more than skin deep. In fact, collagen plays an important role all the way through your skin down to your bones and blood vessels. It is the basic substance for healing wounds, mending broken bones, and preventing bruises. By supporting your circulatory system, collagen keeps your veins from losing strength and tone.

Vitamin C is necessary for your body to make collagen. Natural sources of vitamin C are citrus, sweet red and green peppers, papayas, kiwis, strawberries, brussels sprouts, and broccoli.

Sweep away varicose veins with butcher's broom

This low evergreen bush may not look like much, but that didn't stop herbalists from experimenting with it more than 2,000 years ago. Today, modern scientists have studied the chemistry of this small plant, and discovered that butcher's broom can reduce inflammation and improve the firmness of your veins. Both of these properties are helpful in treating varicose veins.

In one study, scientists found that symptoms of varicose veins improved when subjects took a drug that included extracts of this herb. Itching, tingling, and cramping, seemed to be greatly helped.

Aromatic oil soothes vein pain

Cyprus is a beautiful little island in the Mediterranean Sea with a history dating back to the Phoenicians and ancient Greeks. At one point in its varied history, the people of this island worshipped a certain tall evergreen tree, now called the cypress. The scent of cypress oil will remind you of the tree, for it smells of spice and the forest. You can use this oil externally to treat varicose veins. It has astringent qualities that cause blood vessels and body tissues to contract.

WEIGHT LOSS

Foods that fill you up fast

Losing weight is easier if you eat foods that make you feel full. You're also less likely to binge or snack constantly. Here's the lowdown on foods, from most filling to least.

Bring on the boiled potatoes. According to a Satiety Index developed by Australian researchers, boiled potatoes are the most satisfying and filling food you can eat.

Hail those high-fiber foods. Fiber fills you up because it absorbs water and swells, taking up more space. Fiber also slows the movement of food through your upper digestive tract, so you don't get hungry as quickly. Good sources of high-fiber foods include fruits; vegetables; legumes; and grains, such as oats, barley, wheat, rice, and rye.

Love those beans and lentils. Also high in fiber, beans and lentils make you feel full and leave you feeling full longer because they are slowly absorbed by the body.

Go the whole grain way. When it comes to bread, whole grain is 50 percent more filling than white bread.

Snack on popcorn rather than Snickers. Popcorn will make you feel twice as full as a candy bar or peanuts will. Cakes, cookies, and donuts also measured up as some of the least filling foods.

Favor fish over beef or chicken. Calorie for calorie, fish fills you up better than beef or chicken.

Opt for oranges and apples. When it comes to filling fruit, oranges and apples outscore bananas every time.

Pick porridge over cold cereal. It's almost always 50 percent more filling and many times it's twice as filling.

Give croissants the cold shoulder. They're the least filling food of all.

Weigh your choices. When trying to decide between two foods of equal caloric value, go with the food that weighs more. Generally, researchers have found the heavier food to be the most filling. Another way to determine how filling a food is likely to be is to look it up in your calorie book and compare the calories to the portion size. Limit foods that have over 250 calories per 4-ounce portion.

Generally, carbohydrates make people feel fuller than any other food. Protein-rich foods, such as fish, meat, eggs, and cheese, come in second. Fruits rank third.

Fat just makes you crave more fat. Guess that old story about Jack Sprat and his wife really did make a valid point. For if you remember, "Jack Sprat could eat no fat and his wife could eat no lean. But between them both, you see, they licked the platter clean." And if you remember that, no doubt you also know that Jack Sprat was skinny and his wife a little more than just pleasantly plump.

Follow your nose to lose weight the easy way

Throw those deprivation diets out the door. Dr. Alan Hirsch says he's discovered the secret to slimming down and staying that way. His formula for success? Your nose.

You stop eating when the satiety center in your brain is satisfied. And you satisfy the satiety center in your brain in a big way through your sense of smell according to Hirsch, the Neurological Director of the Smell and Taste Research Foundation in Chicago and author of *Dr. Hirsch's Guide To Scentsational Weight Loss.*

If your nose and satiety center are working well together, your brain can determine the amount of food you've eaten by the amount of odors that reached your satiety center via your nose. However, Hirsch and his team of researchers have also found that it's possible to fool your satiety center just by smelling certain scents. The scents they've found to be most helpful: peppermint, green apple, and banana.

Smelling the scents before you eat and anytime you have a craving can dramatically reduce your calorie consumption. Each time you use the scents, sniff three times in each nostril. Switch odors every day. If you become bored with the smells, they're less likely to be effective.

Even though you're eating less, don't deprive yourself of food. Eat three small meals and two small snacks. Otherwise, you'll likely get so hungry you'll end up stuffing yourself, which defeats the purpose of using the scents.

People who participated in trials to test the scent theory lost an average of five pounds a month, without restricting food or engaging in a lot of exercise. The scents simply helped their satiety center register fullness faster so they ate less and lost weight.

The only side effect so far from this smell therapy has been excess weight loss. However, the researchers do caution that people with asthma or people who have migraines triggered by different odors probably shouldn't participate in this particular weight loss plan.

Some herb shops and drugstores carry the different scents. If you can't find any in your area, a company called Slim Scents offers these products. Call 1-800-825-2261 for more information.

Natural appetite suppressants

Savor some psyllium. Psyllium, the husk of the plantago plant's seed, may work well as an appetite suppressant. In a small study of 17 women, those who took 20 grams of plantago seed granules along with a glass of water three hours before a meal felt significantly fuller one hour after the meal than women who had taken a placebo (fake psyllium). In addition, the women who used the psyllium ate less fat.

Researchers think psyllium works as an appetite suppressant because it holds water and swells, creating a feeling of fullness. Although the evidence supporting psyllium as a weight loss aid is scant, you may want to try it. It won't harm you unless you take more than recommended or are allergic to it. Other benefits include regularity and cholesterol control. You can find psyllium seeds at most health food stores.

Opt for some orange juice. Studies suggest OJ is an effective appetite suppressant. In a Yale University study, overweight men who drank OJ ate nearly 300 fewer calories at lunch. Overweight women consumed an average of 431 fewer midday calories. Their intakes were compared with similarly overweight men and women who drank plain water before lunch.

To reap these benefits, drink a glass of OJ a half-hour to an hour before a meal. You'll eat fewer calories during the meal and still feel comfortably full. Just don't forget to include that glass of orange juice when figuring total calories for the day.

Fight flab with these bulge busters

Break the fast. A good time to eat the majority of your calories is in the morning. Adults who eat breakfast every day tend to weigh less and have lower cholesterol levels. Also, the body's ability to burn calories is greater in the morning than in the afternoon or evening. People who skip breakfast tend to eat more high-fat snacks, too. Some nutrition specialists recommend that 20 to 25 percent of your daily calories come from breakfast. This is also a good meal to focus on fruit.

Turn off the tube. Don't eat while watching television. The average person eats eight times more food watching prime time TV than any other time.

Give chromium a chance. Chromium appears to aid weight loss by burning fat more quickly as well as helping your body build muscle. Chromium also works with insulin in the body to keep blood sugar levels even, so your energy level remains stable and you burn food more efficiently.

Research indicates that supplementing your diet with chromium picolinate is safe, but consult your doctor before trying it. If you'd rather get your chromium from food, some good sources include apples with skins, asparagus, brewer's yeast, liver, mushrooms, nuts, prunes, oysters, fish, and other seafood.

Make nutritional choices if you're a nighttime eater. It's not when you eat that counts as much as what you eat. No doubt you've heard everything you eat after 8 p.m. goes straight to your hips. Well, a new study says it's just not so. Researchers found a calorie counts the same no matter when you eat it. However, women who ate most of their calories at night got less vitamin C, vitamin B6, folic acid, and carbohydrates from their diet than women who spread their calories out over the day. Nighttime eaters were also more likely to get more calories from fat, protein, and alcohol. This could be because they were so hungry by the time they ate they made poor nutritional choices.

Count calories and fat grams. Even though it would be easier just to count one or the other, research suggests you'll get better results from your weight loss efforts if you count both.

A study from Indiana University found that overweight people ate about the same amount of calories as lean people. However, the plump people ate more fat and added sugar while the lean people ate more fiber. This seems to suggest that you can eat more food if you just change the form of the calories from fat and sugar to fiber.

Although Americans have significantly reduced their fat intake in recent years, they're still packing on extra pounds. Thinking that low-fat or fat-free means low-calorie, Americans are eating too many calories. And anytime you eat more calories than you need — whether from fat or carbohydrates — your body stores them as fat.

Don't skip meals. Meal-skipping is a big factor in falling off the diet bandwagon and into an eating binge. Giving your body fuel at regular intervals keeps blood sugar levels stable and helps your body burn calories more efficiently.

Watch yourself in social situations. People eat more when they are with other people, says a study at Georgia State University. When you're counting calories, be careful when eating in a group.

Tailor your diet to your style of eating. If you are a constant nibbler, plan healthy meals and snacks ahead of time to meet your calorie goals. If you eat more when you're bored or frustrated, plan pleasant activities to distract you from overeating. If the vending machines at work are a constant temptation, take healthy snacks with you from home.

Many people eat unconsciously out of habit while watching TV or preparing a meal. At home, pick a specific spot for eating and eat there only. This will help you keep better track of what you're eating and may eliminate some of that unconscious eating.

Make your cheddar better. Don't want to give up your favorite high-fat cheese? Make a low-fat version by zapping it in the microwave for a minute or two. Heating will make the fat separate somewhat from the cheese. Any oil you can pour or blot off will significantly reduce the cheese's fat content. This method also works well for pizzas, fajitas, cheese sandwiches, or cheese toppings on casseroles.

The healthy road to weight loss

- **Balance your diet.** You should eat a wide variety of foods and not deprive yourself of your favorites. Moderation is the key. There are no "good" or "bad" foods. You can enjoy the foods you love in reasonable amounts. In fact, depriving yourself of your favorite foods may result in cravings and binge eating, which will make you gain weight. Balance your diet over several days. That way, if you have a special occasion and want to eat cake, you can cut back a little on other days. What counts is the overall picture.

- **Take a supplement.** If you're eating less than 1,500 calories a day, you're probably not getting all the nutrients your body needs. To keep yourself in tip-top shape, take a multivitamin/mineral supplement just to be sure you're meeting your body's nutritional needs.

- **Shoot for 70 grams of protein a day.** You can get this much from five or six ounces of lean meat and two glasses of skim milk. You also get some protein from grains, fruits, and vegetables.
- **Count your calcium.** Make sure you take in 1,000 milligrams (mg) of calcium a day. If you're older, shoot for 1,200 to 1,500 mg. The body has more trouble absorbing calcium after women turn 60 and men turn 70.
- **Buy dairy with D** — vitamin D, that is. Look for dairy products that have vitamin D added to them, or help your body produce vitamin D by spending 15 minutes a day in the sun. Vitamin D helps your body absorb calcium.
- **Fill up with fluids.** Drink plenty of fluids while dieting, especially if you're taking diuretics.

The essential weight loss supplement

It's free. It's available to absolutely everybody. And it's essential to every weight loss program. What is it?

Exercise, of course.

Without exercise, even the best weight loss plan won't give you the results you're hoping for. As an added bonus, exercise helps you lose weight faster and keep it off longer.

It's best to exercise at your target heart rate for 20 minutes with a 10-minute warm-up and a 10-minute cool-down. To get your target heart rate, subtract your age from 220 and multiply the result by 0.6.

Always check with your doctor before beginning an exercise program.

Making friends with fat

When you're trying to lose weight, it's common to want to flee from all fats. Fat is not your enemy — excess consumption of it is. In fact, without some fat in your diet, your body wouldn't be able to make nerve cells or hormones or absorb the fat-soluble vitamins — A, D, E, and K.

Eat a little fat to feel full. Some researchers believe eating small amounts of fat can actually keep people from overindulging on total calories. Ohio State University nutrition scientist John Allred points out that dietary fat causes your body to produce a hormone that tells your intestines to slow down the emptying process.

This could explain why adding a little peanut butter to your rice cake may satisfy your hunger longer and prevent you from wolfing down the whole bag of rice cakes later.

Certain fats, like olive oil and the omega-3 fatty acids found in cold water fish like salmon, may help prevent heart disease. And most people say a little fat simply makes food taste, look, and smell more appetizing.

Know your limits. The U.S. Department of Health and Human Services recommends that you limit the fat in your diet to 30 percent or less of total calories.

One way to figure this is to make sure all the food you eat meets this 30 percent guideline. No food you choose to eat should have more than 3 grams of fat for every 100 calories. If you decide to splurge on a favorite high-fat food, you can compensate by limiting your fat calories for the rest of the day or week.

Learn to recognize which fats are OK. The easiest rule to remember is to stay away from saturated fats such as those in cheese, butter, and meat. Less than 10 percent of your calories should come from saturated fats.

You should also limit the polyunsaturated fats you eat to less than 10 percent of your calories. Common sources are safflower oil, soybean oil, sunflower oil, and hydrogenated or partially hydrogenated margarines. During the hydrogenation process, fats are changed to trans fatty acids, which have much the same effect on the body as saturated fats.

Pass the prune puree, please. Many people find that the worst part of weight loss is cutting back on favorite foods or feeling guilty when they do indulge a little. Here's where a little prune puree can come in handy. Use it as the butter, shortening, or oil substitute in your favorite brownie, cake, cookie, or bread recipe.

One cup of prune puree has 407 calories and one gram of fat, while one cup of butter has 1,600 calories and 182 grams of fat, and one cup of oil has 1,944 calories and 218 grams of fat. Using prune puree, you save a bundle in fat and calories while indulging your sweet tooth.

To make enough prune puree for several recipes, mix one pound of dried, pitted prunes with one cup of hot water and puree in a food processor. Keep your puree refrigerated in a covered jar.

Stay away from stressor foods

Many people crave so-called "stressor" foods when they're dieting. Although you may find yourself fantasizing about a stressor food feast, don't give in. Stressor foods rob your body of essential nutrients rather than nourishing it.

To give your body the good nutrition it needs while you're working your way toward your weight loss goals, limit stressor foods, such as refined sugars, flours, and pastas; cola; processed fats, such as cheese; and hydrogenated fats like margarine and deep-fried foods.

Livin' low-fat and lovin' it

Part of any successful weight loss plan is learning how to live a low-fat lifestyle. Not only are low-fat foods healthier for your body, eating low-fat lets you eat a little more food without a lot more calories. That's because all fats contain nine calories per gram. All carbohydrates contain four calories per gram.

The best news of all is that low-fat living doesn't have to be a tedious, torturous ordeal. In fact, studies show that as you reduce the amount of fat you eat your cravings for them actually decline. Researchers at the Fred Hutchinson Cancer Research Center in Seattle found that people who switch from high-fat to low-fat foods soon develop a preference for lower-fat foods.

Here are some tips to help you make a smooth transition to a low-fat lifestyle:

- Use low-fat or nonfat dairy foods to replace cream in sauces. Substitute skim milk for whole milk.
- Steam, poach, roast, broil, grill, microwave, or bake foods rather than sauté or pan-fry them. Cook meat on a rack so the fat drains off.
- Skim the fat off soups or stews. If possible, cook the broth in advance, chill, then remove the hardened layer of fat.
- Season vegetables with herbs, spices, chicken broth, or lemon juice instead of high-fat butter and sauces. Experiment with new seasonings.
- Perk up flavors with balsamic vinegar, sun-dried tomatoes, Dijon mustard, Tabasco sauce, salsa, catsup, green chilies, or

small amounts of sesame or hot chili oils.

- Make your own reduced-fat dressing by using more vinegar and less oil. Use lemon juice and Italian herbs for fat-free flavor. When buying mayonnaise, opt for the reduced fat or fat-free version.
- Cut back the fat in your favorite recipes by a third and replace the fat in baked recipes with applesauce or pureed prunes.
- Take advantage of healthful cookware, such as microwave ovens, vegetable steamers, pressure cookers, and nonstick pots and pans. These help foods preserve nutrients and make cooking a little easier as well.
- Limit red meat and other animal products to once or twice a week. When choosing meat, keep in mind that those cuts labeled "select" tend to be lowest in fat. Always trim away fatty edges and remove skin from chicken before cooking.
- Substitute olive or canola oil for other vegetable fats.
- Go for burgers made without grease. Microwave your patties for one to three minutes; pour off the liquid; and then fry, broil, or grill them. This cuts the fat content by almost one-third.
- Drink water or fruit juice without added sugar instead of soda or other sweetened drinks.
- Buy tuna packed in water instead of oil.

Shrink your stomach the natural way

Desperate dieters demand extreme measures. Some people find controlling their appetites so difficult that they have their stomachs surgically stapled so they'll eat less and lose weight.

The bad news for those people is that there's no need to have surgery to shed pounds. Your stomach will shrink naturally — if you just put less food into it.

The trick is to stick to a regular meal plan — typically one that focuses on eating smaller meals more frequently. Just remember that because you eat more meals doesn't mean you get more calories. You simply divide them more evenly throughout the day so you're less likely to get hungry and overeat. You want to avoid large meals and stuffing yourself because you'll undo all your good work and increase your stomach size again.

The skinny on fat substitutes

When nothing will do but the flavor of fat, a fat substitute can save the day. They let you enjoy the taste of fat without the guilt of sabotaging your diet. However, not all fake fats are created equal. Here's the low-down on the major ones on the market these days:

Simplesse. In use since 1989, Simplesse is made from protein particles. Food manufacturers are fond of substituting it in frozen desserts, butter, cheese, mayonnaise, and other refrigerated foods. It may not be listed by name on the product label but may instead be described as a protein complex. Major drawback: It can't stand up to heat so you can't use it for frying or baking. Also, if you are on a protein-restricted diet, you may not be able to eat Simplesse.

Oatrim. Oatrim is one of the healthier choices when it comes to fat substitutes. Early studies suggest it lowers cholesterol as well as blood pressure. It also helps keep blood sugar levels constant, a big plus for diabetics and others who have trouble controlling their blood sugar. You can also use Oatrim for cooking, including baking. Some health food stores carry it or you can order it from Bob's Red Mill, 5209 S.E. International Way, Portland, OR 97222. Phone number: 503-654-3215.

Olestra. Olestra, trade name Olean, looks and tastes just like real fat and can be used for frying and baking. Its unique combination of sugar and vegetable oil prevents it from being absorbed by the body. Major drawback: It can cause stomach cramps and diarrhea. It also interferes with your body's ability to absorb important nutrients such as beta carotene and vitamins A, D, E, and K. In fact, the FDA requires food companies to add vitamins A, D, E, and K to any foods containing olestra.

Z-trim. Developed by Dr. George E. Inglett, a chemist with the USDA's Agricultural Research Service, Z-trim is made from agricultural byproducts, such as the hulls of oats, soybeans, peas, rice, and the bran from corn or wheat. Since it's made from natural fibers, it won't upset your digestive system if you eat normal amounts.

While eating foods made with fat substitutes can sometimes help you conquer your cravings for the smooth, creamy taste of high-fat foods, they can also wreck your diet and add to your weight loss woes if you eat too many of them. Despite being lower in fat, they still contain calories and all calories — low-fat or not — still count.

SUPER FOODS

APPLES

A nutritious and versatile food

What could make a better quick snack? It's naturally sweet, contains no cholesterol, no salt, and no fat to speak of. It's packed with vitamins, minerals, and fiber. It's easy to find at the market, handy to carry in your lunch bag, and requires little or no preparation. Just wash it well and you're ready to bite right in and enjoy this juicy fruit.

Raw apples are good in fresh fruit salads or chopped up and added to cold or hot cereal. And neither Halloween nor the county fair would be the same without a candied apple on a stick.

That's just the beginning. The choices seem endless. Cooked treats range from baked apples to applesauce, from apple pies to apple jelly. Choose fresh apples or dried, canned or frozen. There are many varieties —Red and Golden Delicious, Granny Smith, Macintosh, Rome, and Jonathan, to name a few of the most popular ones. They range in flavor from quite tart to very sweet.

And you can do more than just eat apples. Drink apple juice or apple cider for flavor and nutrition. Sniff the scent of green apples to help with weight loss or migraine headaches. (For more information about the scent of green apples, see the *Headache* and *Weight loss* chapters.) Red, gold, or green, they look pretty sitting in a bowl. However you like them, in one form or another, you can enjoy apples all year long.

Befriend your bowels

Is your medicine cabinet stocked with over-the-counter remedies for bowel discomforts — laxatives for constipation and that pink stuff for diarrhea? What if one natural product could relieve both? Not likely, you say? Well, as strange as it may seem, apples help manage both diarrhea and constipation.

Apples contain pectin, a soluble fiber, that absorbs water in your stomach and intestines. It swells and forms a gummy mass that moistens and softens the stool and helps ease difficult bowel movements.

On the other hand, the bulk formed by pectin firms up the watery stool of diarrhea, changing it to a more manageable consistency. So, whichever condition begs for relief, reach into the fruit bowl to avoid discomfort at the toilet bowl.

Apples warm the heart

The smell of apple pie baking in a hot oven may make you feel all warm and cozy. But apples do more than warm the heart. They help protect the heart by keeping the blood flowing smoothly through unclogged arteries.

The pectin in apples forms a gel that seems to bind LDL, the "bad" kind of cholesterol, and take it out of your body. This cholesterol can build up in the arteries and form plaque that hardens and damages arteries and slows down the blood flow to the heart and other organs.

Apples also contain flavonoids. These are compounds that act as antioxidants in the bloodstream. They help keep the arteries clear, preventing heart attacks and strokes. The flavonoids are mainly in the skins, so don't peel away this protection.

Another heart-helper in apples is potassium. If you have high blood pressure, you are at a higher risk of a heart attack. Potassium lowers blood pressure and also helps keep your heartbeat regular.

Did you know that you can replace fat with applesauce in some recipes? Fats are one of the greatest dangers to a healthy heart. Finding substitutes can be a big help. At least one commercial brownie mix gives both regular and low-fat directions on the box. The low-fat version calls for applesauce rather than oil.

An apple ... keeps cancer away

Some of the same qualities that make apples so healthy for your heart also make them good cancer fighters. The fiber helps move foods quickly through your digestive tract. This reduces the length of time toxic chemicals that might cause cancer stay in your system. This is helpful particularly in preventing colon and rectal cancers.

The antioxidant quality of vitamins C and E and the flavonoids, especially quercetin, helps prevent the damage to cells that makes them more susceptible to cancer. Vitamin E also helps the body get rid of chemicals created when the body breaks down fats. One apple provides 13 percent of the RDA for vitamin C, about 9 percent of the RDA for vitamin E, and almost 15 percent of the RDA for fiber.

(For more information about antioxidants and cancer, see the *Cancer* chapter.

APRICOTS

The healthy appeal of apricots

If you're looking for a quick delicious snack, it's hard to do better than the little apricot. This golden fruit is jam-packed with fiber, vitamin C, iron, boron, silica, and potassium. That means you can help your heart, fight fatigue and infection, improve your skin, hair, and nails, regulate your blood pressure, keep your digestion moving smoothly, and even help produce estrogen, all in only about 16 tiny calories.

What's more, if you are an ex-smoker, you may want to make apricots part of your daily routine. Because they are rich in beta carotene, they can cleanse your system of any nicotine left-overs. This helps fight off both larynx and lung cancer.

If you're short on ways to add apricots to your menu, try these appetizing ideas: slice them up in fruit salads, puree them for sauces, make preserves, peel and slice them in yogurt or on ice cream, or whip up an apricot tart.

Nutrition on the go

This is one case where fresh is not the best. Dried apricots beat fresh apricots hands down when it comes to important nutrients, since the dried variety have more than three times the amount of fiber and vitamin A. That's a lot of punch in one chewy, portable package. Notice in the following chart that the nutrition information is comparing different weights. It takes far fewer grams of dried apricots to give you about the same amount of fiber and vitamin A as fresh.

It's interesting to note that apricots lose over 50 percent of their water when they are dried. This means that it takes six pounds of fresh to make one pound of dried apricots.

Did you know?

Apricot kernels are full of oil that is used to flavor various sweets and liqueurs, but if you feel inclined to chew on one, don't. Apricot pits actually contain cyanide and are considered poisonous until they are roasted.

Nutritional know-how

	(10 dried)	**(3 fresh)**	**(1 cup canned)**
Carbohydrates	22 grams	12 grams	31 grams
Fiber	3 grams	3 grams	3 grams
Vitamin A	2,534 IU	2,769 IU	4,194 IU
Vitamin C	8 mg	11 mg	12 mg
Potassium	482 mg	314 mg	409 mg
Calcium	16 mg	15 mg	30 mg
Phosphorus	41 mg	20 mg	50 mg
Magnesium	16 mg	8 mg	25 mg

RECIPES

Orange-apricot cookies

I cup all-purpose flour
3/4 cup whole-wheat flour
1/4 cup sugar
2 teaspoons baking powder
1/2 teaspoon ground cinnamon
1/4 teaspoon salt

3/4 cup dried apricots, chopped
1/2 cup fresh orange juice
1/4 cup oil
I teaspoon grated orange rind
I egg, beaten

Preheat your oven to 375 degrees. Mix all the dry ingredients thoroughly. Add the remaining ingredients and mix well. Drop the dough by teaspoonfuls onto an ungreased baking sheet, about one inch apart. Bake for about 11 minutes or until lightly browned. Remove the cookies from the baking sheet while still warm and cool them on a rack. Makes 4 dozen cookies.

Per cookie:
40 calories
1 gram fat

6 mg cholesterol
29 mg sodium

Garden couscous salad

Couscous is a crushed grain that is delicious when used as a base for salads or as a side dish. This pretty combination of couscous, finely chopped vegetables and dried fruit can be served as an appetizer or a first course on a crisp lettuce or cabbage leaf, or served in a large bowl.

> 3 cups couscous cooked according to package directions
> 3 carrots, chopped
> 2 celery stalks, finely chopped
> 2 tomatoes, finely diced
> 1/2 cucumber, seeded and finely chopped
> 1 small Bermuda (purple) onion, finely chopped
> 1 large garlic clove, finely minced
> 1 cup fresh parsley, finely minced
> 2 scallions (use white and green portions), finely chopped
> 1 cup fresh mint, finely minced (or 1/4 cup dried mint or
>   you may substitute parsley)
> 1/4 cup dried apricots, finely chopped
> 1/4 cup dates, finely chopped
> 2 tablespoons olive oil
> 1 tablespoon lemon juice, or to taste
> 1/2 teaspoon ground allspice, or to taste
> 1/8 teaspoon white pepper
> 1/4 teaspoon salt (optional)

Prepare couscous according to package directions. Set aside and cool. In a large bowl, combine the remaining ingredients and couscous. The vegetables and fruit can be chopped in a food processor or blender to ease preparation. Chill before serving. Best if made and served the same day.

16 servings, 1/2 cup each
Calories: 84 per serving
Fat: 1.9 grams per serving
Calories from fat: 20%

Raisin apricot oatmeal bars

Looking for a healthy, high-fiber treat to take to your next party or offer guests? Raisin apricot bars are delicious and nutritious. The apricots give them a tart bite while the raisins are sweet. You'd never think these bars are actually a healthier alternative to high-fat cookies and desserts.

FILLING

I cup dried apricots, chopped
I cup raisins, chopped
1/4 cup sugar

I tablespoon cornstarch
1-1/4 cups water

CRUST

1-1/2 cups quick cooking
  oatmeal, coarsely ground
1/3 cup margarine
I cup brown sugar

2 tablespoons honey
1-1/2 cups whole wheat flour
1/2 teaspoon baking soda
I tablespoon water

ICING

I cup confectioner's sugar
  or powdered sugar

1-1/2 tablespoons skim milk
1/4 teaspoon cinnamon

Preheat oven to 350 degrees. Filling: In saucepan, combine chopped apricots, raisins, sugar, cornstarch, and water. Cook over medium heat until thickened and bubbly. Cool. Crust: Grind oatmeal in food processor or blender and set aside. Cream together in processor, blender, or with hand mixer, margarine, sugar, water and honey. Add flour and baking soda and mix until well blended. Stir in oatmeal. Firmly press one-half of mixture in lightly oiled 9 x 13- inch pan. Spread fruit mixture over top. Add one tablespoon water to remaining oatmeal mixture and sprinkle on top of filling. Bake for 25 minutes or until light golden brown. Cool.

Icing: With processor, blender, or hand mixer, whip together confectioner's sugar, cinnamon and milk until mixture reaches a drizzling consistency. Add more milk if needed. Drizzle over baked mixture and cut into 30 bars.

Variation: Two cups of any chopped dried fruit can be used. Try dried apples and dates.

Calories: 124 per bar
Fat: 2.3 grams per bar
Calories from fat: 17%

Avocados

A well-rounded fruit

Some avocados are almost round, but most of them are pear-shaped. When it comes to nutrition, however, the avocado may be the most well-rounded fruit you can eat.

- **Fruitful fiber.** If you want to boost your fiber intake, but don't like the typical fiber fare, avocados provide a fruitful alternative. They have more fiber than almost any other fruit, about 4.7 grams in a medium avocado. That's about as much fiber as you'll get in a cup of raisin bran cereal.

- **B vitamins.** The B vitamins work together to keep you healthy and energized. Avocados contain all these important vitamins, but they are a particularly good source of folic acid. Folic acid is a B vitamin that may help prevent heart disease and certain birth defects. Folic acid is found in many plant foods, but much of it is destroyed during cooking or processing. Since avocados are usually eaten raw, they provide a healthy dose of folic acid, as well as the other B vitamins.

- **Extra antioxidants.** Antioxidants in your diet may protect against a variety of potential ailments, including cancer. Avocados are a rich source of potent antioxidant vitamins E and C.

- **A medley of minerals.** To round out their nutritious contributions to your diet, avocados provide several essential minerals. They are particularly high in potassium, a mineral that helps regulate your heartbeat and your breathing. Avocados can also add iron, magnesium, manganese, phosphorus, zinc, and copper to your mineral stores.

Avocado facial

Avocados may be good for the outside of your body as well as the inside. For years, people have used avocado as a natural facial treatment. Mash some up and mix it with a little milk or oatmeal and smooth it on for smoother skin.

Cutting cholesterol with avocados

If you care about your heart, you try to keep your cholesterol level under control. Research finds that avocados in your diet could help. One study gave people with slightly high cholesterol levels and people with normal levels of cholesterol a diet enriched with avocados. After seven days, even the healthy people who received the avocado diet had 16 percent lower cholesterol levels, and the people with high cholesterol had an even greater improvement in their cholesterol levels.

History of the avocado

The avocado was reportedly first eaten by a Mayan princess around 291 B.C. It was introduced into southern Florida in the 1830s. Americans called the fruit the "alligator pear" because of its skin color and texture, and because they couldn't pronounce the Spanish word for it, "aguacate." Aguacate came from an Aztec word, "ahuacatl," which meant "testicle." The word avocado was first used for the fruit in 1669, although some people still refer to them as "alligator pears."

The fat of the matter

You may have heard that you shouldn't eat avocados because they are high in fat. Avocados do contain more fat than most fruits, around 30 grams compared to less than one gram for most fresh fruits. So if you are on a low-fat diet, avocados may not be the best choice for your daily fruit. However, most of the fat in avocados is monounsaturated fat, which is healthier for you than saturated fat. Studies find that replacing saturated fats with unsaturated fats in your diet can reduce your risk of heart disease. If you use avocado to replace mayonnaise or butter, you may actually be cutting your fat intake. If you are on a low-fat diet, keep in mind that if you cut your fat intake too low, you run the risk of not getting enough vitamin E. Avocados can provide a natural source of vitamin E and a healthier type of fat.

Buying and storing avocados

You're an expert at thumping melons and picking just the right bunch of bananas, but you're not sure how to shop or care for avocados. Here's some information to help you make the most of this unusual fruit.

Ripe avocados are still firm, but yield to gentle pressure when squeezed in your palm. However, most avocados available at your store are not yet ripe. Choose ones that are heavy for their size and have no dark sunken spots or cracked or broken surfaces. For speedy ripening, place them in a paper bag at room temperature. For slower ripening, store in the refrigerator.

Once you cut into an avocado, the flesh tends to turn brown rapidly. Add avocado to your dishes just before serving if possible. You can also put the peeled fruit in lemon or lime juice to help prevent discoloration.

Comparing coasts

When it comes to nutrition, all avocados are not created equal. Whether your avocado was grown on the East Coast or the West Coast of the United States can make a difference. Here's a comparison of average avocados grown in California and those grown in Florida. How does your coast stack up?

	California avocado	Florida avocado
Weight	100 grams	100 grams
Calories	177	112
Fat	17.3 grams	8.87 grams
Vitamin A	612 IU	612 IU
Vitamin C	7.9 mg	7.9 mg
Folic acid	65.5 mcg	53.3 mcg
Calcium	11 mg	11 mg
Potassium	634 mg	488 mg
Iron	1.18 mg	.53 mg

Working avocados into your diet

If the avocado's nutrition appeals to you, but the thought of munching one like an apple doesn't, here are some tips on using avocados.

- Toss some fresh avocado slices in your tossed salads.
- Replace the mayonnaise in your favorite sandwich with mashed avocado for a change of pace.
- Dice them up and drop them onto an omelette.
- Add cubes of avocado to your salsa for extra flavor.
- Use in place of cream cheese or butter on bagels or toast.
- Try it on a baked potato instead of butter or sour cream.

RECIPES

Guacamole dip

6 avocados	1-1/2 tablespoons vinegar
Juice from half a lemon	1 tablespoon low-fat mayonnaise
1/2 cup chopped tomato	1 tablespoon olive oil
1 hot pepper	

Mix together and then refrigerate

California guacamole — diabetic diet

2 medium California avocados	3 tablespoons tomato, chopped
3 tablespoons fresh lemon juice	1/2 teaspoon salt
1/2 cup onion, diced	2 tablespoons cilantro, minced

Cut the avocados in half and remove the seeds. Scoop out the pulp and place in a bowl. Drizzle with the lemon juice and mash. Combine with the remaining ingredients; mix well and serve. Makes 12 servings.

Calories per serving: 55
Fat per serving: 5 grams

Citrus salad with California avocado

3 medium corn tortillas	2 tablespoons raspberry vinegar
3 medium oranges	I medium California avocado,
3 medium grapefruit	peeled and sliced
I tablespoon honey	
6 sprigs fresh mint for garnish (optional)	

Slice the tortillas into very thin strips. Dry the strips by placing them on a cookie sheet and baking them in a preheated 225-degree oven for approximately 15 minutes. Set aside.

Grate the rind of the three oranges. Set aside. Peel, section, and seed the oranges and grapefruit, removing the bitter white membrane. Set the sections aside.

In a large bowl, mix honey, raspberry vinegar, and the orange and grapefruit sections. Add the grated orange rind and toss gently. Top with avocado slices, tortilla strips, and a sprig of fresh mint for garnish. Makes 6 servings.

Calories per serving: 169
Fat per serving: 6 grams

California avocado tacos

I ripe California avocado,	I cup fresh cilantro, finely chopped
peeled and seeded	I-1/2 cups fresh tomato salsa
I medium onion, julienned	(see below)
I large green pepper, julienned	12 flour tortillas
I large red pepper, julienned	nonstick cooking spray

Spray your skillet with cooking spray. Lightly sautè the onion and green and red peppers. Cut the avocado into 12 slices. Warm the tortillas in the oven and fill with peppers, onion, avocado slices, and salsa. Fold the tortillas and serve. Makes 12 servings.

Fresh tomato salsa

I cup tomatoes, diced	1/3 teaspoon jalapeno peppers,
1/3 cup onions, diced	chopped
1/2 clove garlic, minced	1/2 teaspoon lime juice
2 teaspoons cilantro	pinch of cumin

Mix together all the ingredients and refrigerate.

Calories per serving: 170
Fat per serving: 6 grams

BANANAS

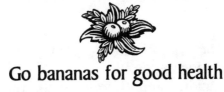

Go bananas for good health

Slipping on a banana peel may make good slap-stick comedy, but the nutrition you get from a banana is no joke. A long time ago it got its scientific name, *Musa sapientum,* which means "fruit of the wise men." And today smart people still take this fantastic fruit seriously. (Did you know it's classified as a berry? But that's another story!)

Bananas are versatile and convenient. Their sturdy skin provides a natural container, so they are easy to carry in your lunch bag or even in your hand.

Eat your bananas plain as a snack or put them in fruit salads, on breakfast cereals, or teamed up with peanut butter in a high-protein sandwich. They can be cooked in banana bread, cream pie, and banana pudding. Thicken and fortify fruit drinks with bananas. And dried banana chips make an easy snack alone or added to trail mix.

Bananas grow in the tropics. Because they are best when picked green, they have a long shelf life. This makes it easy to ship them all over the world, all year long. If you like your bananas really sweet, wait until the skin turns very yellow with brown specks before you eat them. Make bananas ripen faster by putting them in a brown paper bag.

But the best news about bananas is how good they are for you: no sodium, little fat, and no cholesterol. They are high in fiber and contain lots of vitamins C, B6. and folic acid as well as the minerals potassium and magnesium. The nutrients found in bananas help fight cancer, heart disease, and a long list of other ailments.

Bananas even help you think clearly as you age. And that alone is reason enough to give them super food status.

Plantain: the vegetable banana

The plantain is a variety of banana used for cooking, especially in the tropics. It's larger and starchier than the common banana. It's not as soft or sweet. People often bake or boil and mash it, serving it more as a vegetable than as a fruit. Latin Americans eat plantain chips like North Americans eat potato chips.

Plantains are high in most of the same vitamins and minerals as regular bananas. In addition, plantains are high in vitamin A. That vitamin makes plantains good for your eyes, bones and teeth, skin, and immune system.

If you have ulcers, you might want to make plantains a regular part of your diet. Doctors in India frequently prescribe flour made from green plantains for peptic ulcers. Studies show, however, that ripe plantains are acidic, and therefore are not ideal for people with ulcers.

You can cook plantains in any state of ripeness. But to eat them raw you'll want them very ripe. They are not fully ripe until the skin is completely black. Plantain skins are quite tough and you'll need a knife to peel them. But it's worth the effort to get at all that nutrition.

Banana skins make good plant food

Don't toss that banana skin into the garbage! It has a lot of nutrients to enrich your plants — calcium, sodium, silica, magnesium, and especially phosphorus and potash. Just cut the skin into small pieces and bury it in the soil around the plants. Your roses and geraniums will love it.

RECIPES

Baked fruit Alaska

Baked fruit Alaska is only 2 percent fat, high in fiber and packed with vitamins. It can be served for any occasion year-round. Its red, white and blue color scheme makes it especially appropriate for the Fourth of July.

I cup blueberries	1/4 cup kirsch or cherry-
I cup strawberries, sliced	flavored brandy
I cup bananas, sliced	5 egg whites
I cup grapes, halved	2/3 cup sugar

Preheat oven to 500 degrees. Mix fruit and kirsch together and chill. Meanwhile, prepare meringue in large bowl by beating egg whites until soft peaks form. Beat until stiff peaks form. Portion fruit into custard or other oven-proof serving dishes. Top and seal each dish with a generous dollop of meringue. With spoon, swirl meringue to a decorative peak. Place on cookie sheet or baking pan and bake for 3 minutes or until meringue is golden. Serve immediately. Makes 6 servings.

Variation: Any combination of 4 cups of fresh or frozen fruit may be used.

Calories: 184 per serving
Fat: .5 grams per serving
Calories from fat: 2%

The banana bread of kings

I cup ready-to-eat bran cereal	1/4 cup + 2 tablespoons boiling
I cup ripe mashed banana	water
(2 or 3)	1/2 cup sifted flour
3 tablespoons applesauce	2 teaspoons baking soda
(replacing shortening)	1/2 teaspoon salt
1/2 cup sugar	

Measure the bran, banana, applesauce, and sugar in a large bowl. Add water and stir. In another bowl, sift together the flour, baking soda, and salt (or don't sift it — stirring it well with fork works also). Add this to the banana mixture, stirring only until combined. Pour it into a bread pan and stick it in the oven. Bake at 350 degrees for about 45 minutes.

Fruity oatmeal cookies

Making these high-fiber, nutritious cookies with kids is a great activity throughout the year.

2 small, very ripe bananas	I cup all purpose flour
2 cups unsweetened applesauce	3/4 teaspoon baking soda
3 tablespoons margarine	1/2 teaspoon salt (optional)
2 eggs	/2 teaspoon ground nutmeg
2 teaspoons vanilla	1/2 teaspoon ground cinnamon
2 cups oatmeal	3/4 cup currants or raisins
I cup whole wheat flour	

Preheat oven to 350 degrees. Combine bananas, applesauce, margarine, eggs, and vanilla. In large bowl, mix together oatmeal, flours, baking soda, salt, spices, and currants or raisins. Add combined fruit mixture to dry ingredients until just blended. Drop by rounded tablespoons onto ungreased cookie sheets. Bake for 25 minutes or until light golden brown. Makes 40 cookies.

Variation: Fruit-n-Sauces (such as Apple-n-Apricot, Apple-n-Pineapple, or Apple-n-Cherry) can be used instead of applesauce.

Calories: 61 per cookie
Fat: 1 gram per cookie
Calories from fat: 20%

Baked banana

We often think of bananas in cold dishes — banana splits, congealed salads, and frozen desserts. But for a warm cold-weather treat, try baking a banana in its skin. Put a whole ripe banana on a cookie sheet. Bake it for 20 minutes at 350 degress. Split the skin with a knife and sprinkle with nutmeg or cinnamon.

BROCCOLI

The best of broccoli

Broccoli is a terrific vegetable with a terrible reputation. Even a U.S. President pronounced it "yucky." Fortunately, new scientific research has shown broccoli to be a star performer in the vegetable world when it comes to fighting vitamin deficiencies and disease. Here are some of broccoli's best points:

- **Vitamin C.** The high level of vitamin C in broccoli makes it a close rival of citrus fruits. It helps protect you from gallstones, cataracts, and the memory loss that often comes with aging. Broccoli's vitamin C may also help lower your high blood pressure. One spear of raw broccoli contains 141 milligrams (mg) of vitamin C, more than twice the RDA of 60 mg.

- **Beta carotene.** If you're a smoker, taking supplements of vitamin A or beta carotene (which your body turns into vitamin A) may be risky, according to recent research. But you really need these nutrients to protect you from lung cancer. Getting your beta carotene or vitamin A from a fresh source such as broccoli is a smart move. Eating lots of vegetables containing beta carotene also lowers your risk of age-related macular degeneration, the leading cause of blindness in older adults. Cook up one cup of frozen broccoli and you'll get a whopping 3,500 IU of vitamin A, three and a half times the RDA for men and more than four times the RDA for women.

- **Selenium.** To fight against free-radical damage and protect your eyes from cataracts, you need a high level of the mineral selenium. Selenium may also fight cancer by boosting your immune system and repairing damaged cells. Lightly cook some fresh broccoli for a good dose of selenium.
- **Calcium.** Your body needs calcium to build and keep strong bones so you don't have to cope with osteoporosis. New research shows it may protect you from colon cancer, too. Dairy products supply the most calcium, but broccoli is a good additional source. In one cup of cooked frozen broccoli, you get 94 mg of calcium, contributing to the 800 mg you need every day.
- **Folic acid.** One of the nutrients that may guard against memory loss is folic acid. It also helps prevent birth defects. Broccoli is a good source of folic acid, but for this nutrient you need to eat it raw. Cooking destroys almost half of the folic acid in broccoli.
- **Fiber.** If you have diabetes, fiber can help you keep your blood sugar on an even keel. Fiber also helps keep your body running smoothly and prevents constipation. One serving of raw broccoli contains 3 to 5 grams of fiber. If you prefer eating your broccoli cooked, it still retains every bit of its beneficial fiber.

An age-old treat

Broccoli appeared in the earliest known cookbook, written by a Roman in the first century A.D. The recipe was for broiled broccoli, a favorite of the son of the Roman emperor Tiberius. By the third century A.D., broccoli was a frequent part of the Roman citizen's evening meal.

Beware of broccoli

As wonderful and nutritious as broccoli is, it does have a couple of small strikes against it. First, it is one of those veggies that may give you that bloated feeling. Because it's rich in carbohydrates and insoluble fiber, it's naturally more gas-producing than many foods. You might try your stalks cooked, rather than raw, to see if cooking cuts down on the gassiness. Eating a small quantity, rather than a huge plateful, might make your broccoli more digestible. And if all else fails, you might try a gas-inhibiting product such as Beano to ward off the unpleasant side effects of a great food.

The other negative aspect of broccoli may affect you if you're a woman going through menopause. Researchers have recently found that broccoli contains a substance that counteracts the hormone estrogen. So if you're trying to get more estrogen in your body, either through diet or replacement therapy, broccoli could be working against you. Try leaving broccoli out of your diet temporarily to see if there's an improvement in your menopause symptoms.

A matter of taste

You know broccoli is full of good things for your health, but you just can't stand the taste. What's a health-conscious person to do? If you like the idea of broccoli, but it just doesn't taste good to you, it may not be a matter of preference. You may have been born with too much taste.

Scientists have discovered that some people actually have more taste buds than others and are more sensitive to flavors, especially bitter or sweet ones. It seems that people can be divided into three categories: nontasters, about 25 percent of the population; medium tasters, about 50 percent; and super-tasters, about 25 percent. People who are super-tasters have far more taste buds per square centimeter of tongue surface compared to nontasters. It's the super-tasters who may be most bothered by the taste of broccoli and other bitter foods like cabbage and grapefruit.

If you are truly troubled by the taste of broccoli, you might want to find some other foods to substitute for the nutrients it contains. And don't fall for those broccoli pills you see in the health food store, which promise a shortcut to all the benefits of broccoli with none of the taste. Researchers have shown that the special qualities that make broccoli so great can't be put in a pill; you have to eat the real thing.

Little sprouts fight cancer

In 1992, scientists at Johns Hopkins University discovered a potent compound, sulfurophane, that may prevent cancer. Sulfurophane triggers enzymes in your body that neutralize cancer-causing substances before they can do any damage. They also found that broccoli was a potent source of this helpful chemical. Now the same researchers have found another food with even more sulfurophane —

broccoli sprouts. Three-day-old sprouts of the broccoli plant contain 20 to 50 times the amount of this cancer-fighting substance as mature broccoli plants.

The sprouts have some big advantages over regular broccoli. They grow in three days instead of the two months it takes to cultivate a mature stem of broccoli, and the amount you have to eat for its cancer-fighting benefits is much smaller. Scientists say the sprouts, a little spicier than alfalfa sprouts, are a tasty addition to salads and sandwiches. And in case broccoli isn't your favorite flavor, they don't even taste like broccoli. The only drawback is that you can't buy them — at least not yet.

Scientists caution that you shouldn't try to grow broccoli sprouts from commercially available broccoli seeds, which are treated with fungicides and pesticides. But keep your eyes open for vegetable growers to soon start investing in this little powerhouse of disease-fighting potential. Broccoli sprouts could be the next real health food.

Broccoli — best cooked or raw?

If you want to get the most from the nutrients in broccoli, should you cook it or eat it raw? Well, it depends. If you want to get vitamin C from your broccoli, it's best to munch on the raw spears. You get somewhat less C when fresh broccoli is cooked, and a lot less when you eat frozen, cooked broccoli. If you want to get lots of vitamin A, you should get frozen broccoli and boil it. Frozen, cooked broccoli has more vitamin A than raw or fresh cooked. For getting the most fiber, eat it any way you like. Broccoli's fiber content isn't really affected by cooking.

RECIPES

Broccoli soup

1-1/2 cups chopped broccoli or
1 box of frozen, chopped broccoli
1/4 cup diced celery
1/4 cup chopped onion

2 tablespoons cornstarch
1/4 teaspoon salt
dash of pepper
dash of ground thyme

1 cup chicken broth, unsalted   1/4 cup Swiss cheese, shredded
2 cups skim milk

Place vegetables and broth in saucepan. Bring to a boil, reduce heat, cover, and cook until vegetables are tender — about 8 minutes. Mix milk, cornstarch, salt, pepper, and thyme; add to cooked vegetables. Cook, stirring constantly, until soup is slightly thickened and mixture just begins to boil. Remove from heat. Add cheese and stir until melted. Makes 4 one-cup servings.

Calories per serving: 110
Fat per serving: 3 grams

Chicken divan

10 oz. fresh or frozen   1/2 teaspoon curry powder
   broccoli spears   1/2 teaspoon pepper
3/4 - 1 lb. chicken,   12 oz. evaporated skim milk
   cooked and deboned   1/4 cup Parmesan cheese, grated
1 tablespoon margarine   2 tablespoons sherry or dry white
2 tablespoons flour   wine - optional

Preheat oven to 350 degrees. Steam broccoli until tender-crisp. Lay on bottom of lightly greased baking dish with flower heads toward sides of dish. Lay chicken on broccoli. Melt margarine with flour, curry, and pepper, stirring into a paste. On low heat, slowly add milk and stir until thickened. Stir in cheese and sherry or wine. Pour over broccoli and chicken. Bake 30 minutes. Makes 4 servings. Quick and easy hint: This is a great recipe for leftover chicken or turkey.

Calories: 354 per serving
Fat: 10 grams per serving
Calories from fat: 25%
Sodium: 324 mg per serving

Serving tip: Serve with brown and wild rice and sliced tomato salad.

Italian chicken stir-fry

4 chicken breast halves (boneless)
2 tablespoons peanut oil
1-1/2 cups broccoli, in small pieces
   (or 1 10-oz. frozen package)
1 large green pepper, in 1-inch squares
1 teaspoon basil

1/4 - 1/2 teaspoon garlic powder
3 medium tomatoes, chopped
   (or 2 - 2-1/2 cups canned, chopped)

To debone chicken, trim off all skin and fat. Remove from bones. (Slide knife between ribs and meat to loosen meat, working toward the breast bone. Pull and cut as needed to separate.) Cut meat into 1-inch cubes.

Heat wok, electric fry pan, or large skillet over high heat for 30 seconds. Add oil, swirl to cover pan bottom and heat 30 seconds. Scatter chicken into pan and turn rapidly and continuously. Cook 1/2 – 1 minute, then add broccoli, green pepper, garlic powder, and herbs. Cook, still stirring, until vegetables are almost to desired stage of crisp-tenderness (about 1/2 – 1 minute). Add tomatoes and stir until heated through and mixed well. Makes 4 servings.

Calories: 255 per serving
Fat: 10 grams per serving

GARLIC

"One must be very suspicious of anyone who does not eat garlic."
Romanian Proverb

A moment in history

This fragrant bulb was valued so highly in ancient Egypt, that not only was it used as a form of currency, but they recorded its qualities on the walls of the Great Pyramid at Giza. The laborers that built the pyramid were fed chickpeas, onions, and garlic to give them the strength to complete their awesome task.

A tasty weapon against heart disease

Several of the separate qualities that make garlic so important to overall health combine to form one big heart disease-fighting package. Because it lowers bad cholesterol, increases good cholesterol, and helps prevent blood clots, you can battle atherosclerosis, heart attack, and stroke in one fell swoop.

There may be no other single food that lowers cholesterol as dramatically as this simple seasoning. In one study, test subjects ate one-half to one clove of garlic every day for eight to 24 weeks. Their cholesterol levels dropped by as much as 9 percent.

Other studies have discovered a compound, ajoene, that thins your blood and helps prevent your platelets from clumping together. This means fewer blood clots that could lead to heart attacks and stroke.

And last, experiments show that eating garlic can lower high blood pressure. Just by adding garlic to your diet, you can reduce the risk of all forms of heart-related diseases.

'Anti-' up with garlic

Antibacterial, antiviral, and antifungal. These are the three big healing properties of garlic. For thousands of years, man has been using garlic in folk remedies to treat all kinds of ailments, everything from leprosy to deafness. But since scientists discovered chemical properties in garlic that fight bacterial, viral, and fungal infections, they are approving many of these ancient cures.

They say that although garlic may not cure leprosy, it will attack strep throat, urinary tract infections, influenza, intestinal disorders, candidiasis, and various bacteria. It goes after *H. pylori,* the ulcer-causing bacteria, and takes out staph and yeast infections. Eat it for diarrhea, bronchitis, asthma, and gallbladder disorders.

If you think that garlic is the super food of the future, you may be pleased to discover that scientists are beginning to think that, too. They are conducting more research than ever before in order to learn all of garlic's healing secrets.

A clove or 2 combats cancer

Perhaps the most exciting area of garlic research is in cancer prevention. The USDA rated garlic as having the highest antioxidant level of all the common vegetables, which means it can really battle those cancer-causing free radicals.

How does it do this? Scientists know that garlic contains selenium, a trace mineral necessary to the antioxidant enzyme, glutathione peroxidase. They also know that selenium can do the same job as vitamin E, another powerful antioxidant. There may be other characteristics of garlic that give it that cancer-fighting one-two punch, but the bottom line is that studies have proven that a diet rich in garlic protects against a variety of cancers by boosting your immune system and reducing the growth of malignant cells.

Did you know?

How much do you love garlic? If you are a true-blue, dyed-in-the-wool fan of "the stinking rose," there are many ways to indulge your passion. You can buy a garlic lover's cookbook; attend a garlic festival, (the largest one is held every year in the garlic capital of the world, Gilroy, California); or talk to other garlic addicts by calling the garlic information hotline at 1-800-330-5922.

To market, to market

Buying garlic can be quite complicated nowadays. There are so many varieties and sizes to choose from. You can select produce grown anywhere from California to Europe, with cloves ranging from bean-size to softball-size. There is the small, young variety called green garlic, which is quite mild in flavor, and the traditional American garlic which is white and very strong-tasting. With a flavor somewhere in between is the pinkish Mexican and Italian garlics. The largest is, of course, the elephant garlic, produced mainly in California. This type can grow to the size of a grapefruit. To find this mild garlic that is really a leek, however, you may have to visit a gourmet food store.

Choose garlic bulbs that are firm, not soft or moldy. The outer white husk should be dry and peel off easily. Avoid garlic that has sprouted or that breaks apart, since this means the bulbs are not fresh. Don't use any cloves that have turned brown.

Garlic will keep for as long as six months if you store it in a cool, dark place with good circulation. However, the sooner you use it, the stronger the flavor will be.

To get the most health benefit and the best flavor, crush or chop the cloves, since this causes a chemical reaction that releases important enzymes and the distinctive garlic odor. To get rid of garlic breath, suck on a lemon or chew a sprig of parsley.

Garlic is inexpensive, abundant, and healthy — so are you cooking with it tonight?

An onion a day

The onion is from the same plant family as the garlic, which means you can get many similar health benefits from either vegetable. Whether you are looking to prevent high blood pressure or battle cancer, the onion is a great natural weapon. In fact, many scientists want to take advantage of today's technology to genetically improve the healing qualities in certain foods, like the onion. Some day you may slice up a "super onion" for your ailments instead of popping a pill.

RECIPES

Cauliflower — northern Italian style

Different than any cauliflower you've had before, this features the red wine and garlic flavors of northern Italy. If you plan to cook less than the full amount of cauliflower in this recipe, do not reduce the quantity of liquids or seasonings for best results.

     I small-to-medium head cauliflower
     2 tablespoons olive oil
     4 cloves of garlic, finely minced
     1/8 teaspoon finely ground pepper
     2 tablespoons red wine vinegar
     2 tablespoons water

Trim cauliflower and separate into small flowerets. Heat large skillet or wok over medium-high heat for 30 seconds, add olive oil, and heat for another 20 – 30 seconds. Reduce heat to medium and sauté garlic in the heated oil, stirring constantly, until just starting to brown. Add cauliflower and stir for 2 – 3 minutes. Add pepper, vinegar, and water. Cook over low heat, covered, about 10 minutes. Makes about 4 one-cup servings.

Calories: 78 per serving
Fat: 5 grams per serving

Tip: Broccoli can also be prepared in this manner.

Sopa de Ajo (Cuban garlic soup)

16 cloves garlic	3 eggs
8 slices bread, no crust,	2 large white onions,
cubed into croutons	coarsely chopped
1/2 cup extra virgin olive oil	salt and pepper to taste
2 quarts chicken stock	

Heat the olive oil in a large, deep skillet. Coarsely chop the garlic and fry it in the oil until it is crisp. Strain the garlic from the oil and set it aside. Return the oil to the skillet and heat. Add the bread cubes, turning frequently and browning until crisp. Remove the croutons and reserve. Return the oil to the heat and add more as needed to sauté your onion. When the onion is translucent, add the chicken stock. Finely chop the crisp garlic and add it to the stock. When the stock is near boil, beat eggs in a small bowl. Pour 1/2 cup of the hot stock slowly into the eggs, continuing to whisk. Remove boiling stock from heat and add the egg mixture to stock, whisking briskly until the eggs cook and thicken. Add salt and pepper to taste. Ladle this delicious, garlicky soup into large serving bowls, add reserved croutons, and enjoy. Makes 6 servings.

Baked Vidalia onion

Peel and core one medium-sized onion per person and place in baking dish just large enough to hold them. Fill cores with 1 tablespoon margarine and 1 tablespoon low sodium soy sauce. Cover and bake in preheated 350 degree oven for 45 minutes. Uncover and continue baking for another 15 minutes.

Calories: 165
Fat: 11.8 grams
Calories from fat: 62%

GRAPE JUICE

You've heard all the press about the benefits of red wine for good digestion and a healthy heart, but what if you aren't a wine drinker? Do you lose out on that extra edge of protection? Not necessarily, says new research. Scientists have studied wine and found out that the actual beneficial compounds, called polyphenolic antioxidants, come from grape skins. This explains why red wine is beneficial, but white wine is not. The grape skins are removed during the production of white wine.

But back to the real dilemma. If you don't drink red wine, how can you get all those eager little antioxidants to zap your nasty free radicals? It's an easy answer: Drink grape juice.

Even though grape juice contains only about one-third the amount of antioxidants as red wine, it still helps prevent the blood clotting that can cause heart attacks. In fact, in a recent study that tested the antioxidant activity of five commercial fruit juices, grape juice ranked the highest. This means you are fighting cancer, heart disease, and stroke with every glass.

So, if you're feeling festive, fill your wine glass with grape juice, but remember it doesn't really matter how you drink it, just as long as it's bottoms up.

A moment in history

Grape juice first became popular during the temperance movement of the late 1800s when teetotalers wanted a nonalcoholic substitute to use during communion. It was called "unfermented wine."

Nutritional know-how

Overall, unsweetened grape juice from a can or bottle is more nutritious.

	1 cup grape juice (from sweetened frozen concentrate)	1 cup grape juice (canned/bottled unsweetened)
Vitamin A	20 IU	20 IU
Vitamin C	60 mg	.25 mg
Potassium	52 mg	334 mg
Calcium	10 mg	23 mg
Phosphorus	10 mg	28 mg
Magnesium	10 mg	25 mg

RECIPES

Fruit juice cubes

I-1/2 tablespoons (I-1/2 envelopes) unflavored gelatin
3/4 cup water
6-ounce can frozen grape juice concentrate

Very lightly grease a 9 x 5-inch loaf pan or plastic ice cube trays. Soften the gelatin in water in a small saucepan for five minutes. Heat over low heat, stirring constantly, until the gelatin dissolves. Remove from heat. Add the fruit juice concentrate and mix well. Pour into your pan. Cover and refrigerate until it is set. Cut into 1-inch cubes or remove from ice cube trays. Keep covered in refrigerator. Makes 45 cubes.

Calories per cube: 10
Fat per cube: trace

Nonalcoholic grape juice cocktail

If plain grape juice isn't your "cup of juice," try adding carbonated soda to increase its appeal.

I part grape juice (red or white)
I part ginger ale

Chill liquids separately and add ginger ale just before serving. Serve in a punch bowl or pitcher.

GRAPEFRUIT

Did you know?

Grapefruit was so named because the fruit grows in clusters, like grapes.

Everyone has heard of the old grapefruit diet. And thousands of people probably lost some weight while they were on it. But now you're going to have to think of the humble grapefruit in a whole new light: as more than just a sunny Florida breakfast fruit. Hold onto your spoon, because grapefruit are the newest weapon against two very serious conditions.

Counter cancer. While you're reading the morning paper and scooping out those delicious sections or downing a glass of that tangy pink juice for a mid-morning pick-me-up, you may be fighting breast cancer at the same time. A recent animal study showed that mice had 50 percent fewer tumors and tumors that spread to other parts of the body when they were given grapefruit juice instead of water. Researchers believe that the flavonoids act with other elements in citrus juices to check breast tumors. Of course, human studies need to be done, but in the meantime, a round of applause for the ruby red.

Combat cholesterol. While scientists were studying the cancer-fighting effects of this tasty citrus, they stumbled upon yet another benefit: grapefruit reduced LDL cholesterol levels by as much as 43 percent in animal tests.

> Try sprinkling a halved grapefruit with brown sugar and broiling until hot and bubbly. A great cold-weather idea for this tasty fruit.

Drugs and grapefruit. Grapefruit may be on the next prescription your doctor writes for you, especially if you have high blood pressure. One test found that a man taking nifedipine and terazosin to lower his blood pressure had remarkable improvement when he simply began drinking grapefruit juice. If an organ transplant is in the cards for you, consider grapefruit as part of your recovery process. Studies have shown that a specific substance found only in grapefruit may help prevent transplant recipients from rejecting transplanted organs.

> Do you like to add grapefruit to your fruit salad? Here's a quick and easy tip for loosening the peel of a whole grapefruit. Drop it into boiling water for 60 seconds.

The best of the crop. If you want the most vitamin A you can get, choose pink grapefruit rather than white. Even though both varieties are full of antioxidants, vitamin C, fiber, and potassium, the yellow-pink to ruby red will give you that little extra nutritional value.

You can enjoy grapefruit at any time of the year, since crops are harvested from California, Arizona, Texas, and Florida. Choose heavy, brightly colored fruit with thin skin. Put them in a plastic bag and store them for up to two weeks in the refrigerator.

Nutritional information: (1/2 fresh grapefruit)
Vitamin A   149 IU
Vitamin C   41 mg

GREEN TEA

The green key to a happy heart

In the Far East, green tea has been a staple of most cultures' diets for more than 2,000 years. Green tea's pleasant taste and aroma, its low cost, and its role in Eastern traditions all have had something to do with its popularity. But now, modern science is proving that tea has a much more tangible, medicinal value. Available just about anywhere, green (and in some cases black) tea is more than just a good drink, it's heart-healthy.

In one recent study, volunteers drank about 3 cups of black tea every day. After four weeks, researchers found that their arteries resisted the build up of cholesterol. The study showed that the flavonoids in tea may help prevent hardening of the arteries and thus guard your body against heart disease. Some health experts even predict that tea flavonoid supplementation might be the wave of the future for heart health. But for now, drinking tea looks like a good way to start.

Another study that followed Japanese tea drinkers over the course of nearly five years showed that having several cups of green tea a day reduced cholesterol and triglyceride levels significantly. This study also showed a direct relationship between how much green tea was consumed and the rate of heart disease. For those people who drank more tea, the incidence of heart disease was much less than for people who did not. It should be noted, however, that the best results were achieved by people who drank 10 cups of green tea per day. Also, the benefits appeared to be greater for men than for women.

It's all in the processing

Green tea is green and black tea is black because of how it's processed. The leaves come from the same plant, but to make green tea, the leaves are merely picked and steamed — almost no processing at all. To get black tea, the leaves must be processed a lot longer and allowed to ferment. There is an in-between tea, too, called Oolong, and its fermentation process is shorter than black tea's. From light and mild to floral and fruity and spicy to classic, there's a tea for every taste.

Your liver will love you for it

Everything you consume finds its way through your liver, in one form or another, the good stuff and the bad. Sometimes it seems like there are a thousand easy ways to damage this vital organ, but not much you can do to give it a boost. Luckily, green tea is a way to show your liver that you still care.

A study of Japanese tea drinkers that showed a reduced incidence of heart disease also showed that green tea can save your liver. Over the course of the study, men who drank green tea every day had much less cell damage to their livers than men who did not. This is good news indeed, since there are so many ways to make life hard on your liver. A few cups of green tea each day might be the way to easy street.

A kick in the cancer

Think you can keep cancer away with a warm beverage? It might sound too good to be true, but the evidence is building. Green tea and tea extract contain strong antioxidants that can help stop the formation and development of some tumors.

Researchers have found that one of the main tannins in green tea is a compound that can prevent the development and growth of various types of cancer. This compound inhibits the growth of some of the worst and most common cancers, including skin, stomach, colon, liver, pancreatic, lung, and breast. This compound can also combat cancer that has already formed, and it has been shown to lengthen the lives of people who have already been diagnosed with cancer.

Maybe the most encouraging news about green tea is that you can start seeing positive effects no matter when you start drinking it. In some studies, the tea was able to attack the growth of stomach cancer even during the later stages of development. These same studies indicated that the protective benefits of green tea were no less significant for people who started drinking it later in life.

Tea time

Most people in Western cultures drink black teas, perhaps because until recently, green teas were hard to find. Today, however, most major tea brands put out green tea varieties, which are available at almost any grocery store.

This is good news for Americans. Although both green and black teas have proven health benefits, green tea is clearly the healthier choice. If you're still not convinced, consider this: Japan, where green tea is a part of a typical daily diet, has twice the smoking rate of the United States, but only half the rate of lung cancer.

LEGUMES

The other 'meat'

Question: What grows in a garden and is packed full of protein? Answer: Peas and beans, better known as legumes. They are blessed with so many essential nutrients, and so few drawbacks, that it's tempting to think of legumes as the perfect food. And in many ways they are.

Legumes are plants whose seeds develop in pods. The most widely consumed of these are beans, peas, lentils, peanuts, and soybeans. Legumes can be eaten raw or cooked in any number of dishes. Cannellini beans, pea pods, and cooked fava beans are delicious when tossed into salads, while lentils and kidney beans are great for adding flavor and thickness to soups, stews, and chilies. Whether you buy them dry or fresh, legumes could very well be your diet's best friend.

Almost all legumes are low in fat, but high in carbohydrates and fiber. And because they contain so many of the vitamins and minerals provided by meats, legumes are generally considered a good dietary replacement for meat.

Protein powerhouse

Is there such a thing as a better meat than meat? Sounds like a silly question, but it's not. In fact, legumes are loaded with many of the same nutrients as meat, without nearly as much fat and calories.

Although a serving of beans might not contain as much protein as a T-bone steak, most experts agree that Americans already get twice as much protein as they need. And an excess of protein, in the long run, can put a strain on your kidneys and liver and make it more difficult for your body to absorb other nutrients. Some studies have even shown that by switching just half of your protein intake from meat to legume sources, you can lower your cholesterol by 10 percent or more.

One of the most popular legumes, the peanut, is particularly high in protein. Unfortunately, it is also high in fat. On the plus side, the vegetable fat from peanut oil is better for your body than animal fat, and contains no cholesterol. So why not go a little nutty? (Sounds better than "legumey," don't you think?)

Fiber-fest

Like their cousins the leafy greens, legumes are a good source of fiber. Beans are especially rich in fiber, whether you prefer them fresh or dried. Kidney beans, lentils, and soybeans will help keep your digestive system up and running. In many cases, legumes have more fiber than foods that are known for their high fiber content. The two tables below show how legumes measure up.

Fiber content of selected legumes (1/2 cup serving)

Kidney beans	7.3 g
Navy beans	6.0 g
Lima beans	4.5 g
Lentils	3.7 g
Peas	3.6 g

Fiber content of selected foods (1/2 cup serving)

Bran flakes	2.7 g
Celery	1.1 g
Brown rice	1.0 g
Spaghetti	0.6 g
Lettuce	0.5 g

Get your vitamin B(ean)

As if being low in fat and calories, yet high in fiber and protein, were not enough, legumes go a big step further. Most peas and beans are packed with vitamins and minerals. They're a good source of vitamins B1, B3, and B6. Most are also a great way to get extra calcium.

Many beans have their own unique nutritional strengths, too. The soybean, for example, is rich in the B vitamins that are so important to the healthy function of your brain and metabolism. If you're looking for a tasty way to put more zinc in your body, try a little black bean soup. For extra iron, a small serving of navy beans will do the trick. Lima beans are particularly rich in potassium, while black-eyed peas are your best bet for magnesium.

All beans contain phytoestrogens, substances that are similar to natural estrogen, and tests show that they ease the symptoms of menopause. Soybeans seem to be the richest source of phytoestrogens.

The soy luck club

Perhaps the most versatile of all the legumes is the soybean. The nutritional value of soybeans can be savored through dozens of soybean and soy-based products, staples of many Eastern diets for thousands of years. In addition to helping with menopause, this little bean is also thought to be able to lower the risk of certain types of cancer.

Although soy-based meat substitutes like "soy burgers" can provide you with some of soy's nutritious benefits, you'll get the greatest benefit from eating the bean itself. Dried soybeans are available in most grocery stores and supermarkets. For fresh soybeans, you might have to visit an Asian market or health food store. For more information about soybeans, see the *Soy* chapter.

Healthy tips for tasty beans

Variety is the spice of life, as they say, and with legumes, you have enough variety to make interesting meals for a long time. Try some of these variations for some spicy good bean-eating.

- Add rice to black beans, then season with chili powder or Cajun spices for a real taste of the islands.
- To make "Hoppin' John," a traditional Southern dish, mix black-eyed peas and rice.
- Take a tip from salad bars and toss kidney beans or chick-peas in with your lettuce.
- For a cool alternative to the same old vegetables, chill green beans, lima beans, kidney beans, great northerns, wax beans, or chickpeas. Drizzle with a vinegar and oil dressing, let marinate for a couple of hours, and serve.

RECIPES

Three-bean chili

2/3 cup dried black beans	I teaspoon olive oil
2/3 cup dried white (navy, pea) beans	28 oz. canned tomatoes in puree or no salt added canned tomatoes
3/4 cup dried red beans	I tablespoon chili powder, may wish to add more or less
8 cups water	
I clove garlic, crushed or finely minced	I teaspoon ground cumin
	1/8 teaspoon ground allspice
I medium onion, chopped	1/2 teaspoon pepper
1/2 green pepper, chopped	I tablespoon brown sugar

Rinse beans. Add to 8 cups boiling water and boil for 2 minutes. Then set aside for 1 hour (beans can be soaked overnight if more convenient). Then simmer beans in soaking water for 1 hour or until beans are tender. In a large saucepan, sauté garlic, onion, and pepper in olive oil until tender. Add remaining ingredients and beans. Add water to bring to desired consistency. Bring to a boil. Reduce heat, cover and simmer for 30 minutes. Makes 4 – 6 servings. This chili is great frozen and reheated on another day.

Calories: 326 (larger serving)
Fat: 3 grams
Calories from fats: 8%
Sodium: 189 mg (larger serving) or 35 mg (larger serving) if low-sodium alternative is used.

Serving tip: Serve with brown or white rice and low-fat cornbread.

Nutritional plus: This dish contains very little fat and is loaded with fiber and minerals.

Quick and easy tip: Canned beans may be used in this recipe, eliminating the time spent soaking and simmering the beans. Canned beans will greatly increase sodium content. Use 16 oz. cans of each type of bean and rinse the canned beans before adding to the mixture.

Quick 'n hearty bean soup

I tablespoon vegetable oil
1/2 - 3/4 cup onion, chopped
2 cloves garlic, minced
3 cups water
I cup quick-cooking brown rice
I 15-1/2-ounce can kidney beans, drained
I 15-1/2-ounce can garbanzo beans (chickpeas), drained
I green pepper, chopped
2 cups tomato puree
I teaspoon instant low sodium chicken bouillon
2 cups raw spinach, coarsely chopped
2 teaspoons basil
I teaspoon oregano
3 tablespoons grated reduced fat Parmesan cheese (optional)

Heat oil in large saucepan or Dutch oven over medium heat. Add onion and garlic; cook 2 minutes until onion has softened. Add all remaining ingredients except parmesan cheese. Increase heat to bring to a boil, then reduce heat and cover. Simmer 5 – 10 minutes until rice is cooked. Ladle into bowls to serve. Sprinkle each with approximately 2 teaspoons grated Parmesan cheese if desired. Makes 4 servings.

Calories: 267 per serving (288 with cheese)
Fat: 5 grams per serving
Calories from fat: 17%

OAT BRAN

The cholesterol cure?

Scientists used to think the only reason oat bran was so good at lowering cholesterol was because people were eating it instead of fatty foods. Through numerous dietary studies, this theory was put to the test. It turns out it was the oat bran that was doing the trick. The secret: a soluble fiber called beta-glucan. Now researchers know that the soluble fiber in oat bran can reduce cholesterol in your bloodstream even when other attempts have failed.

In one study, 59 people who had not been able to reduce their LDL cholesterol using a conventional low-fat diet were able to lower their levels an average of 9.5 percent when given an oat bran supplement. This effect is not common to all kinds of bran, however. When put up against wheat bran in another study, for instance, oat bran decreased LDL cholesterol by 12 percent, while wheat bran had no effect at all.

So then, just how good is oat bran for you? As a cholesterol fighter, at least, it can't be beat. The beta-glucan found in oat bran is so good, in fact, that researchers are working to perfect a concentrated form so it can be added to other foods.

Soluble fiber's secret

There's a good reason why oat bran's soluble fiber is so good at lowering cholesterol. Insoluble fiber — like that found in wheat germ and brown rice — goes through your body quickly, not breaking down much and absorbing up to 15 times its weight in water. But soluble fiber like beta-glucan moves more slowly and binds with water to form a gel as it travels through your system. Some researchers think that this gel cleans up your blood by binding to bile acids, which the body produces to digest fats. Once the soluble fiber takes them out of your body through your intestines, your body has to make new bile acids from its cholesterol stores in the liver. Pulling from these reserves results in lowered cholesterol.

Help oat bran help your heart

Although it can help reduce the amount of cholesterol in your blood, you shouldn't count on oat bran alone to improve your cardiovascular health. Many doctors complain that some of their patients eat bacon and donuts and french fries all week, and then expect that a bran muffin on Sunday morning will undo the damage. This simply isn't so.

Oat bran is a great tool to help fight cholesterol, but it can't save your heart by itself. For a safe cholesterol level and sound cardiovascular health, you should watch how much cholesterol you put into your body, as well as what you do to get rid of it. Most experts recommend a diet high in fiber, yes, but also one low in salt and saturated fat. The more seriously you follow your sensible, low-fat diet, the more good oat bran will do you ... and your heart.

Diabetes super food?

Oat bran's fiber might work wonders for your blood in more ways than one. Although they aren't sure exactly how it works, doctors are sure that oat bran can help control Type II diabetes.

In one study, people with Type II diabetes ate white bread for 12 weeks and then oat bran concentrated bread products for 12 weeks. The oat bran products not only improved their insulin levels, but also reduced their cholesterol ratios by 24 percent. In other studies, diets rich in oat bran have lowered blood glucose levels and insulin production in diabetics as well as people without diabetes.

Controlling diabetes over the long haul is the most important concern of diabetics, so finding a diet that helps control blood sugar and insulin levels on a permanent basis is a top priority. Fortunately, long-term studies have also shown oat bran to be a diabetes super food. Over a six-month period, oat bran concentrate products benefited all aspects of Type II diabetes, reducing blood sugar and slowing insulin release after meals.

Just remember that altering your blood sugar through dietary changes is serious business. Starting a program of eating lots of oat bran is something that you should discuss with your doctor, especially if you are on diabetic medication.

It's more than just oats

Well, no, that's actually not true. The only true source of oat bran is, well, oats. However, if the mention of oats makes you think of a feedbag around Mr. Ed's neck, think again. There are a good number of tasty ways to put oat bran into your diet.

Of course, nothing is easier than good old-fashioned oatmeal. Quaker Oats come with recipes right on the box, and many other instant oatmeals are available, often packaged in ready-to-eat, single-serving pouches. Oat bran itself can be purchased at health and natural food stores, as well as some supermarkets. You can add oat bran to almost any recipe for bread, rolls, or biscuits, or buy bread made with oat bran at the store.

Oats for sale! Know what you're getting

The American Heart Association warns that store-bought foods claiming to be rich in oat bran often are not. Many of these products contain very little actual oat bran, and instead may be rich in things such as fat and sodium. Always take a minute to read the labels on the foods you buy to be sure you know what you're getting and what you're not.

Oatmeal vs. oat bran: which is better?

Researchers were curious about which would do a better job of lowering cholesterol, oatmeal or oat bran. So they gave 148 people either oatmeal, oat bran, or another grain for 12 weeks. It turns out that it takes 3 ounces of oatmeal to lower cholesterol as much as 2 ounces of oat bran.

Next question: cooked or raw?

Although it's fun to find ways to add it to recipes, oat bran loses a lot of its nutritional value when it's cooked. Luckily, cooking doesn't break down the soluble fiber — so it keeps its cholesterol-fighting strength — but it does rob oat bran of some of its vitamins.

The table below shows how much of a group of valuable nutrients is satisfied by a half-cup of raw oat bran vs. a half-cup of cooked.

	Raw	Cooked
Protein	8 g	3 g
Potassium	266 mg	101 mg
Calcium	27 mg	11 mg
Phosphorus	344 mg	103 mg
Magnesium	110 mg	44 mg

RECIPES

Currant bran muffins

I cup whole wheat flour	I/4 cup vegetable oil
I cup oat bran	I cup low-fat buttermilk
I/2 teaspoon salt	I/2 cup mashed banana or
I teaspoon cinnamon	sweetened applesauce
I/4 teaspoon ground allspice	I/4 cup brown sugar
I teaspoon baking soda	I egg (or egg substitute
I/2 cup currants or raisins	equivalent)

Preheat oven to 425 degrees. Mix together whole wheat flour, oat bran, salt, cinnamon, allspice, baking soda, and currants or raisins in a mixing bowl. In another bowl, mix together oil, buttermilk, banana or applesauce, sugar, and egg. Blend into dry ingredients, using a minimum of strokes. Fill lightly oiled muffin tins or paper-lined tins three-fourths full. Bake for 15 minutes. Makes 12 muffins. Serving tip: Serve with apple butter

Calories: 152 per muffin
Fat: 5 grams per muffin
Calories from fats: 30%
Sodium: 186 mg per muffin

Half-the-fat carrot cake

Traditional carrot cake gets about half of its calories from fat, but this recipe lets you have your cake and eat it too! This carrot cake is 25 percent fat, rich in beta carotene, and unbelievably scrumptious.

CAKE

2 cups carrots, shredded	2 cups cake flour *
I/2 cup golden raisins, chopped	I cup oat bran flour *
I/2 cup vegetable oil	2-I/2 teaspoons baking soda
2 teaspoons vanilla	I-I/2 cups sugar
I II-oz. can mandarin oranges,	3 teaspoons cinnamon
undrained	I/2 teaspoon ground nutmeg
5 egg whites	I/2 teaspoon salt, optional

  * **Variation:** 1-1/2 cups cake flour and 1-1/2 cups whole wheat flour may be used.

ICING
4 oz. Neufchatel or light cream cheese

I teaspoon vanilla
2 cups confectioner's sugar or powdered sugar

Cake: Preheat oven to 350 degrees. Combine in food processor or large bowl the carrots, raisins, oil, vanilla, mandarin oranges, and egg whites; mix together. In another large mixing bowl, sift together flours, baking soda, sugar, cinnamon, nutmeg, and salt. Add carrot mixture to dry ingredients and beat until well blended. Pour into two 9-inch, lightly oiled cake pans. Bake 40 minutes or until cake tester comes out clean. Cool.

Icing: Blend together Neufchatel or light cream cheese, vanilla, and confectioner's sugar. Frost only the middle and top layers of the cake. Serves 16.

Half-the-fat carrot cake	**Traditional carrot cake**
Calories: 312 per serving	Calories: 573 per serving
Fat: 8.9 grams per serving	Fat: 32.8 grams per serving
Calories from fat: 25%	Calories from fat: 51%

SOY

The joy of soy

Eastern cultures have long boasted some of the best overall health records in the world. For centuries, the people of such countries as Japan, China, Thailand, and Vietnam have enjoyed delicious, exotic meals, while managing to avoid many of the pitfalls of the Western diet. The lower-fat, higher fiber makeup of these diets, combined with more active, physically demanding lifestyles, offer a much better defense against heart disease. People from Asian nations also enjoy lower rates of many types of cancer.

But how can you enjoy the health benefits of the Asian diet without moving to China? The answer is as simple as one little bean.

The soybean is actually a legume, like a pea or lentil, and is a common staple of almost all Asian diets. Like other beans, the soybean is rich in essential B vitamins, which help to keep your metabolism, blood, and brain in good working order. Soy also packs a powerful protein punch, which makes it a good weapon against bone and muscle loss. In some forms, such as fresh soybeans and sprouts, soy is also an excellent source of fiber.

Slash cancer risk with Asian eating

Researchers at the University of Alabama have learned that soy may significantly reduce the risk of certain types of cancer. Recent studies show that people who regularly eat soy foods are less likely to get hormone-related cancers, such as breast and prostate cancers. The reason for this is that soybean products contain high levels of hormone-like substances called phytoestrogens. One of these substances, called genistein, is similar enough to human estrogen that it interferes with the cancer-causing activities of your body's own hormones.

Although genistein shows some promise as a cancer-fighter, it is more effective as a preventive measure. Doctors warn that genistein works 10 times better in preventing cancer growth in healthy cells than in cells already showing cancerous activity. The American Cancer Society reports that the cancer-inhibiting effects of phytoestrogens in animal testing are encouraging and recommends soybeans as a good alternative to meat.

Isoflavone (genistein) content of soy products per 1/2 cup:

Soy flour	50 mg
Miso	40 mg
Tempeh	40 mg
Tofu	40 mg
Soybeans (cooked)	35 mg
Soy milk	20 mg

Is soy sauce soy-less?

When you hear the word "soy," you probably think of soy sauce, the salty brown condiment you sprinkle over chop suey. True, soy sauce comes from soy, but it is not the only, nor even one of the best, soy-based products.

Soy sauce is the most popular soy product in America. But don't think you're going to boost your phytoestrogens by sprinkling it on rice or into stir fry. Soy sauce has an extremely low concentration of the cancer-fighting genistein and is usually high in salt. If you want to use it anyway, doctors advise using one of the low-salt varieties that are available.

Tidings of comfort and soy

Besides soy sauce, tofu is probably the most well-know soybean product. Tofu usually comes in block form and has about the same weight and consistency as a soft cheese. These blocks can be cut into strips or cubes for use in stir fry or soups, or blended into shakes and salad dressings. One of the remarkable properties of tofu is that it has almost no taste. Instead, the tofu absorbs the flavor of whatever it is cooked with. You can use tofu as a substitute wherever meat, cheese, or yogurt is called for. Or simply add a few cubes to a recipe to give it an extra, healthful kick.

Tofu comes in several textures, ranging from soft to extra firm. Be sure to buy the right kind for the type of cooking you want to do. For example, extra firm tofu works best for grilling, while softer varieties are better suited for blending into dressings. Nutritionists recommend that you buy refrigerated, individually wrapped tofu, because it has less chance of being contaminated. At home, tofu will keep in your refrigerator for up to a week. Keep the tofu submerged in water, and change the water once a day.

A quick warning: Some brands of tofu can be fatty, so be label conscious when you're shopping. Low-fat varieties are almost always available. In addition, tofu can be a great source of calcium if you look for calcium-enriched brands. This is particularly important if you plan to use tofu in a recipe as a replacement for cheese, milk, or yogurt.

Tempeh is another popular soy product. This Japanese delicacy comes in a firmer, cake-like form and has a more distinct taste than tofu. Like tofu, tempeh can be grilled, stir-fried, served as shish kebab, or simply served plain. Tempeh is a little less common, however, so you might have to visit a health food store or Japanese market to find it.

The soy of cooking

Much the same way you might substitute tofu for less-healthy ingredients in a recipe, health food companies are marketing a wide range of traditional foods made from soybeans. These items include soy burgers, hot dogs, margarine, cream cheese, and soy milk. Many of these items are available at your local supermarket or health food store.

Soy flour is a great way to boost the protein content of your home-cooked breads, muffins, and cakes. Try substituting soy flour for up to 25 percent of a recipe's white or wheat flour content. (You can't use

100 percent soy flour in recipes that include yeast because it has no gluten to make the dough rise properly.) And here's a new egg substitute you wouldn't guess: one tablespoon of soy flour plus one tablespoon of water equals one whole egg, with no cholesterol. To enhance the natural nutty flavor of soy flour, you can "toast" it in a dry skillet over medium heat for a few minutes before adding it to your recipe.

Miso is a salty, tangy paste made from soybeans and is often used to make soup. You can make a tasty, healthful treat by melting miso to taste in hot water and adding some diced green onion. Miso is an excellent source of the phytoestrogens that make soy such a good cancer stopper. Better health food stores might carry it, but you'll probably have to visit an Oriental market to get your hands on some miso.

Powdered soy protein is available at almost all health food stores and can be mixed into juices, milk, yogurt, and just about anything else. While powdered protein does give you many of the benefits of soy, it does not carry the full nutritional value of eating soybean products as part of your daily diet.

You shouldn't have much trouble finding many delicious soy products to add to your menu. You might have to look a little harder, but the potential health benefits are more than worth the extra effort. A diet that includes low-fat, protein-rich soy products can reduce your risk of heart disease, breast cancer, and prostate cancer.

The soy of sex

It's starting to look like soy might have more healing powers than was ever thought possible. Although still in early stages, some research is beginning to suggest that soy can help combat the symptoms of menopause, such as vaginal dryness and tissue damage. In one recent study at Bowman Gray School of Medicine, menopausal women who used a daily dose of 20 grams of soy protein powder for six weeks found that their hot flashes and night sweats became much less severe.

These encouraging results hint at the possibility that a conscientious diet of soy protein could someday eliminate the need for hormone replacement therapy.

Soy to the world

If you're looking to add soy to your diet, it's probably a better idea to stay home for dinner. Although soy is very common in the diets of most Asian cultures, you're not likely to get too much of it eating out. The truth is, many restaurants that claim to serve authentic Oriental food really do not. Traditional Western tastes tend to prefer saltier, heavier foods than those found in a typical Asian diet. For this reason, many Asian restaurants add more salt and extra meat to the dishes they serve. While this might make such meals taste more familiar, it also robs them of much of their nutritional value.

RECIPES

Tofu and veggie stir-fry

2 cups tofu cubed
2 tablespoons olive oil
3/4 cup onion, chopped
I cup green pepper, cut in strips
I cup mushrooms, sliced

1/4 cup soy sauce, low sodium
I-1/4 cups bean sprouts
1/2 cup bamboo shoots
2-1/2 tablespoons cornstarch

Heat olive oil in a large skillet. Add green pepper and onions and cook until onion is translucent. Add mushrooms and cook until tender, about 2 minutes. Scoop out vegetables from the pan and set aside. Add tofu to the skillet and brown. Add sautéed vegetables to tofu mixture, including bean sprouts and bamboo sprouts. In a small bowl, blend soy sauce and cornstarch and pour into skillet. Cook for several minutes and serve over rice. Makes 4 servings.

Calories: 194 per serving
Fat: 12 grams
Calories from fat: 51%

Surprise zucchini brownies

These brownies are much lower in fat (approximately half of the fat and calories are gone) than traditional brownies and have the added benefit of more fiber — but remember, everything in moderation!

4 egg whites
I cup grated zucchini (about I medium zucchini)
I cup whole wheat flour *
I cup sugar
1/3 cup cocoa powder
1/2 teaspoon baking powder
1/3 cup vegetable oil

I teaspoon vanilla extract
1/4 cup walnuts
* You can use 1/4 cup of soy flour and 3/4 cup of whole wheat flour instead.

Preheat oven to 350 degrees. In food processor or blender, whip egg whites together. Then add grated zucchini. Sift dry ingredients together in a mixing bowl. Stir in oil, vanilla, nuts, and zucchini-egg white mixture just until blended. Don't overmix. Pour into lightly oiled 8-inch square pan and bake for 30 - 35 minutes. Cool and cut into 16 squares. Makes 16 servings.

SPINACH

Spinach tips

When buying spinach, look for dark green leaves that are crisp and have a fresh fragrance. Don't buy leaves that are limp, wilted, or have yellow spots. You can refrigerate fresh spinach in a plastic bag for up to three days. Spinach tends to be gritty, so rinse well before cooking. You can use spinach raw, in salads, or you can boil or sauté it. Eat it alone or use it in recipes to give your dishes an extra nutritional punch.

Give spinach a spin

If you're looking for a vegetable with nutritional panache, try some spinach. This leafy green is packed with vitamins A and C; it's high in disease-fighting carotenoids; and has lots of iron, potassium and calcium. The only trouble is that it contains oxalic acid, too, which decreases your body's absorption of these minerals. This takes some of the nutritional punch out of spinach, but it still provides a good source of other nutrients. Studies find that it may provide protection from some diseases.

- **Sight protection.** Age-related macular degeneration (AMD) is the leading cause of new cases of legal blindness in the United States. This disorder, which affects part of the retina, can take away your ability to drive a car, read a book, or recognize your best friend from across the street. There is no known cure for AMD. However, research shows that people who eat foods high in carotenoids are less likely to develop AMD. One study found that people who ate the greatest amount of carotenoid-rich foods were 43 percent less likely to develop AMD. This study also found that spinach and collard greens were the foods most closely associated with decreased risk of AMD. If you want to keep your eyes sharp for the rest of your life, eating lots of spinach could be a very wise choice.

- **Cancer prevention**. Eating your spinach could also help protect you from some deadly forms of cancer. Studies find that spinach may help prevent colorectal, stomach, prostate, bladder, and lung cancers. This protective effect may come specifically from the vitamin A found in spinach or from its high carotenoid content.

The power of Popeye

Everyone knows how strong Popeye became when he popped open a can of spinach. He was an unlikely Superman, able to take care of Bluto in a single punch. He was also a very powerful salesman for spinach. In the years just after the cartoon sailor made his first appearance in 1929, spinach consumption in the United States increased by 33 percent. Children rated it as one of their favorite foods. Spinach growers were so grateful that they erected a statue of Popeye in Crystal City, Texas, in 1937.

Spinach nutrition

	Raw	Boiled	Canned	Frozen
Serving size	about 2 cups	about 1/2 cup	about 1/2 cup	about 1/2 cup
Calories	22	23	23	28
Fat	.35 g	.26 g	.50 g	.21 g
Vitamin A	6715 IU	8190 IU	8776 IU	7784 IU
Vitamin C	28.10 mg	9.8 mg	14.3 mg	12.3 mg
Magnesium	79 mg	87 mg	76 mg	69 mg
Calcium	99 mg	136 mg	127 mg	146 mg
Folic acid	194 mcg	145 mcg	97.8 mcg	107 mcg
Potassium	558 mg	466 mg	346 mg	298 mg
Iron	2.7 mg	1.5 mg	2.3 mg	3.5 mg

Did you know?

À la Florentine is French for "in the style of Florence (Italy)," and refers to food that is served on a bed of spinach and topped with Mornay sauce. If you see "Florentine" on a restaurant menu, it usually means that the dish contains spinach.

RECIPES

Spinach and lentil soup

6 cups water
I cup lentils
2 bay leaves
I tablespoon olive oil
I bunch spring or green
   onions, sliced

2 cloves of garlic, finely chopped
1/2 teaspoon cumin powder
1/2 teaspoon salt
pinch of freshly ground pepper
I lb. spinach, chopped

Boil lentils in 4 cups of water with bay leaves until soft. Heat olive oil in another pan and gently fry green onion for 2 minutes, stirring frequently. Add garlic, cumin powder, salt, pepper, and spinach; mix well and add to lentils. Add remaining 2 cups of water and cook an additional 15 minutes. Makes 6 servings.

Calories: 110 per serving
Fat: 3 grams per serving
Calories from fat: 25%

Spinach pita pizzas

Company at the last minute? Kids or grandchildren are bored? These spinach pizzas are quick, easy, and fun for kids to make. Enjoy this appealing all-time favorite year-round.

5 mini pitas
8 oz. tomato sauce *
I cup fresh spinach, sliced into thin strips
1-1/2 cups skim milk mozzarella cheese, shredded

Preheat oven to 450 degrees. Toast pitas. Slice around the edge of the pitas to open pockets (be careful not to burn yourself from the steam inside). Place pita halves on a baking sheet with the inside of the pita upward. Cover the pita with about 1-1/2 tablespoons tomato sauce. It's best to top pitas with tomato sauce shortly before baking, otherwise they become soggy. Then sprinkle with spinach and cheese. Bake for 9 to 10 minutes or until cheese is melted. Cut into quarters for appetizers. Serve warm. Makes 40 pizza appetizers.

Calories: 27 per appetizer
Fat: .8 grams per appetizer
Calories from fat: 27%
Cholesterol: 2.4 mg

* Tomato sauce: use either your own homemade tomato sauce or a commercial sauce. Or, you can quickly blend this one together:

8 oz. canned tomato sauce
1/4 teaspoon "Italian" spices or "fine herbs," or more to taste
1/8 teaspoon garlic powder
1 teaspoon onion, finely chopped
pinch of sugar
dash of pepper

SWEET POTATOES

How sweet it is

The lowly sweet potato masquerades as a humble root, but it's actually a standout in the world of vegetables. Its biggest claim to fame is the sweet potato's generous dose of vitamin A, but sweet potatoes are strong in the vitamin C and fiber departments, too. Their store of nutrients helps protect you from a number of problems.

- **All about A.** Vitamin A, often found in the form of beta carotene, is vital to your body. It's necessary for good eyesight, helps your body's immune system work, and fights cancer and heart disease as a powerful antioxidant. It can also help protect you from ulcers and from losing your mental abilities with age. If you have diabetes, vitamin A plays an important role in controlling your insulin levels. Vitamin A may also be able to counteract some of the damage to the liver and muscles caused by alcoholism. What a bounty of benefits from this one nutrient! Sweet potatoes pack plenty of vitamin A per serving. One-half cup of mashed, fresh sweet potato contains 21,822 International Units of vitamin A, more than twice the RDA for an adult male.

- **Consider some C.** Vitamin C is another big hitter on your body's vitamin team. Vitamin C helps produce collagen, the protein that holds your body together. It also protects your eyes, your memory, and your mood, and fights colds and flu, cancer, heart disease, stroke, and diabetes. Vitamin C is something your body can't get along without, and sweet potatoes help you get it. One-half cup of mashed sweet potatoes has about as much vitamin C as one-half cup of broccoli or brussels sprouts.

- **Find out about fiber.** You may not realize it, but fiber is a fighter for your body's health. In addition to preventing constipation and hemorrhoids, the fiber in foods helps protect you from cancer, heart disease, gallstones, diverticular disease, and hiatal hernia. If you have diabetes, fiber helps keep your blood sugar under control. A half-cup serving of sweet potatoes has 3 grams of fiber, as much as two-thirds of a cup of oatmeal or shredded wheat cereal, and more than a bran muffin or a cup of popcorn.

Sweet potato or yam?

Technically, yams and sweet potatoes are not the same; they even come from different plant families. The yam is a tuber and the sweet potato is the root of a particular type of flowering vine, in the same family as the morning glory. But if you're talking about a moist potato with orange-colored flesh, you're talking about an American sweet potato. The word "yam" comes from the African word "nyami." Yams come from the Caribbean or Africa and can grow to 100 pounds.

If you ever have to choose between an authentic yam and a sweet potato, choose the potato. It has thinner, smoother skin; a sweeter taste; and a softer texture. A sweet potato also has a high beta carotene (vitamin A) content, but a yam has almost none.

Keeping potatoes sweet

If you want your potatoes to be really sweet, you need to "cure" them. When sweet potatoes come fresh from the field, they should be stored in a warm (85 to 90 degrees), dark, and very humid place for about a week. This process "cures" the potatoes of any cuts and bruises and changes some of the starch in the potato to sugar.

After curing, the potatoes will taste much sweeter and will last longer. Store the potatoes in a cool, humid place, but not in the refrigerator. If they are stored below 50 degrees, they will suffer cold damage and will rot. If you store them properly, however, they will last for months.

Potatoes: regular or sweet?

When you're choosing between potatoes as a side dish for your meal, there are some things you might want to consider. One-half cup of mashed potatoes, either regular or sweet, has a little over 100 calories and just under 2 grams of protein. But that's where the similarities end. When it comes to nutrients, sweet potatoes have the advantage over regular potatoes hands down. Here's how things stack up in one-half cup of mashed potatoes:

- **Vitamin C.** Sweet potatoes have four times the vitamin C of regular potatoes. (24.6 mg compared to 6.1 mg)
- **Vitamin A.** Here the sweet potato really shines, with more than 10 times the vitamin A of regular potatoes. In one-half cup of mashed sweet potatoes, you get 21,822 International Units (IU) of vitamin A, more than twice your Recommended Dietary Allowance (RDA) for the day. Regular potatoes have 169 IU of vitamin A.
- **Folic acid.** There's almost three times as much in sweet potatoes as in regular ones. Sweet potatoes contain 22.6 micrograms (mcg) compared to 7.9 mcg.
- **Minerals.** Potassium, phosphorus, and magnesium all have a greater presence in sweet potatoes than in regular potatoes.
- **Dietary fiber.** Regular potatoes have 2 grams of fiber; sweet potatoes have 3 grams.

So which potato do you want to put on your plate?

RECIPES

Sweet potato and apple rings

40 ounces sweet potatoes	I tablespoon cinnamon
3 whole apples, peeled	1/4 cup margarine
1/2 cup brown sugar	I cup maple syrup

Preheat the oven to 350 degrees. Lightly grease a shallow casserole dish. Cook sweet potatoes until tender or use canned sweet potatoes. Core and peel apples. Then slice sweet potatoes and apples. Place slices in casserole, alternating the potatoes and apples. Mix brown sugar and cinnamon and sprinkle over the sliced layers. Cut the margarine into small pieces and dot the layers. Add maple syrup and bake, covered, for 30 minutes. Remove the cover and bake for about 1 hour more. Makes 8 to 10 servings.

Calories: 293 per serving (smaller size)
Fat: 5 grams
Calories from fat: 15%

Cooking tips

Sweet potatoes are versatile vegetables. They can be cooked a number of ways for different textures and flavors. Experiment by adding your own touch of spice.

- **To bake:** Wash and dry the potatoes, then rub with oil. Prick the skin in a few places with a fork and place on a cookie sheet. Bake at 400 degrees for about 30 to 50 minutes.
- **To microwave:** Wash and dry the sweet potatoes and pierce with a fork in a few places. Place in the microwave on a dry paper towel about one inch apart. Turn the potatoes halfway through cooking. The cooking time will vary. Potatoes are done when they pierce easily with a fork. Allow them to stand after microwaving to finish cooking.
- **To boil:** Drop clean potatoes into a pot of boiling water. Cover the pot and bring to a boil again. Turn down the heat and cook the potatoes until they are tender. Peel and slice them, then season with butter or salt to taste.

TOMATOES

History of the tomato

The Aztec emperor Montezuma offered Spanish conquistador Hernando Cortés tomatoes, reportedly the first experience Europeans had with tomatoes. Cortés apparently ignored this friendly gesture, as he went on to conquer Mexico for Spain. Spanish explorers took tomato seeds back with them to Europe as part of their plunder. Tomatoes received a mixed reaction in Europe. The French called them "love apples" and considered them an aphrodisiac. Some people, however, thought that tomatoes were poisonous, but still grew them for their ornamental beauty. Eventually the tomato's flavor, as well as its appearance, made it a favorite of people all over the world.

Cancer protection from tomatoes

You say to-MAY-to, I say to-MAH-to. Any way you slice it or say it, the tomato is chock full of cancer protection. Tomatoes contain a carotenoid called lycopene that gives the tomato its cheerful red color. Lycopene may also give you protection from several types of cancer.

- **Prostate cancer.** A large study from Harvard University found that men who ate at least 10 servings of tomato products a week cut their risk of prostate cancer almost in half. Tomato sauce had the strongest protective effect, followed by tomatoes and pizza. Tomato juice did not seem to have any effect on cancer risk. Researchers think that heating tomato products in oil may make the lycopene easier for you to absorb, which could explain why tomato sauce was so effective. Chopping and cooking your tomatoes may also make the lycopene easier for your body to absorb.
- **Digestive tract cancers.** Several studies have found that the

lycopene found in tomatoes may reduce your risk of digestive tract cancers like stomach, esophageal, colon, and rectal cancers. One study found that eating tomatoes at least once a week resulted in a 40 percent reduction in the risk of esophageal cancer. Another study on cancers of the mouth, throat, esophagus, stomach, colon, and rectum found that people who had a high intake of lycopene were less likely to develop any of these cancers, but it was particularly protective against cancers of the stomach, colon, and rectum.

Eating tomatoes is no guarantee that you won't get cancer, but it's a delicious, nutritious way to "hedge your bets" and maybe sidestep a deadly disease.

The right way to ripen

You may want the tomatoes on your sandwich or in your salad to be chilled, but don't put that tomato in the refrigerator until it is fully ripened. The cold temperature may keep your tomato from ripening properly and might ruin its flavor. To speed up the ripening process, place your tomatoes in a paper bag or wrap them in newspaper. As they start to ripen, the tomatoes will give off a gas called ethylene, which in turn helps them ripen faster. The paper will keep the gas concentrated around them, resulting in a ripe, red tomato in a fraction of the normal time.

Genetically engineering the perfect tomato

Gardeners have been trying to grow what they consider the perfect tomato for years: big, round, juicy, richly-colored and tasty. Scientists, however, have been working on their own version of the perfect tomato, full of disease-fighting carotenoids.

Scientists at Royal Holloway, University of London, have created a tomato that has either twice as much lycopene or four times as much beta carotene as an ordinary tomato. They did this by inserting a gene that helps the plant produce the carotenoids. According to the researchers, the genetically-altered tomatoes taste the same as any other tomato, but they may be a bit more colorful.

Since lycopene and beta carotene have both been shown in scientific studies to help prevent certain diseases, increasing their content in foods could help people get more protection from cancer and heart disease while eating the same quantity of fruit or vegetables. Scientists in other parts of the world are working on similar projects involving peppers and rice.

While it may be some time before any genetically-altered foods appear in your grocery store, this scientific approach to agriculture may someday help make people a little healthier.

Fruit or vegetable?

The tomato is a versatile food indeed. In fact, some confusion exists as to whether it is a fruit or a vegetable. Botanically speaking, a fruit is the part of the plant that contains the seeds, and a vegetable comes from the root, stem, or leaves of a plant. Tomatoes have seeds, so a tomato is a fruit — more specifically, a berry. In 1893, however, the U.S. government classified the tomato as a vegetable for trade purposes. That brings back the original question: Is the tomato a fruit or a vegetable? The answer may depend on whether you consider botanists or the government the authority, but perhaps now you'll look at cherry tomatoes in a whole new light.

Tomato nutrition

	1 raw tomato	1/2 cup canned tomatoes	1/2 cup tomato sauce
Calories	26	33	37
Fat	.40 g	.17 g	.20 g
Vitamin A	76 RE	70 RE	120 RE
Vitamin C	23 mg	17 mg	16 mg
Potassium	273 mg	305 mg	452 mg
Folic acid	18 mcg	7 mcg	11 mcg

RECIPES

Salsa

8-ounce can "no salt added" tomato sauce

1 tablespoon chili peppers, canned, drained, chopped

1/4 cup green pepper, finely chopped

2 tablespoons onion, finely chopped

1 clove garlic, minced

1/4 teaspoon oregano leaves, crushed

1/8 teaspoon ground cumin

Mix all ingredients thoroughly. Chill before serving to blend flavors. Serve with toasted pita bread, breadsticks, or raw vegetables pieces. Makes about 1 cup.

Calories per tablespoon: 5
Fat per tablespoon: Trace

Pasta ruffles and beef

3/4 lb. extra-lean ground round or sirloin beef

1/2 onion, chopped

10 oz. pkg. frozen chopped spinach

7 oz. uncooked pasta ruffles

16 oz. tomato sauce or no-salt-added tomato sauce

6 oz. tomato paste or no-salt-added tomato paste

1/2 teaspoon dried basil

1/2 teaspoon oregano

1/4 teaspoon pepper

1-1/2 tablespoons Parmesan cheese, grated

Brown beef and onion in a large saucepan. Drain any remaining fat. Prepare pasta according to package directions. Add frozen spinach, tomato sauce, tomato paste, basil, oregano, pepper, and pasta to meat mixture. Heat thoroughly until spinach is dispersed in mixture. Simmer for 5 to 10 minutes. Sprinkle Parmesan cheese on each portion before serving. Makes 4 to 6 servings. Serving tip: Serve with a fruit salad and warm whole wheat or pumpernickel rolls.

Calories: 442 (larger serving)
Fat: 10 grams (larger serving)
Calories from fat: 20%
Sodium: 875 mg or 260 mg if low sodium alternatives used

Quick and easy hint: Before serving, remove portion wanted for leftovers and place in a freezer container. Sprinkle with cheese and freeze for later meal. When you need a quick meal or don't wish to cook, reheat in a microwave or conventional oven.

New England casserole

4 thin pork chops or cutlets, trimmed of all outside fat
I cup uncooked brown rice
I medium onion, sliced
I cup cabbage, shredded
1/2 large green pepper

1/2 teaspoon dried sage
1/2 teaspoon pepper
28 oz. canned tomatoes in heavy puree or stewed tomatoes
I cup water

Preheat oven to 375 degrees. In deep baking dish, place 2 pork chops or cutlets; sprinkle rice, half the onion, all the cabbage, then add the remaining pork. Sprinkle with the rest of the onion and all of the green pepper. Mix sage and pepper with tomatoes and water, then pour over pork. Bake 1-1/2 hours or until rice is done. Makes 4 servings.

Calories: 451 per serving
Fat: 14 grams per serving
Calories from fat: 28%
Sodium: 394 mg per serving

Fresh tomato chutney

3 tomatoes, cut into 3/4 inch cubes
3/4 cup onions, finely sliced
I tablespoon mustard oil
1/2 tablespoon grated jaggery (unrefined sugar)
2 tablespoons lemon juice

I to 3 small green chilies, chopped
2 tablespoons fresh coriander leaves (or any green herb), chopped
1/4 teaspoon freshly ground black pepper

Toss all ingredients in a large bowl and serve. Makes 6 servings.

Calories: 68 per serving
Fat: 5 grams per serving

WATER

The nutrient that does it all

Water is more essential to life than any other single nutrient on this planet. You could live without food for a month or more, but you can only live a couple of days without water.

Water has no calories, no fat, and no sugar; does not need processing by your digestive system; and is gentle, even helpful, to most of your body's functions. It's everywhere, part of every living thing, and the world's most perfect beverage.

You need about eight servings of water (one serving equals eight ounces, or one cup) each day, yet most Americans drink less than half that amount. Most people think water is just for quenching thirst, but it does much more than that. Hundreds of systems and processes in your body need water to work properly.

For instance, water helps control your body's temperature. That's why you should drink plenty any time you exercise and especially when you have a fever. You'll not only replace the fluids you've sweated out, you'll cool your body down as well.

If you're watching your weight, water is a dieter's dream. In fact, one of the first things many weight loss programs give you is a large water jug. Experts know that drinking water is an easy but important way to curb your appetite. Drink up about an hour before you eat, and drink lots with every meal. You will feel more full and eat more slowly because of it. And, don't forget, drinking water is more natural than diet pills and safer on your body.

Your joints especially love water because it helps keep them cushioned and working properly. Arthritis sufferers need to remember that dehydrated joints mean sore knees, painful fingers, and achy backs. In many cases, drinking more water will relieve the pain and swelling of this crippling disease.

If your digestive system is plagued with problems, you need to make water your number one priority. Whether it is constipation, heartburn, irritable bowel syndrome, or just plain indigestion, lots of water will soothe your system and get things moving in the right direction.

Would you believe that drinking enough water can help you escape three painful conditions? Urinary tract infections, kidney stones, and gallstones are all helped by this fabulous fluid. Water dissolves the calcium in your urine that can turn into kidney stones. Plus it helps the bile in your liver dissolve cholesterol that could become painful gallstones.

So fill your glass, add a twist of lemon, and drink a toast to the best thing you can do for your body.

Did you know?

If you weigh 150 pounds, and do one hour of moderate exercise, your water intake for the day should be 10 eight-ounce servings. That's two extra servings!

The dangers of dehydration

When the percent of water in your body begins to fall below normal, you start becoming dehydrated. It is a vague condition to most people — you may think of dehydration as simply feeling thirsty. However, by the time you actually feel thirsty, you're already in need of water and will soon start feeling the effects, some of which can be dangerous.

Besides feeling like you need a drink, you may have any of these other symptoms: dizziness, dry lips and mouth, a faster heart rate, rapid breathing, confusion, and dark urine. If your dehydration is severe enough, you could lapse into a coma.

You may think you could never get into that much trouble simply by not drinking enough water, but dehydration can be a sneaky condition, creeping up without much warning. This is especially true for older people.

As you age, you lose some of your feelings of thirst, and so might not notice that you need a drink. In addition, your kidneys are older, too, and not as efficient at keeping water in your body. Statistics prove how serious this condition can be. Back in 1991, Medicare spent over $1 billion on hospital care for people who had become dehydrated.

So, even if you don't feel thirsty, you need to drink, drink, drink. Some experts recommend a pint of water every hour during the hot summer months.

Did you know?

Your brain is 75 percent water. This is why even slight dehydration can cause headaches and dizziness.

The water dilemma: bottle or tap?

Spring or mineral. Deionized or distilled. Bulk or artesian. How many types of commercial H2O are there, and are they really anything more than just filtered tap water? The International Bottled Water Association (IBWA), which has represented 85 percent of the industry since 1958, wants you to know that if you choose to drink something besides the water from your faucet, either for quality or taste, you are getting a good, safe product.

First, bottled water must meet all federal and state standards regulated by the FDA and state officials. Furthermore, the IBWA requires its members to meet even tougher standards, ensuring that all their bottled water is of high quality. The U.S. Centers for Disease Control and Prevention claims that bottled water has never caused an outbreak of waterborne illness.

Bottled water cannot contain sweeteners, chemicals, or calories, but may contain spice or fruit flavors. This means an endless variety of refreshing, healthy choices. So, read your labels, check the bottler's credentials, and then decide if you prefer sparkling or still, natural or purified.

For more information, call or write:
International Bottled Water Association
1700 Diagonal Road, Suite 650
Alexandria, VA 22314
Tel: (703) 683-5213
Fax: (703) 683-4074
1-800-WATER-11 (1-800-928-3711)

Soft means salty

If you are on a low-sodium diet, be careful of home water softener systems and bottled mineral water. Both can allow high levels of sodium.

YOGURT

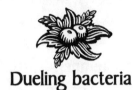

Dueling bacteria

When you hear the word bacteria, you probably think of germs and infections. It's enough to make you run to your doctor, or at least to your sink to wash your hands with a disinfecting soap. However, bacteria aren't all bad for you. Some bacteria are essential for life, and some will even do battle for you against the bad bacteria that cause infections. Yogurt contains "good" bacteria, *Lactobacillus acidophilus, Lactobacillus bulgaricus* and/or *Streptococcus thermophilus,* that may help protect you from some of the "bad guy" bacteria.

- **Vanquish vaginal infections.** Yeast may make bread soft and fluffy, but a yeast infection makes you itchy and irritable. A bacteria called *Candida albicans* can cause this annoying vaginal infection, but the *Lactobacillus* bacteria in yogurt may help fight it. Women have used yogurt to remedy vaginal infections for many years, not only by eating it, but also by applying yogurt directly to the affected area. Studies have found that yogurt is one home remedy that works. In one study, women who had recurrent vaginal infections ate 8 ounces of yogurt daily for six months. During the time they were eating yogurt these women had three times fewer infections. Another small study tested the direct application of yogurt on women who had vaginal inflammation. After three days, more than half of the women were completely well.

- **Ditch diarrhea.** You're trying to have a good time on your vacation, snapping pictures of Aztec ruins or sunning yourself on the beach, but your stomach is cramping and you can't get far from a bathroom. You have traveler's diarrhea, and you probably have a bottle of chalky-tasting pink stuff in your hotel room. But wouldn't it be nice if you could just eat some creamy sweet yogurt instead? According to research, yogurt can kill *E. coli* bacteria that is often responsible for your frequent runs for the restroom. Yogurt also battles *Salmonella typhimurium* bacteria that can sneak into your body through raw or undercooked foods. So if you plan to eat raw oysters on your vacation, make sure you eat plenty of yogurt too ... though they might not taste so good together.

To make sure you get bacteria-fighting "good guys" in your yogurt, read the label. Look for the words "active cultures," "live active cultures," or "contains viable cultures." Don't buy heat-treated yogurt. This treatment makes yogurt last longer, but it also kills those helpful bacteria you need.

Tangy yogurt popsicles

For an easy, healthful snack that even kids will appreciate, combine 6 fluid ounces of undiluted frozen fruit juice concentrate with 8 ounces of plain low-fat yogurt and freeze in small paper cups. Put a popsicle stick in the center when the mixture is partially frozen. When it's completely frozen, just tear away the paper cup, and you have a cold, refreshing yogurt treat.

Cholesterol-soaking sponge

Yogurt has been prized since it was discovered more than 4,000 years ago. In ancient Persia, today known as Iran, a woman's dowry was determined by how much yogurt her prospective husband could buy. In ancient Assyria, the word for yogurt was lebeny, which also meant life.

One of the many health benefits associated with yogurt is reduction of cholesterol. Linking yogurt and cholesterol causes more controversy than consensus, but early research shows some strains of the *Lactobacillus* bacteria may indeed lower cholesterol. Researchers at Oklahoma State University have found that certain strains work like sponges and actually soak up cholesterol in the intestines before it can be absorbed by the body. Since this research is still in the early stages, however, you won't find any of these cholesterol-clobbering yogurts at your local grocery.

Other scientists have explored whether yogurt can reduce blood cholesterol levels. Studies of Masai warriors in East Africa found that when the Africans ate large quantities of yogurt, they lowered their cholesterol levels even though they gained weight. But beware, the American Heart Association doesn't agree with these results. It says the key to lowering your cholesterol levels is to reduce the amount of saturated fat in your diet.

Try a little tolerance

Milk may do most bodies good, but for people with lactose intolerance, milk and other dairy products can cause stomach pain and cramps. Lactose, a sugar found in milk, can be hard for some people to digest because they don't have enough of certain digestive enzymes. Yogurt may provide a high-calcium alternative that eases the pain of lactose intolerance. Yogurt contains less lactose than many dairy products, and new research finds that the bacteria in yogurt may help process that hard-to-digest milk sugar. Yogurt may not be the answer for every person with lactose intolerance, but give it a test run. Try dipping into some smooth yogurt and see if your stomach tolerates it better than milk.

Fat-slashing yogurt tips

- Use plain low-fat yogurt as a substitute for sour cream in dips or salad dressings.
- For dessert, top frozen low-fat yogurt with an unsweetened or lightly sweetened fruit sauce.
- Add unsweetened fruit to plain yogurt for a dessert or snack.
- Whip up a tasty, nutritious drink by combining fresh fruit, yogurt, and low-fat milk.
- Mix minced fresh dill and slivered almonds into plain low-fat yogurt and spoon on top of broccoli, brussels sprouts, or asparagus.
- Dip a peeled banana in any flavor yogurt (strawberry is a good choice). Roll it in crushed breakfast cereal, then freeze for a crunchy, cold snack.

Yogurt packs a powerful protein punch

You probably know that yogurt is crammed full of bone-building calcium. Yogurt can also provide you with muscle-building protein. Yogurt has as much protein as milk, but because of the way yogurt is processed, its protein is easier to digest and absorb. Many brands of yogurt are also fortified with extra protein, so for strong bones and strong muscles, yogurt may be the best body-building food around. Does Arnold Schwarzenegger know about this?

Make your own yogurt cheese

Yogurt cheese can be a natural, low-fat alternative to cream cheese. You can make this tasty cheese by removing the liquid from yogurt. Put 8 ounces of plain low-fat or nonfat yogurt that doesn't contain gelatin into a strainer lined with cheesecloth or three coffee filters. Don't try to use yogurt with fruit because the fruit tends to clog the strainer. Place the strainer over a bowl to catch the draining liquid. Cover and refrigerate for 24 hours. The liquid will drain into the bowl and what is left behind in the strainer is versatile yogurt cheese. You can season it with herbs and spread it on a bagel or use it as a dip for chips, crackers, or veggies. You can even use it in place of cream cheese in your favorite cheesecake recipe. Cheese made from lemon yogurt gives cheesecake a tangy twist.

Shopping for yogurt

The vast array of yogurts in your grocery store can be confusing. The dairy case displays dozens of containers with brightly-colored labels: fruit-flavored yogurt, fruit-on-the-bottom yogurt, low-fat yogurt, nonfat yogurt, vanilla yogurt, chocolate yogurt, plain yogurt, even dessert yogurt. You're trying to watch your weight, limit your fat intake, and boost your calcium and protein intakes, and yogurt is an excellent choice. But which kind do you choose? The best way is to turn those containers around and read the backs of the labels carefully to make sure you know what you're getting. However, for those of you who just scan the front, the U.S. Food and Drug Administration, which controls how food is labeled, has divided yogurt into three main categories according to fat content:

- **Whole milk yogurt (regular)** contains at least 7 grams of fat per one-cup serving, or at least 3.25 percent fat.
- **Low-fat yogurt** contains 1 to 6 grams of fat, or .5 percent to 2 percent fat per cup.

- **Nonfat yogurt** contains 1 gram of fat or less, making it less than .5 percent fat per cup.

While you're checking out the fat content, don't forget to look for those live active cultures that make yogurt a truly super food.

The history of yogurt

With all the new yogurt products popping up, you may think of it as a popular, new health food, but this is one health food that's no fad. It's been around for about 4,000 years. Middle Eastern civilizations used the fermenting process as a way to help their milk supply last on long desert journeys. The ancient Assyrian word for yogurt, lebeny, also meant "life." The next time you spoon up some soothing yogurt, close your eyes and imagine how it would taste even better eaten from a goatskin bag under a scorching desert sun. Suddenly, you're not eating a fad food, you're eating history.

A fat and calorie sampler

Yogurt by any other name could have twice as many calories. Different brands and types of yogurt vary widely in calorie and fat content. Here's a small sample:

	Serving size	Calories	Fat grams
Borden, cherry vanilla	8 oz	270	2 g
Breyers, peach	6 oz	270	5 g
Colombo, Bavarian chocolate	5 oz	270	11 g
Dannon, light plain	8 oz	110	0 g
Dannon, plain	8 oz	150	4 g
Lite n' Lively, fat-free, strawberry	4.4 oz	50	0 g
Weight Watchers, all flavors	8 oz	150	1 g
Yoplait, cherry	6 oz	190	4 g
Yoplait, New Lite, raspberry	4 oz	60	0 g
Frozen yogurt			
Dannon, chocolate	1 cup	190	3 g
Dreyer's, nonfat, vanilla	3 oz	80	0 g
Haagen-Dazs, peach	3 oz	120	3 g
Sealtest, strawberry	4 oz	100	2 g
Soft-serve frozen yogurt			
Colombo low-fat	1/2 cup	99	2 g

Colombo nonfat	1/2 cup	95	0 g
TCBY nonfat, small	5.9 oz	162	<1 g *
TCBY small	5.9 oz	192	4 g
TCBY sugar-free, small	5.9 oz	118	<1 g *

* The symbol < means less than.

RECIPES

Curry vegetable dip

8-ounce carton plain low-fat
  yogurt
1/4 cup carrots, shredded
2 teaspoons green onions,
  minced

I teaspoon sugar
1/4 teaspoon curry powder
dash of pepper
I tablespoon salad dressing,
  mayonnaise-type

Mix ingredients in a bowl, chill, and serve with raw vegetable, such as celery, carrots, or summer squash sticks. Makes about 1 cup.

Calories per tablespoon: 15
Fat per tablespoon: 1 gram

Keep it cool

When using yogurt for cooking, keep in mind that heating may destroy those friendly bacteria.

Madras vegetable stew

I-inch piece fresh ginger, peeled
  and coarsely chopped
1/4 cup fresh coriander leaves
  and stems (or flat-leaf parsley)
I to 4 fresh hot green chilies,
  stemmed, split, and seeded
  (optional)
3/4 pound yellow squash, trimmed
  and cut into 1/2-inch slices
I medium red onion, thinly sliced

I-1/2 teaspoons ground cumin
I-1/2 teaspoons cornstarch
I teaspoon curry powder
1/2 teaspoon cumin seeds
I teaspoon mustard seeds
I cup plain low-fat yogurt
2 tablespoons vegetable oil
I pound broccoli, trimmed and
  cut into 2-inch florets

Place the ginger, coriander, chilies, yogurt, ground cumin, and cornstarch in a blender or food processor and process until combined; then set aside. Heat the oil in large, heavy-gauge saucepan over medium-high heat. When the oil is hot, add the curry powder and let it sizzle, shaking the pan constantly for about 10 seconds. Add the broccoli, squash, and onion and toss to coat them with the spices. Cook for 1 minute. Add the yogurt sauce and stir to combine. Pour 1 cup of water into the blender or food processor container, shake to rinse it, and pour the water over the vegetables; stir to combine. Increase the heat to high and bring the mixture to a boil. Reduce the heat to medium-low and cook, covered, for 5 minutes. Uncover the pan, increase the heat to high, and boil rapidly for 1 minute. Then turn off the heat. Meanwhile, heat a small, heavy frying pan or a wok over medium heat for 2 minutes. Add the cumin and mustard seeds; roast the seeds, stirring and shaking the pan to prevent burning. Cook for a few minutes, until browned. When the vegetable mixture is ready, add the roasted seeds, stir in quickly, and serve. Makes 4 servings.

Calories per serving: 150
Fat per serving: 9 grams

Potatoes with mustard-tarragon stuffing

    4 baking potatoes
    I cup plain low-fat or nonfat yogurt
    2 tablespoons Dijon-style mustard
    2 teaspoons dried tarragon

Scrub the potatoes and puncture each once with a fork. Bake the potatoes in microwave oven: place on a paper towel and cook on high for 10 to 12 minutes (6 to 8 minutes for two potatoes; 12 to 13 minutes for six). Turn and rearrange the potatoes halfway through if possible. Meanwhile, blend the remaining ingredients in a small bowl until smooth. When the potatoes are done, cut them in half lengthwise like boats, or cut off just a small oval on each long side. Scoop out the flesh. Combine it with the yogurt mixture. Heap the mixture back into the potato shells. After stuffing the potatoes, reheat them in microwave on high for about 1 minute to serve immediately, or if preparing ahead, refrigerate them until serving time and reheat them for about 1 to 3 minutes. Makes 4 servings.

(This can also be prepared in a conventional oven by baking the potatoes at 400 degrees for 45 to 60 minutes and then reheating them for 10 minutes or briefly under the broiler.)

Calories per serving: 194
Fat per serving: 1 gram

VITAMINS
AND
SUPPLEMENTS

CALCIUM

Bone-building powerhouse

Calcium is one of the most abundant and important substances in your body. It plays a critical part in the strength and health of your bones and teeth. Your bones are constantly being reformed; old bone cells are replaced by new ones around the clock. Think of your bones as a savings account, and calcium is the money they store for the rest of the body to borrow from. When another part of your body needs calcium, it makes a "withdrawal" from your bones. You need a daily supply of calcium going back into the account to keep up with demand. If you don't get enough calcium, you will eventually pay the price with fragile bones that break easily.

About 99 percent of your calcium is stored in your skeleton. Only one percent is in bodily fluids like blood. However, that tiny bit of calcium plays extremely important roles. It helps nerve impulses travel around, helps keep your blood pressure normal, and helps in clotting your blood. Your muscles, including your heart, need calcium to contract. Without it your heart would be unable to keep beating regularly.

Food sources

Yogurt, plain low-fat, 1 oz	415 mg
Sardines, canned, 3 oz	371 mg
Milk, low-fat, 1 cup	297 mg
Oysters, raw, 1 cup	226 mg
Cheddar cheese, 1 oz	204 mg
Turnip greens, cooked, 1 cup	197 mg
Salmon, canned, 3 oz	167 mg
Beet greens, cooked, 1 cup	164 mg
Cottage cheese, low-fat, 1 cup	155 mg
Refried beans, canned, 1 cup	141 mg
Peanuts, 1 cup	125 mg
Kale, cooked, 1 cup	94 mg
Pinto beans, cooked, 1 cup	86 mg

Deficiency

A calcium deficiency can silently creep up on you, producing no noticeable symptoms for years. Your body regulates the calcium in your blood very carefully, taking it from your bones as it's needed, so you don't realize that you are deficient. But eventually your body takes so much calcium from your bones that they become porous and weak, snapping at the smallest impact. A person with advanced osteoporosis, caused by a calcium deficiency, can break a bone simply by stepping down too hard off a curb.

RDA

Males	ages 11-24	1,200 mg
	ages 25-up	800 mg
Females	ages 11-24	1,200 mg
	ages 25-up	800 mg

Cautions

There are some big differences of opinion on how much is enough calcium for older people. Some scientists at the National Institutes of Health say that for optimal health, postmenopausal women on estrogen should take 1,500 mg of calcium. They recommend that men over 65 also take 1,500 mg. In fact, most people can safely take up to 2,000 mg of calcium a day. However, too much calcium can cause serious side effects. Calcium toxicity might start with vague symptoms like loss of appetite, constipation, drowsiness, and a dry mouth. In more advanced cases it can cause depression, high blood pressure, nausea, vomiting, increased sensitivity to light, and a slow or irregular heartbeat.

Did you know?

Many medicines you take may contain the words "take with food" on the label. However, if you are taking calcium supplements, the best time to take them is between meals. Some foods contain substances which may compete with calcium for absorption in your body.

CAROTENOIDS

Color me healthy

When you think carotenoids, think color. Carotenoids are pigments that brighten up your garden by giving fruits and vegetables distinctive colors, ranging from light yellow to purple. There are more than 500 different types of carotenoids present in fruits and vegetables. They are fat-soluble, and about 50 of them convert to vitamin A in your body. The most well-known of these is probably beta carotene. Other healthful carotenoids include lycopene, lutein, and alpha carotene.

Carotenoids do more than just add color to your dinner plate. Carotenoids like beta carotene that are converted into vitamin A in your body have the same benefits as vitamin A. They protect your vision, strengthen your immune system, and also provide benefits of their own. They are powerful antioxidants, fighting free radical damage in your body. Researchers are discovering that carotenoids can protect you against a variety of diseases. For example, studies find that beta carotene may protect against some forms of cancer, and lycopene may protect against prostate disease.

Food sources

The amount of carotenoids in foods can be judged by the intensity of their color. Fruits and vegetables that have a deep, dark color are richer in carotenoids than pale-colored ones. Even the same type of vegetable can vary in carotenoid content. Sweet potatoes are rich in beta carotene, but light-colored sweet potatoes have less beta carotene than dark orange sweet potatoes. The table below shows some common fruits and vegetables and which carotenoids they contain:

	Alpha carotene	Beta carotene	Lutein	Lycopene
Carrot (raw)	•	•	•	
Sweet potato		•		
Apricot (dried)		•		•
Tomato (raw)		•	•	•
Spinach		•	•	

	Alpha carotene	Beta carotene	Lutein	Lycopene
Broccoli		•	•	
Mango		•		
Cantaloupe	•	•		
Watermelon		•	•	•
Cress leaf (raw)		•	•	
Collard greens		•	•	
Parsley		•	•	
Pumpkin	•	•	•	

RDA

The government has not set an RDA or safe and adequate intake level for carotenoids, but the Alliance for Aging Research recommends that you get 10 to 30 mg of beta carotene a day.

Cautions

Do you love carrots? Go ahead and pig out, or rabbit out, on all the carrots you can eat. You might turn a little yellow, but that's the only known side effect of too many carotenoids. Carotenemia causes a yellowish discoloration of your skin that goes away when you reduce your carotenoid intake.

Natural wart removal

Do you have an unsightly wart that you'd love to get rid of? Try some beta carotene. A dermatologist in Ohio recommends large doses of beta carotene to combat warts. One of his patients, a dentist who had tried conventional wart remedies with no success, took eight 15 milligram capsules of beta carotene daily. After two months, the warts were smaller, and by the end of the fourth month, they were completely gone.

CHROMIUM

Boost blood sugar control

Chromium products are showing up everywhere, from health food stores to grocery and department stores. Advertisements for chromium promise quick and easy weight loss, extra energy, and no-sweat muscle building. But don't fall for all that pretty packaging. Get the facts and then decide if chromium supplements are for you.

Chromium is a trace mineral that works with insulin to move glucose (sugar) out of your blood and into your cells, where it is needed for energy. Studies have found that this function of chromium may make it helpful in the treatment or prevention of diabetes.

Some studies have also shown that chromium supplementation improves cholesterol levels, which may help prevent heart disease.

While some early studies suggested that chromium's ability to convert sugar into energy was useful in weight loss and muscle building, more recent studies which use more accurate methods of measurement have not confirmed those findings.

Food sources

The amount of chromium in foods is difficult to measure, partly because amounts tend to vary according to the soil in which the food was grown and how the food was processed and packaged. The following foods and condiments are good sources of chromium:

Oysters
Fish
Eggs
Cheese
Dairy products
Beef, chicken, and calves' liver
Fresh fruits
Potatoes with skin
Black pepper
Thyme

Deficiency

If you eat a lot of processed foods like most Americans, you probably aren't getting enough chromium in your diet. Much of the chromium in foods is lost during processing. According to one estimate, over 90 percent of Americans get less than 50 mcg of chromium daily, which is the low end of the recommended amount. A low intake of chromium may make it harder for the insulin in your body to work properly, and thus may increase your risk of developing adult-onset diabetes.

RDA

There is no RDA for chromium. However, the National Research Council's Estimated Safe and Adequate Daily Dietary Intake is 50-200 mcg for adults.

Pick the picolinate

If you decide to take a chromium supplement, be sure that you get chromium picolinate. It might also be called GTF (Glucose Tolerance Factor) chromium. These formulations make it much easier for your body to absorb the chromium. Store the tablets in a cool, dry place away from light, and don't freeze them.

Cautions

The amount of chromium that you could normally get in foods and supplements probably won't cause your body any harm. However, people who are exposed to large amounts of chromium on their jobs have experienced serious side effects including skin problems, liver and kidney damage, and lung cancer. While it is not known for sure if large doses of supplements taken over a long period of time could have the same effects, it is a possibility. As with most supplements, exercise caution, and don't exceed the recommended safe amount of 200 mcg daily.

COPPER

A brilliant blood-builder

Copper is a trace mineral that can be found in all the tissues in your body. It helps your body absorb iron and assists in building healthy blood. Because of this, it helps prevent anemia. It also aids in the formation of collagen, a protein that is an important part of bones and connective tissue. The table below shows the copper content of various foods.

Food sources

Oysters, canned, 3 oz	3.792 mg
Brazil nuts, 1 oz	.502 mg
Baked potato, with skin	.474 mg
Lima beans, boiled, 1 cup	.442 mg
Mushrooms, boiled, 1/2 cup	.393 mg
Avocado, Florida, 1/2 cup pureed	.288 mg
Wheat germ, 1 oz	.176 mg

Deficiency

You need very little copper, and your body stores it in your cells, so a deficiency rarely occurs. Symptoms of a copper deficiency include breathing difficulties, skin sores, and weakness.

RDA

There is no RDA for copper, but the Estimated Safe and Adequate Daily Dietary intake is 1.5 to 3.0 mg for adults.

Cautions

Too much copper can cause nausea, vomiting, headache, weakness, diarrhea, dizziness, and a metallic taste in your mouth. You are unlikely to get too much copper from food sources, but copper supplements may cause side effects. Serious cases of copper toxicity are rare but can result in rapid heartbeat, high blood pressure, coma, and even death.

FLUORIDE

A mineral that makes you smile

If your water supply doesn't contain fluoride, your toothpaste probably does. Fluoride is a mineral that helps build healthy teeth. Fluoride also helps build strong bones, partly because it helps your body retain more calcium. It also makes the structure of your bones and teeth harder, larger, and more resistant to decay.

Fluoride isn't just for children who are forming new teeth. Doctors sometimes prescribe it to treat older people with osteoporosis. It may also help prevent hearing loss in older people by helping maintain the inner bone structure of the ear.

Food sources

Usually your water supply is your main source of fluoride. However, you can also get it in your diet. The fluoride content of foods varies. It is higher in foods grown in areas where the fluoride levels in the soil and water are higher. Some foods that are usually good sources of fluoride include apples, eggs, tea, seafood (especially canned salmon and sardines) and beef organ meats like liver and kidneys.

Deficiency

If you don't get enough fluoride, you can expect to have plenty of unattractive and perhaps painful cavities in your teeth. Otherwise, a deficiency of fluoride produces no problems.

RDA

There is no RDA for fluoride, but the Estimated Safe and Adequate Daily Dietary Intake for adults is 1.5 to 4.0 mg.

Cautions

Water that contains too much fluoride can cause discolored, mottled teeth. However, although the teeth may be unattractive, they will most likely be cavity-free.

Although fluoride is usually harmless, if you take an overdose of fluoride supplements, the results can be fatal at amounts more than 2,500 times the recommended amount. Early symptoms of fluoride toxicity include stomach cramps, diarrhea, vomiting, black stools, faintness, shallow breathing, and tremors. If your doctor prescribes fluoride supplements for you, never take more than the recommended dosage.

FOLIC ACID

Fabulous heart protector

Folic acid, folate, folacin, vitamin B9, tetrahydrofolic acid. What do these substances have in common? A lot, because they're just different names for the same basic substance. Maybe folic acid deserves to have so many different names because of the extremely important roles it plays in your health.

Folic acid affects your health even before you are born. It is essential in regulating the development of nerve cells in fetuses. Studies show that folic acid supplements taken during pregnancy may reduce birth defects like spina bifida by 70 percent.

Perhaps folic acid's most important role in your health is protecting your heart. High levels of a chemical called homocysteine in your blood can increase your risk of heart disease and blood clots. Folic acid helps lower homocysteine levels.

Your body also needs folic acid to manufacture DNA that is essential to creating new cells all over your body. It plays a particularly important role in the production of red blood cells.

Food sources

Folic acid's name came from the word foliage, so as you might expect, it's found mostly in plant foods, especially green leafy vegetables and legumes. Cooking and processing can reduce the amount of folic acid in your food, so stick to fresh and raw foods whenever possible.

Chicken liver, cooked, diced, 1 cup	1,078 mcg
Pinto beans, boiled, 1 cup	294 mcg
Kidney beans, boiled, 1 cup	229 mcg
Spinach, boiled, 1 cup	262 mcg
Avocado, Florida, 1 raw	162 mcg
Green peas, boiled, 1 cup	101 mcg
Asparagus, boiled, 4 spears	87 mcg
Orange juice, 1 cup	80 mcg
Cauliflower, raw, 1 cup	57 mcg
Broccoli, raw, flowerets, 1 cup	50 mcg

Deficiency

Studies show that American women generally don't get anywhere near the proper amount of folic acid. One study revealed that only seven percent of women eat even one folic acid-rich leafy green vegetable in a four-day period.

Because folic acid is needed for red blood cell formation, not getting enough can lead to anemia. A deficiency of folic acid is also associated with arthritis. Symptoms of folic acid deficiency include weakness, weight loss, forgetfulness, irritability, digestive problems, sore or burning tongue, and diarrhea.

Other things that can deplete the body's stores of folic acid include alcoholism, tobacco use, stress, pregnancy, and breastfeeding. Drugs can also interfere with folic acid absorption. The worst offenders are anticonvulsants, aspirin, antacids, and oral contraceptives.

RDA

Males	ages 11-14	150 mcg
	ages 15-up	200 mcg
Females	ages 11-14	150 mcg
	ages 15-up	180 mcg
Pregnant		400 mcg

Cautions

Taking folic acid rarely causes any direct side effects, even in large doses. However, taking too much folic acid (1,000 mcg daily or more) may mask a deficiency of vitamin B12. If a B12 deficiency goes undetected and uncorrected for a long time, it can cause permanent nerve damage.

IRON

Pump up your blood cells

If you're an energetic, red-blooded American, you're probably getting plenty of iron. Iron is a critical part of the hemoglobin in your red blood cells. Hemoglobin allows the red blood cells to carry energizing oxygen through your blood to the parts of your body that need it. It also picks up carbon dioxide and other cell waste products and carries them away.

Iron is the substance that makes your red blood cells red. It plays an important role in energy production, helps manufacture collagen, and helps keep your immune system strong.

Food sources

Cream of Wheat cereal, cooked, 1 cup	10.9 mg
Beef liver, fried, 3 oz	5.3 mg
Lima beans, cooked, 1 cup	4.4 mg
Baked potato, with skin	2.7 mg
Sirloin steak, broiled, 3 oz	2.6 mg
Chicken, fried breast, 4.9 oz	1.8 mg
Broccoli, cooked, 1 cup	1.4 mg
Tuna, canned, 3 oz	1.3 mg
Turnip greens, cooked, 1 cup	1.2 mg
Egg, scrambled, 1 whole	0.7 mg

Deficiency

Maybe you aren't so energetic all the time. Do you think you have iron-poor blood? Iron deficiency is the most common nutritional deficiency in the world. It is most likely to affect women of child-bearing age because they lose blood every month through menstruation. If your iron levels go low enough, you will develop iron-deficiency anemia. Your red blood cells won't have as much hemoglobin, so your body cells will become starved for oxygen. Symptoms include fatigue, pale skin, and headache. Some anemic people also develop a behavior called pica, in which they eat strange substances like clay soil, paste, or ice.

Another thing that contributes to deficiency is the fact that iron is not absorbed very well from the foods you eat. To help with absorption, some iron pills also contain vitamin C. Drugs such as antibiotics and calcium carbonate antacids also affect how much iron you can absorb from pills and from your diet. If you need to take an antacid while you're taking an iron supplement, take calcium citrate tablets instead of calcium carbonate.

RDA

Males	ages 11-18	12 mg
	ages 19-up	10 mg
Females	ages 11-50	15 mg
	ages 51-up	10 mg

Cautions

Iron deficiency is common, but iron overload can be deadly. Too much iron is toxic, and it isn't difficult to accumulate large amounts, especially for men. Symptoms of iron toxicity include nausea, diarrhea, vomiting blood, pale skin, and bluish nails and lips. Extreme cases of iron overdose can cause convulsions, coma, and even death.

Too much of a good thing

Because it is so critical to your health, your body literally hoards iron. It recycles iron by removing it from used-up blood cells and sending it back into your bone marrow to be used again. The only time your body loses iron is when you get a haircut, trim your nails, or bleed from a wound. Because you don't excrete excess iron like you do some nutrients, it's easier to get an overload.

People whose bodies hoard too much iron can develop a serious blood disease called hemochromatosis. They have so much extra iron in their bodies that they have a golden skin tone all the time. This perpetual suntan comes from the toxic amount of brownish-red pigment in iron that accumulates in their skin and organs. This disease can be treated by giving blood frequently, which reduces iron stores.

Cut your risk of heart disease

Another serious side effect of too much iron is that it raises homocysteine levels in the blood. Homocysteine, a form of the amino acid cysteine, increases your risk heart disease, heart attack, and stroke. If you already eat a healthy diet and take a multivitamin supplement with iron, you should take note of how much additional iron you are getting in your diet. Some food manufacturers are now adding iron to their products like cereals and breads. You could be getting iron from three sources: the natural iron in foods, the iron in your vitamins, and the iron in prepared foods. So take a minute to add these numbers up and avoid undue risk to your heart.

MAGNESIUM

Magnificent energy mineral

Magnesium is a major mineral, which means that your body needs relatively large amounts of it. Fortunately, it is present in a wide variety of foods, so if you eat a balanced diet you should be getting enough magnesium. Unfortunately, most of us don't eat a balanced diet.

Your body stores some magnesium in your bones, to be used whenever dietary levels fall too low. Your kidneys also help regulate the amount of magnesium in your body, absorbing more when blood levels are low, and releasing more into your urine when blood levels are high.

Your body needs magnesium in order to use calcium, vitamin D, and potassium. Magnesium is important in energy production, and helps you build strong bones and teeth. It also helps keep your teeth healthy by holding calcium in your teeth, discouraging tooth decay.

Magnesium enables your muscles, including your heart, to relax after contracting, and it helps transmit nerve impulses.

Food sources

Magnesium is easily lost during washing, peeling, and processing, so choose fresh or minimally processed foods whenever possible.

Avocado, Florida	104 mg
Sunflower seeds, 1 oz	100 mg
Pinto beans, boiled, 1 cup	95 mg
Oysters, steamed, 3 oz	93 mg
Black-eyed peas, boiled, 1 cup	91 mg
Almonds, raw, 1 oz	83 mg
Spinach, boiled, 1/2 cup	79 mg
Baked potato, with skin	55 mg
Broccoli, boiled, 1 cup	47 mg
Acorn squash, baked, 1/2 cup	43 mg
Oatmeal, cooked, 2/3 cup	40 mg

Deficiency

People who live in areas where the water has a high magnesium content are less likely to die from a heart attack. That may be because a magnesium deficiency makes your heart unable to stop spasms once they start.

Even if you get enough magnesium in your diet, vomiting, diarrhea, alcoholism, or the use of diuretics can cause you to become deficient in this important mineral. And, if you don't get enough magnesium, your levels of other minerals like calcium and potassium will also drop.

Symptoms of a magnesium deficiency include nausea, confusion, depression, and muscle tremors. A prolonged deficiency can produce more severe symptoms including high blood pressure, irregular heartbeat, hair loss, skin sores, and muscle spasms.

RDA

Males	ages 11-14	270 mg
	ages 15-18	400 mg
	ages 19-up	350 mg
Females	ages 11-14	280 mg
	ages 15-18	300 mg
	ages 19-up	280 mg

Cautions

Magnesium is an ingredient in many over-the-counter medications, including many laxatives and antacids. If you are taking a supplement containing magnesium, and you take other medicines that also contain magnesium, you could overdose. Too much magnesium can cause drowsiness, weakness, nausea, and diarrhea. Severe cases of magnesium toxicity can cause irregular heartbeat, breathing difficulties, coma, and sometimes death. If you have a medical emergency, always tell your doctor all the medicines you are taking, even vitamin supplements and over-the-counter medicines like antacids.

Label check could save your life

If you don't think it's important to check labels on your over-the-counter medications, you should know what happened recently to a 69-year-old woman taking seemingly-harmless antacids. She ended up paralyzed, in a coma, on life support, and doctors couldn't figure out why. Then routine blood work revealed that she had dangerously high levels of magnesium in her blood. The two bottles of antacids she had been taking every day for several months contained magnesium. Because the symptoms of magnesium overdose included nausea and constipation, she had continued taking more and more of the antacid, attempting to get relief. Luckily for her, doctors identified the problem and she was soon back on her feet.

Don't let this happen to you. Become a label reader and know what is in the medicines you are taking. It could save your life.

MANGANESE

A tireless team player

You know how good vitamin C is for you, but did you know that manganese, a trace mineral, enhances your use of vitamin C and several other vitamins? Manganese also helps your body make and process proteins, including collagen, which is a protein that is important for healthy skin. It aids in proper bone formation and in processing sugar, fat, and cholesterol.

Food sources

Beef liver, fried, 3.5 oz	.423 mg
Blackberries, raw, 1/2 cup	.930 mg
Lima beans, boiled, 1 cup	.970 mg
Pineapple juice, canned, 8 oz	2.475 mg
Pinto beans, boiled, 1 cup	.951 mg
Sweet potato, baked	.638 mg
Turnip greens, boiled, 1/2 cup	.243 mg

Deficiency

There are no known cases of manganese deficiency in humans. However, since you need manganese for proper processing of sugar, not getting enough could possibly lead to diabetes.

RDA

There is no RDA for manganese, but the Estimated Safe and Adequate Daily Dietary Intake for adults is 2 to 5 mg.

Cautions

Too much manganese can interfere with your body's ability to absorb iron and lead to iron-deficiency anemia. If you overdose on manganese supplements, you could experience symptoms like depression, sleep problems, impotence, breathing difficulties, hallucinations, and leg cramps. Notify your doctor right away if you have any of these symptoms.

NIACIN

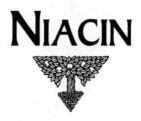

Cholesterol cruncher

Watching your cholesterol? Maybe you need to beef up your niacin intake. Niacin is a B vitamin that is often prescribed by doctors to lower LDL ("bad") cholesterol and triglycerides. It helps treat dizziness, ringing in the ears, and premenstrual headaches. Every cell in your body needs niacin for energy metabolism, and it is vital for healthy skin and proper functioning of your nerves and digestive system.

Most protein-rich foods contain tryptophan, an amino acid that helps raise your niacin level naturally. Tryptophan can be converted into niacin in your body. That's why you will often see the amount of niacin in foods expressed in NE or niacin equivalents. The food either contains pre-formed niacin or tryptophan for your body to convert to niacin.

You might also see niacin referred to as nicotinic acid or nicotinamide. They are both forms of niacin, but they aren't related to the drug nicotine.

Food sources

Beef liver, fried, 3 oz	12.3 mg
Chicken breast, roasted, 3 oz	11.7 mg
Tuna, canned in water, 3 oz	11.3 mg
Salmon, canned, 3 oz	5.6 mg
Ground beef, lean, broiled, 3 oz	5.0 mg
Pork chop, center loin, fried, 3 oz	4.8 mg
Potato, baked	3.3 mg
Kidney beans, canned, 1 cup	1.3 mg
Green peas, canned, 1 cup	1.2 mg

Deficiency

Symptoms of pellagra, a disease caused by niacin deficiency, include the four Ds — diarrhea, dementia, dermatitis, and, if uncorrected, death. About a hundred years ago, pellagra affected hundreds of thousands of people in the midwestern and southern United States. These people were thought to have a contagious illness until health workers realized that well-fed people never got the disease. Today, pellagra still occurs in areas of the world where poor nutrition is common.

Cooking destroys some of the niacin in foods, but you can get some of it back by using the cooking water in your recipes.

RDA

Males	ages 11-14	17 mg
	ages 15-18	20 mg
	ages 19-50	19 mg
	ages 51-up	15 mg
Females	ages 11-50	15 mg
	ages 51-up	13 mg

Cautions

High doses of the nicotinic acid form of niacin can cause flushing, itching, rash, and abdominal pain. Take it with meals to lessen your chances of these side effects. You can also try taking 325 mg of aspirin or 200 mg of ibuprofen about 45 minutes before taking nicotinic acid to lessen its side effects. Avoid alcohol and hot liquids right after taking nicotinic acid. Nicotinamide, the other form of niacin, doesn't cause these kinds of side effects.

You should let your doctor know if you plan to take niacin to try to lower your cholesterol or triglycerides. People with liver problems, diabetes, ulcers, gout, or heart problems should only take niacin under a doctor's care because it can worsen these conditions.

PHOSPHORUS

First-rate protection for bones

Most of the phosphorus in your body is combined with the calcium in your bones and teeth. However, this mineral is present in every cell of your body.

Phosphorus works with calcium to keep your bones and teeth strong and rigid. Because it's part of the genetic material in each of your cells, it's necessary for the growth, maintenance, and repair of all body tissues. Phosphorus also works with enzymes and vitamins to process energy from the nutrients you take in.

Food sources

Peanuts, dry roasted, 1 cup	522 mg
Ricotta cheese, part-skim, 1 cup	499 mg
Sunflower seeds, dry roasted, 1 oz	328 mg
Yogurt, plain, low-fat, 8 oz	325 mg
Kidney beans, canned, 1 cup	268 mg
Chicken, fried, half-breast	259 mg
Milk, skim, 1 cup	247 mg
Sirloin steak, broiled, 3 oz	188 mg
Salmon, smoked, 3 oz	139 mg
Egg, scrambled, 1 egg	102 mg

Deficiency

People very rarely become deficient in phosphorus. However, animals with a phosphorus deficiency exhibit symptoms including loss of appetite, stiff joints, fragile bones, and weakness. Similar symptoms have occured in people who took antacids for a long time. The antacids caused them to be unable to absorb phosphorus.

RDA

Males	ages 11-24	1,200 mg
	ages 25-up	800 mg
Females	ages 11-24	1,200 mg
	ages 25-up	800 mg

Cautions

While phosphorus is not toxic, too much of it can affect your body's ability to absorb and use calcium. Soft drinks and convenience foods may contain particularly high amounts of phosphorus.

POTASSIUM

Puts the brakes on high blood pressure

Your very life depends on a delicate balance of potassium in your cells. Your heartbeat, your breathing, and other vital organ functions require the right amount of potassium for regulation. Because this balance is so important, your body usually maintains tight control, but it is possible to upset the balance.

Potassium helps keep your heartbeat regular by helping your muscles contract, helps supply oxygen to your brain, and assists your kidneys in removing waste from your body. Potassium also helps maintain the water balance in your cells.

Food sources

Dried apricots, 1 cup	1,791 mg
Avocado, Florida	1,484 mg
Figs, dried, 1 cup	1,416 mg
Acorn squash, baked, 1 cup	895 mg
Baked potato, with skin	844 mg
Kidney beans, canned, 1 cup	657 mg

Cantaloupe, diced, 1 cup	482 mg
Banana	467 mg
Orange	237 mg
Peach	193 mg

Deficiency

A dietary deficiency of potassium is unusual in healthy people. However, diarrhea, vomiting, kidney disease, fasting, and the use of diuretics or laxatives can cause you to become deficient.

Dehydration causes you to lose potassium from your cells. This can be especially dangerous because the loss of potassium from brain cells can make you unaware of your need for water. If you are taking diuretics (water pills) that cause you to lose potassium, make sure you eat plenty of potassium-rich foods to make up for the loss.

Potassium deficiency can cause confusion, weakness, drowsiness, dizziness, kidney damage, paralysis, irregular heartbeat, and death.

RDA

There is no RDA for potassium. The estimated minimum requirement for adults is 2,000 mg a day.

Cautions

Too much potassium can be as dangerous as too little. Fortunately, it is difficult to get too much potassium through your diet. Certain disorders, like kidney disease and Addison's disease, can make you more likely to accumulate potassium. If you take potassium supplements or if you use a salt substitute containing potassium chloride, it is possible to get too much. Symptoms of potassium overdose include nausea, diarrhea, weakness, paralysis, kidney damage, irregular heartbeat, and death.

SELENIUM

Super defender

Selenium is a mineral that is required by your body only in very small amounts. However, don't mistake small for unimportant. Selenium helps carry out many vital functions in your body.

Selenium works as an antioxidant, protecting your body from free radical damage. Selenium and vitamin E sometimes team up to protect your cells from oxidation. Selenium also helps your body conserve vitamin E, because it sometimes stands in for the vitamin's antioxidant duties.

Studies show that selenium may help prevent cancers of the esophagus, lung, stomach, prostate, colon and rectum. What's more, it may also help prevent heart disease.

Food sources

Because the selenium content of foods varies according to the soil in which it was grown, it is difficult to give the exact amount found in various foods. However, the following foods are generally high in selenium.

Bran
Broccoli
Cabbage
Celery
Chicken
Cucumbers
Eggs
Garlic
Milk
Mushrooms
Wheat germ

Deficiency

A deficiency of selenium may cause a specific type of heart disease. This was first discovered in China among people who lived in areas where the soil was deficient in selenium. Selenium deficiencies rarely occur in the United States and Canada, where the selenium content of the soil is usually adequate.

RDA

Males	ages 11-14	40 mcg
	ages 15-18	50 mcg
	ages 19-up	70 mcg
Females	ages 11-14	45 mcg
	ages 15-18	50 mcg
	ages 19-up	55 mcg

Cautions

People who take excessive amounts of selenium to fight cancer run the risk of toxicity. Too much selenium can result in symptoms like hair loss and diarrhea. If you continue to take toxic levels, you could suffer liver damage and heart problems. Never take more than 200 mcg of selenium a day unless advised by a physician.

VITAMIN A

Ammunition against infections

Vitamin A was the first fat-soluble vitamin to be discovered, earning it the honor of the first letter of the alphabet for its name. Vitamin A exists in several forms in your body, including retinol, retinal, and retinoic acid, collectively called retinoids. Carotenoids (like beta carotene) are substances which may be turned into vitamin A in your body.

Your body needs vitamin A for many important functions. Your eyesight depends on an adequate supply of vitamin A. It is also needed by your epithelial tissues, which include your skin and the internal linings of your body. Vitamin A assists in bone growth and it helps keep your immune system healthy, so you can fight off infections.

Should you buy natural or synthetic vitamins?

Does the word "natural" on a label mean there's a better product inside? When it comes to vitamins, not usually. Natural simply means that the vitamin was made from natural substances. For example, natural vitamin C may be made from rose hips, and natural vitamin E may come from vegetable oil. Synthetic vitamins are made in a laboratory. A vitamin is a vitamin no matter what the source, and some vitamins that are labeled "natural" may be mostly synthetic anyway. They could just be mixed with natural substances. According to research, the only vitamin that may be better in its natural form is vitamin E because your body absorbs it better than the synthetic form. If a vitamin costs more because it's labeled "natural," it's probably not worth the extra expense.

Food sources

The active form of vitamin A is found only in animal sources like meat and dairy products. However, beta carotene, which is converted into vitamin A in your body, can be found in plant sources like leafy green vegetables. (For more information about beta carotene, see the *Carotenoids* chapter.)

Beef liver, fried, 3 oz	9,120 RE	30,690 IU
Butter, 1 tbsp	107 RE	434 IU
Chicken liver, cooked, 1 cup	6,878 RE	22,925 IU
Cottage cheese, 1 cup	100 RE	342 IU
Egg yolk, 1	97 RE	323 IU
Milk, whole, 1 cup	75 RE	307 IU
Ricotta cheese, 1/2 cup	166 RE	607 IU

Deficiency

Vitamin A depends on fat for absorption, so very-low-fat diets as well as any disorder that interferes with fat absorption (such as celiac sprue) can cause vitamin A deficiency. Diabetics may develop a deficiency because they don't convert carotene to retinol as well as most people. A kind of permanent bumpy skin or "gooseflesh" called keratinosis is an early sign of deficiency. Other symptoms include night blindness, weight loss, reduced resistance to infection, stunted growth, and crooked teeth and poor dental health. A more serious vitamin A deficiency can lead to other vision problems, including total blindness.

RDA

The RDA for vitamin A is expressed in retinol equivalents (RE). This is the amount of retinol that your body will get from a food containing vitamin A. However, you may sometimes still see vitamin A expressed in international units (IU) on some food labels.

Males	1,000 RE	5,000 IU
Females	800 RE	4,000 IU

Cautions

Too little vitamin A can blind you, but too much can kill you. Because vitamin A is fat-soluble, it can be stored in your body over long periods of time. This makes it easier for you to accumulate toxic amounts. Too much vitamin A can cause vomiting; hair loss; bone abnormalities; weight loss; joint pain; and cracked, dried out, or bleeding lips. Extremely high doses (five times or more over the RDA) can cause irreversible or fatal liver damage. Fortunately, it is difficult to get too much vitamin A from food sources. If you ate liver every day, you might build up too much vitamin A, but the danger comes from over supplementing. If you take a vitamin A supplement, you probably shouldn't exceed the RDA.

VITAMIN B1
THIAMIN

Leader of the pack

Thiamin, like all B vitamins, is water-soluble, which means that your body doesn't store it on a long-term basis like the fat-soluble vitamins A, D, E, and K. Excess amounts leave your body every time you go to the bathroom. So it's really important to keep up your daily intake of all water-soluble vitamins. As a safety net, your body stores small amounts of thiamin in your heart, liver, kidneys, and brain to provide a temporary reserve if you neglect your intake for a few days.

If you're feeling tired and a little forgetful, you may need more thiamin in your diet. Thiamin is required by every cell in your body to process energy. It also plays important roles in the function of your nerves, muscles, and heart. You need thiamin for your nerves to carry signals from your brain to other parts of your body, so it helps keep your brain and your body working efficiently.

Food sources

Pork chop, 3 oz	.97 mg
Pork tenderloin, broiled, 3 oz	.82 mg
Oatmeal, instant, 1 cup	.70 mg
Wheat germ, toasted, 1 oz	.47 mg
Black beans, 1 cup	.42 mg
Black-eyed peas, cooked, 1 cup	.38 mg
Avocado, Florida	.33 mg
Brazil nuts, 1 oz	.28 mg
Rice, white cooked, 1 cup	.26 mg
Pecans, 1 oz	.24 mg

Polishing off the thiamin

Thiamin deficiency, also called beriberi, was seen in the Far East as early as the 1600s when the custom of polishing rice, or removing the outer hull, was invented. Unfortunately, the hulls contain all the thiamin in rice. As more and more people began to eat polished rice, beriberi quickly became widespread, but no one caught on to the cause. Finally, right around the turn of this century, a doctor realized the relationship between thiamin and polished rice, and he devised a cure using the hulls.

Deficiency

Mild symptoms of a thiamin deficiency include irritability, tiredness, and sleep disturbances. If a mild thiamin deficiency develops into beriberi, you would begin to experience weight loss, fatigue, weakness, and loss of appetite. If beriberi isn't treated, your symptoms would worsen and soon include nausea, depression, numbness, or paralysis.

Alcoholics are more likely to become deficient in thiamin because they substitute alcohol for nutritious foods. To make matters worse, alcohol decreases the absorption of thiamin in the intestines and increases the loss of thiamin in your urine.

Elderly people who don't eat a well-balanced diet are particularly at risk for a deficiency of thiamin. Unfortunately, their symptoms may be mistaken for normal changes associated with aging and may go untreated.

RDA

Males	ages 11-14	1.3 mg
	ages 15-50	1.5 mg
	ages 51-up	1.2 mg
Females	ages 11-50	1.1 mg
	ages 51-up	1.0 mg

Cautions

Thiamin causes no side effects whether you get it from your diet or from a supplement. The only reported side effect from too much thiamin is anaphylactic shock (severe allergic reaction) from repeated injections of the vitamin.

VITAMIN B2
RIBOFLAVIN

A remarkable ally

Riboflavin, also known as vitamin B2, is a real team player. It works with the other B vitamins to provide you with energy and healthy skin and eyes, and it may help your body absorb iron better.

People who have low iron often have low levels of riboflavin, too. Riboflavin also helps your adrenal glands produce hormones.

Riboflavin may help in the treatment of several disorders, including stomach and liver disorders, alcoholism, burns, and infections.

Food sources

Beef liver, fried, 3 oz	3.50 mg
Milk, 1 cup	.40 mg
Cottage cheese, 1 cup	.37 mg
Oysters, fried, 6 pieces	.35 mg
Yogurt, 8 oz	.32 mg
Egg, scrambled, 1 whole	.28 mg
Turkey, roasted, chopped, 1 cup	.25 mg
Ricotta cheese, 1/2 cup	.24 mg
Mushrooms, cooked, 1/2 cup	.23 mg
Asparagus, 1 cup	.22 mg
Salmon, canned, 3 oz	.15 mg

Deficiency

Riboflavin deficiency usually occurs along with a deficiency of other nutrients, especially other B vitamins. It doesn't cause a specific disease, like many other vitamin deficiencies. However, too little riboflavin is associated with certain symptoms, including depression, cracks at the corners of your mouth, dry scaly skin, and red, itchy, burning eyes.

Unfortunately, riboflavin isn't very stable in foods. Cooking removes some of it from vegetables and meats. To reduce the loss of riboflavin from milk, buy it or store it in opaque containers. Vegetables should be stored in a dark, cool environment to maintain riboflavin content.

RDA

Males	ages 11-14	1.5 mg
	ages 15-18	1.8 mg
	ages 19-50	1.7 mg
	ages 50-up	1.4 mg
Females	ages 11-50	1.3 mg
	ages 50-up	1.2 mg

Cautions

Riboflavin has no known side effects, even in high doses. Taking large amounts in supplements may be a waste of time and money, though, since riboflavin can't be stored in your body. Excess amounts simply pass out of your body in your urine.

VITAMIN B6
PYRIDOXINE

A busy 'B' of a nutrient

If you eat lots of meat and beans, you also need to get lots of vitamin B6. Vitamin B6 helps your body process protein, so the more protein-rich foods like meat and beans that you eat, the more B6 you need. It turns amino acids, which are the building blocks of protein, from a form that you have in abundance into forms that you need more of. It also helps convert tryptophan into niacin, another example of how B vitamins work together to keep you healthy.

Vitamin B6 helps build healthy blood and helps regulate your blood sugar. It gives you energy and strengthens your immune system. The production of neurotransmitters like serotonin requires vitamin B6. If you don't get enough B6, neurotransmitter production could be affected, causing problems with your mood, sleep patterns, and brain function.

Your body also depends on B6 to help it utilize some important minerals including selenium, calcium, and magnesium.

Food sources

Avocado, Florida	.85 mg
Baked potato, with skin	.70 mg
Banana	.66 mg
Chicken breast, roasted	.55 mg
Corn flakes cereal, 1 cup	.48 mg
Lima beans, boiled, 1 cup	.30 mg

Mackerel, canned, 1 cup	.40 mg
Pinto beans, boiled, 1 cup	.27 mg
Prunes, 10 dried	.22 mg
Spinach, boiled, 1 cup	.43 mg

Deficiency

Vitamin B6 deficiency is not associated with a specific disorder. However, because it affects so many functions of your body, a deficiency can cause general wide-ranging symptoms including weakness, insomnia, irritability, confusion, nervousness, and skin problems. A severe deficiency can cause convulsions.

RDA

Males	ages 11-14	1.7 mg
	ages 15-up	2.0 mg
Females	ages 11-14	1.4 mg
	ages 15-18	1.5 mg
	ages 19-up	1.6 mg

Cautions

Although most water-soluble vitamins don't build up to toxic levels in your body, vitamin B6 is an exception. A group of women who took vitamin B6 supplements for their premenstrual syndrome (PMS) symptoms found that out the hard way. The women were taking 2 grams (2,000 mg) of B6 daily, more than 1,000 times the RDA. After a couple of months the women began to develop numbness in their hands and feet and eventually became unable to work. Although these women took very large amounts, doses as small as 200 mg a day can produce side effects over a long period of time.

VITAMIN B12
COBALAMIN

Nature's feel-good supplement

If you're feeling a little depressed, you may just need a jolt of vitamin B12 to snap you out of it. Vitamin B12, also called cobalamin, helps your body manufacture neurotransmitters, chemicals that help carry messages between nerves and your brain. This can be helpful in preventing depression and other mood disorders.

The delicate sheaths that cover the nerve fibers in your body require vitamin B12 to keep your nervous system healthy. Without vitamin B12 to help protect them, your nerves and muscles would soon begin to malfunction.

Vitamin B12 also works along with folic acid to build healthy red blood cells, and it may play a role in building bone tissue.

Food sources

Vitamin B12 can only be found in foods of animal origin, so strict vegetarians may become deficient. If you are a vegetarian, ask your doctor if you need to take vitamin B12 supplements.

Beef liver, fried, 3.5 oz	95.03 mcg
Sardines, 3.75 oz	8.22 mcg
Crab, steamed, 3 oz	6.20 mcg
Salmon, smoked, 3 oz	2.77 mcg
Ground beef, broiled, 3 oz	2.31 mcg
Sirloin steak, broiled, 3 oz	2.28 mcg
Cottage cheese, 1 cup	1.40 mcg
Clams, fried, 3/4 cup	1.10 mcg
Oysters, fried, 6 pieces	1.01 mcg
Yogurt, plain, 1 cup	.91 mcg
Milk, whole, 8 oz	.87 mcg

Deficiency

A deficiency of vitamin B12 can result in pernicious anemia. A clue to the seriousness of this condition lies in the name. Pernicious means "causing great injury, destruction, or ruin." Symptoms include fatigue, pale skin, dizziness, sore tongue, confusion, loss of appetite, loss of muscle control, and paralysis.

Some people who get plenty of vitamin B12 in their diet may still develop pernicious anemia because their stomachs don't secrete enough intrinsic factor, a compound needed for your body to absorb B12. This condition can be corrected by getting injections of intrinsic factor. Others likely to develop pernicious anemia include vegetarians and people who have had part of their stomach or intestines surgically removed.

RDA

Males	ages 11-up	2 mcg
Females	ages 11-up	2 mcg

Cautions

If you take in too much vitamin B12, the excess just passes out of your body in your urine. The only possible complication occurs if you take B12 along with large doses of vitamin C. That combination may cause a dry mouth, nosebleeds, or bleeding from your ears.

VITAMIN C

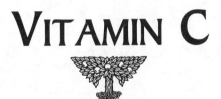

A top-notch antioxidant

If you want to fight wrinkles, then you need to make vitamin C your ally. Vitamin C helps make and maintain collagen, the fibrous substance that keeps your skin looking young. Collagen also holds muscle tissue and bone together and forms the scar tissue that heals wounds. Vitamin C also helps strengthen small blood vessels to help prevent bruising.

Vitamin C has strong antioxidant properties. As a water-soluble vitamin, it protects water-soluble substances in your body from damaging oxidation in the same way that vitamin E protects fats from free radical damage.

Folic acid and iron need vitamin C to be processed properly by your body. Vitamin C keeps iron from becoming oxidized, making your iron intake more effective. Even if you get plenty of iron, if you don't also get enough vitamin C, you may still become anemic.

People have long believed that vitamin C can prevent colds. While that may have not been proven, studies find that it may reduce the length of time you suffer cold symptoms. It also plays a role in your immune system, so it may help prevent infections.

And if all that isn't enough, vitamin C can help you fight off at least three major diseases: cancer, diabetes, and heart disease. The antioxidant properties of vitamin C fight cancer cells in the colon, mouth, esophagus, and cervix. Insulin is secreted more slowly by the pancreas when vitamin C is present, resulting in better control of blood sugar. And perhaps most importantly, vitamin C helps prevent damage to the heart and promotes thinner blood.

Food sources

Sweet red peppers, 1 raw	226 mg
Orange juice, 1 cup	120 mg
Green peppers, 1 raw	106 mg
Strawberries, 1 cup	86 mg
Cantaloupe, 1 cup	66 mg
Brussels sprouts, 1/2 cup	48 mg
Tomato juice, 1 cup	45 mg
Grapefruit, 1/2 medium	44 mg
Collard greens, 1 cup	35 mg
Broccoli, 1 spear	28 mg
Cabbage, raw, 1 cup	22 mg

Limes to the rescue

Vitamin C's other name, ascorbic acid, means "no-scurvy acid." Many sailors died of this disease when they were deprived of fresh fruit on long voyages, long before scientists discovered what caused the disorder. Once the link was established, the British Navy began to require its sailors to carry lime juice on every voyage to fight scurvy, thus earning them the nickname "limeys."

Just what is an antioxidant anyway?

Every time you breathe, you take in invigorating oxygen. As your body processes this oxygen, it produces chemicals called free radicals. Free radicals are unstable molecules that lack an electron. They travel through your body like a band of pickpockets, trying to steal electrons from stable, healthy cells. When they succeed, they leave the cell irreversibly damaged. One damaged cell is not a big deal. But over time, lots of these pickpocket molecules can cause so much damage that your body becomes weak, and you're more likely to fall prey to cancer and heart disease. This cell damage is called oxidation, and it is similar to the oxidation of metal that produces rust.

Don't feel betrayed by your body because it creates these roving thieves. Luckily, your body also produces antioxidants, which neutralize free radicals. You also get them from your diet in the form of antioxidant vitamins. They fight oxidation by combining with free radicals to form a harmless substance or by contributing an electron to the free radical, making it stable. Like the local policeman, antioxidants like vitamin C are always patrolling, protecting your health and arresting oxidation wherever it happens.

Deficiency

A mild deficiency of vitamin C can result in fatigue, bruising, joint pain, dry eyes and mouth, and depression. If untreated, these symptoms can worsen and result in scurvy. Symptoms of scurvy include bleeding or swollen gums, loose teeth, swollen ankles and wrists, weakness, poor wound healing, and hysteria. Scurvy rarely occurs today, because of the easy availability of fruits and vegetables. However, if you neglect your fruit and vegetable intake, it is still possible to become deficient in vitamin C.

Cigarette smokers need more vitamin C than nonsmokers because smoking interferes with the use of vitamin C in the body. Alcoholics may also be more vulnerable to vitamin C deficiency.

The stress connection

Did you ever wonder why some vitamins include the word "stress" in their brand name? It's because of vitamin C. Some studies have shown that vitamin C is used up quickly during times of stress. So vitamin makers made up formulas of mostly vitamin C with some B vitamins to fight stress. But the truth is, you don't really lose that much vitamin C, and the deficit can be made up easily through your diet.

Stave off sore muscles

Do you love to exercise, but hate having sore muscles the next day? Research finds that vitamin C may help head off some of those muscle aches. One study found that people who took 400 mg of vitamin C before doing one hour of aerobic exercise woke up the next day feeling less sore than usual.

RDA

Males	ages 11-14	50 mg
	ages 15-up	60 mg
Females	ages 11-14	50 mg
	ages 15-up	60 mg

Cautions

Many people take supplements containing mega-doses of vitamin C, as much as 1,000 mg a day or more. Although too much vitamin C probably won't kill you, large doses may cause kidney stones, nausea, abdominal cramps, and diarrhea. A recent study found that your body has trouble absorbing more than 400 mg at a time, and you lose the rest in your urine. To make matters worse, chewable vitamin C tablets can erode your tooth enamel. You can easily get enough vitamin C if you eat the recommended five fruits and vegetables a day. So before you invest a lot of money in mega-dose supplements, see if you can't just eat more oranges or broccoli or brussels sprouts. That's a much cheaper, healthier, and safer alternative.

VITAMIN D

'The sunshine vitamin'

Soaking up some sunshine may make you feel happier. It may also make you healthier, because sunshine is an important source of vitamin D. Your body can manufacture vitamin D from sunlight on your skin, earning it the nickname "the sunshine vitamin."

Vitamin D's most important role is helping your body absorb calcium and phosphorus. These minerals are essential for strong bones and teeth. However, your body can't use their bone-building abilities without some help from vitamin D. This makes vitamin D as important as calcium in maintaining strong bones and preventing osteoporosis.

Vitamin D also helps your immune system resist infections, and research indicates that it may play a part in preventing colorectal cancer. One study found that people who got more than 3.75 mcg of vitamin D daily were half as likely to get colorectal cancer.

Food sources

Sunlight is the main source of vitamin D for most people. However, if you don't get out in the sun much, you can still get vitamin D in your diet, especially in fortified milk.

Egg, 1 whole	.65 mcg
Fortified margarine, 1 tsp	.5 mcg
Fortified milk, 1 cup	2.5 mcg
Shrimp, boiled, 3 oz	3.0 mcg

Deficiency

Centuries ago, children with bowed legs, knock knees, and protruding chests were a fairly common sight. They had rickets, which is caused by a vitamin D deficiency. Even before vitamin D was discovered, doctors realized that rickets could be cured by cod liver oil, which happens to be high in vitamin D, or by spending time in the sunshine. Adult rickets is called osteomalacia, and it causes your bones to become soft and easy to break.

You absorb less vitamin D as you get older, so elderly people may be more likely to become deficient. People with dark skin may need more vitamin D in their diet because they absorb less sunlight than other people. Anyone who doesn't get enough sunlight, like night workers or people in nursing homes, may become deficient. Smog, fog, clouds, and window glass can block out the UV rays that help you make vitamin D and could contribute to a deficiency.

RDA

Males to age 25	10 mcg	400 IU
Males over age 25	5 mcg	200 IU
Females to age 25	10 mcg	400 IU
Females over age 25	5 mcg	200 IU

Cautions

Vitamin D is the most toxic of all the vitamins, so be cautious with supplements. If you take as little as four to five times the RDA for vitamin D, you may experience toxicity symptoms including headache, nausea, and diarrhea. If you continue to get too much vitamin D, the level of calcium in your blood can become too high. Your body may then deposit the excess calcium in your heart or kidneys. This can cause irreversible kidney damage or heart disease.

You probably can't get too much vitamin D from food or sunlight. Some vitamin D is stored in your fat for the darker days of winter, but your skin breaks down any excess. Just remember not to overdo it: too much sunlight does increase your risk of skin cancer.

VITAMIN E

Free-radical fighter

When vitamin E was discovered, researchers named it toco-pherol, from the Greek word "tokos," meaning "offspring." That was because researchers found that rats who didn't have enough of this substance were unable to reproduce. It was later called vitamin E and includes four different forms. The active and most common form is alpha tocopherol. The others are beta tocopherol, gamma tocopherol, and delta tocopherol.

Vitamin E may be the most effective antioxidant in your body. It works along with other antioxidants like vitamin C and selenium to protect your cells from damaging free radicals. Vitamin E is espe-cially important to your lungs, helping protect them from the harm-ful effects of pollution.

As far back as the 1940s, researchers realized that vitamin E could significantly improve angina symptoms at 200 to 600 mg a day. More recent studies have shown that vitamin E can make your blood less sticky and help prevent heart and artery disease. It may also reduce your risk of cancer by preventing free radical damage to your DNA, and it strengthens your immune system, making your body more able to fight off infections and disease.

Food sources

Wheat germ oil, 1 tbs	26.17 mg
Sunflower seeds, roasted, 1 oz	14.25 mg
Sunflower oil, 1 tbs	6.88 mg
Almonds, blanched, 1 oz	5.74 mg
Safflower oil, 1 tbs	4.70 mg
Mango, 1 raw	2.32 mg
Peanuts, dry roasted, 1 oz	2.10 mg
Olive oil, 1 tbs	1.67 mg

Deficiency

You may not be getting enough vitamin E to prevent heart disease, but you're probably not deficient. Because vitamin E is widespread in foods, true deficiency rarely occurs in humans. However, people who eat a very-low-fat diet or have a disorder that interferes with their fat absorption may become deficient. A vitamin E deficiency may sometimes cause fibrocystic breast disease, which involves painful non-malignant lumps in your breast. Vitamin E deficiency may also cause intermittent claudication, a disorder that causes leg pains when you walk.

Heat and cooking quickly destroy vitamin E in foods, so try to eat vitamin E-rich foods raw whenever possible.

Are vitamins and minerals ever harmful?

According to an old Hindu proverb, "Even a nectar is a poison if taken in excess." That can certainly be the case with vitamins and minerals. For example, vitamin A is vital for the health of your eyes and the growth of skin, bones, and reproductive organs. In large doses, however, vitamin A can cause headache, vomiting, peeling skin, loss of appetite, and swelling of your bones.

Be sure to read the cautions in this book to avoid turning nature's prescription for health into a life-threatening poison.

RDA

The following amounts of vitamin E are recommended by the U.S. government for healthy individuals. However, most studies that have found health benefits (like a reduction in heart disease) from vitamin E have used doses from 200 to 400 IU (132 to 264 mg) daily. The Alliance for Aging Research recommends a much higher amount than the RDA, 100 to 400 IU (66 to 264 mg) daily.

To convert milligrams (mg) of vitamin E to International Units (IU), multiply the mg by 1.5. For example, 10 mg x 1.5 = 15 IU.

Males	10 mg	15 IU
Females	8 mg	12 IU

Cautions

Although most fat-soluble vitamins can be dangerous, vitamin E is relatively safe. Side effects are rare, even at a daily intake as high as 3,200 mg. However, people who are taking blood-thinning medication and those with a vitamin K deficiency shouldn't take high doses of vitamin E because it would thin their blood even more, which could lead to uncontrolled bleeding.

VITAMIN K

The healing hero

The K in vitamin K stands for the Danish word koagulation, which means clotting. Your blood needs vitamin K to clot properly. Doctors sometimes give people vitamin K before surgery to help reduce bleeding during the operation.

Vitamin K also helps your body produce a protein necessary for building bones. It works along with vitamin D to make sure you have strong, healthy bones.

Food sources

You usually think of bacteria in your body as undesirable, but bacteria in your intestines provides a major source of vitamin K. Vitamin K is also found in many foods, especially leafy green vegetables. The list below shows the amount of vitamin K contained in 100 grams (about 3.5 ounces) of the food listed.

Beef liver	104 mcg
Cabbage	149 mcg
Cauliflower	191 mcg
Egg yolk	147 mcg
Garbanzo beans (chickpeas)	264 mcg
Milk, nonfat dry	10 mcg
Soybean oil	540 mcg
Spinach	266 mcg
Turnip greens	650 mcg

Deficiency

A deficiency of vitamin K is rare because your body can produce it from intestinal bacteria. However, a deficiency might occur if you have a liver disorder or chronic diarrhea or if you take antibiotics that kill the bacteria that produce vitamin K. A deficiency of vitamin K can cause nosebleeds, excessive bleeding from wounds, and bruising.

RDA

Males	ages 25-up	80 mcg
Females	ages 25-up	65 mcg

Cautions

Natural forms of vitamin K have no known side effects. However, the synthetic version found in supplements can quickly reach toxic levels. Vitamin K toxicity can cause your red blood cells to rupture, which may turn your skin a yellowish color. It can also cause brain damage. Because of the dangers of overdosing, you can't get vitamin K supplements without a doctor's prescription.

ZINC

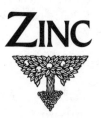

A safeguard for your senses

If you want to keep your senses sharp, make sure you get enough zinc in your diet. Zinc plays a part in sense functions, including your sense of taste and smell. It also helps keep your vision keen by helping maintain levels of sight-saving vitamin A. It is particularly important in night vision.

Zinc is found in more than 60 enzymes in your body and assists those enzymes in performing many important tasks. It is needed for your body to produce DNA for cell growth, which helps speed wound healing. Zinc also strengthens your immune system, helps produce sperm, and is essential for proper growth and development.

Food sources

Oysters, fried, 6 medium	15.60 mg
Chicken livers, cooked, 1 cup	6.07 mg
Dark meat turkey, roasted, 5 oz	5.82 mg
Crab, cooked, 3 oz	3.58 mg
Beef, tenderloin, roasted, 3 oz	3.37 mg
Lobster, cooked, 3 oz	2.48 mg
Pork, tenderloin, broiled, 3 oz	2.45 mg
Black beans, boiled, 1 cup	1.92 mg
Lima beans, boiled, 1 cup	1.79 mg
Cheddar cheese, 1 oz	.88 mg
Baked potato, with skin	.65 mg
Whole wheat bread, 1 slice	.54 mg

Deficiency

Zinc deficiency is likely to affect elderly people, particularly women. About half of all adult women in the United States get substantially less than the recommended amount of zinc daily. Most cases of deficiency are caused by poor nutrition, but alcohol abuse, kidney disease, and sickle cell disease can all increase your risk of becoming zinc deficient. Zinc deficiency can damage your sense of taste and smell, which can lead to a loss of appetite. Other symptoms include poor wound healing, weakness, increased susceptibility to infections, and skin, hair, and nail changes.

RDA

Males	ages 11-up	15 mg
Females	ages 11-up	12 mg

Cautions

Most people can take 50 to 100 mg of zinc without any serious problems. However, high doses of zinc taken over time can interfere with levels of other minerals in your body, including copper and iron. If you take high-dose supplements (2 grams or more), zinc toxicity can result. Symptoms include drowsiness, dizziness, vomiting, poor muscle coordination, anemia, and kidney failure.

COOKING FOR HEALTH

Veal with orange slices

> 2 oranges, peeled and thinly sliced
> 2 teaspoons grated orange rind
> 6 veal cutlets, thinly sliced
> 1-1/2 tablespoons vegetable oil
> 2 tablespoons brandy, warmed
> 1/2 cup beef bouillon
> 1/2 teaspoon salt (optional)
> 1/8 teaspoon white pepper
> 1/4 cup orange juice

Place orange slices in a covered baking pan in a warm oven, 200 degrees. In large frying pan, sauté the veal in hot oil until lightly browned. Add the warmed brandy and flame until the alcohol is completely burned off. Stir in the bouillon, salt, pepper, orange juice, and orange rind. Simmer, covered, for 8 minutes. Remove lid and raise heat to reduce sauce for 4 additional minutes. Serve the veal on a heated platter, covered with sauce and garnished with warm orange slices. Makes 6 servings.

Calories: 250 per serving
Fat: 12 grams per serving

Sherried peas and mushrooms

> 1 4-oz. can sliced mushrooms
> 1 tablespoon margarine
> 1/8 teaspoon marjoram
> 1/8 teaspoon nutmeg
> 2 tablespoons dry sherry
> 1 10-oz. package frozen peas

Drain mushrooms, reserving liquid. In frypan, melt margarine and sauté mushrooms slightly. Stir in marjoram, nutmeg, and sherry. Break apart frozen peas and pour into the pan with the mushrooms. Turn off heat; cover, and let stand for several minutes. Just before serving, add 2 tablespoons of reserved mushroom liquid and bring to a boil, stirring occasionally. Makes 4 servings.

Calories: 94 per serving
Fat: 3 grams per serving

Sicilian pepper steak

1 tablespoon lemon juice
2 teaspoons olive oil
1-1/2 teaspoons fresh mint, chopped
1/4 teaspoon fresh garlic or shallot, minced
1/4 teaspoon peppercorns, crushed
1/2 lb. top round steak

In shallow dish, combine lemon juice, olive oil, mint, and garlic or shallot to make marinade. Marinate steak, covered, in refrigerator for 1/2 to 1 hour. Remove from marinade and press crushed peppercorns into steak. On rack in broiling pan, broil steak 2 inches from heat source, turning once, for about 3 minutes on each side or until done to taste. Remove to warmed platter; serve immediately. Makes 2 servings.

Calories: 230 per serving
Fat: 9 grams per serving

Risotto

1 tablespoon plus 1 teaspoon margarine
1/2 cup onion, chopped
2 cloves garlic, minced
4 oz. uncooked arborio rice (or any medium- or short-grain rice)
1 cup chicken bouillon
1 medium tomato, blanched, peeled, seeded, and chopped
Dash salt
Dash pepper

In 10-inch skillet, heat margarine until bubbly; add onion and garlic and sauté until onion is soft (do not brown). Add rice and cook, stirring frequently, until golden, about 3 minutes; stir in 1/4 cup bouillon and cover skillet. Cook over medium heat until rice begins to absorb liquid, about 3 minutes. Stir in tomato, salt, pepper, and about 1/4 cup more bouillon; cover skillet and cook, checking rice frequently, until liquid is almost absorbed. Continue cooking and adding remaining broth until rice is tender but still moist, about 15 minutes. Makes 3 servings.

Calories: 205 per serving
Fat: 5 grams per serving

Lemon chicken oregano

1 tablespoon lemon juice
1 teaspoon olive oil
1 small clove garlic, mashed
1/2 teaspoon oregano leaves
1/4 teaspoon salt (optional)
1/4 teaspoon pepper
2 chicken cutlets (5 oz. each)
2 lemon slices (garnish)
1 teaspoon fresh parsley, chopped (garnish)

In shallow glass or stainless steel bowl, combine lemon juice, oil, garlic, oregano, salt ,and pepper. Add chicken and turn to coat with marinade. Cover and refrigerate at least 1 hour. Transfer chicken to shallow baking pan that is large enough to hold chicken in a single layer; brush with half of the marinade and broil for 4 minutes. Turn chicken over, brush with remaining marinade, and broil until browned, about 4 minutes longer. Serve garnished with lemon slices and parsley. Makes 2 servings.

Calories: 260 per serving
Fat: 7 grams per serving

Gazpacho

4 cups chicken broth, fat-skimmed, chilled
4 medium tomatoes, chopped
1/2 teaspoon seasoned pepper
2 teaspoons olive oil
6 tablespoons fresh lime juice (about 3 limes)
1 small, red onion, finely chopped
2 green bell peppers, finely chopped
2 stalks celery, finely chopped
Salt to taste
Lime slices (optional garnish)
Watercress sprigs (optional garnish)

Mix broth and tomatoes (including juices), pepper, oil, lime juice, salt, and chopped vegetables. Chill thoroughly and serve garnished with lime slices and watercress. Makes 4 servings.

Calories: 110 per serving
Fat: 4 grams per serving

Oriental cucumber salad

> 1 lb. cucumbers (about 2 medium)
> 1/4 cup plus 2 tablespoons white vinegar
> 1/4 cup plus 2 tablespoons water
> 2 tablespoons soy sauce (reduced-sodium type, if desired)
> 1 tablespoon sugar

Cut off end of cucumber and discard. Peel or leave skin on as you prefer; cut in half lengthwise and scoop out seeds. Cut halves crosswise into thin slices. Stir together all remaining ingredients in a nonmetal bowl. Add cucumber slices, stir to coat well, cover, and let marinate at least 20 minutes (overnight if preferred). Makes 4 servings.

Calories: 28 per serving
Fat: 0 grams per serving

Barbecued pork

> 1 lb. pork tenderloin or thick, boneless loin chops
> 1 teaspoon salad oil
> 1/4 cup onion, sliced
> 1/3 cup prepared barbecue sauce
> 2 tablespoons orange juice
> Hot sauce to taste (optional)

Cut pork across the grain into thin slices; cut each slice into thin strips. Heat oil over medium heat in a large nonstick skillet (if skillet is not nonstick, a bit more oil will be needed) about 30 seconds. Add pork and sauté for 2 to 3 minutes, stirring frequently. Add onions and continue cooking another 3 to 5 minutes or until cooked through. (If using pork chops, a fair amount of juices may accumulate in pan; drain these off before mixing in sauce below.) Meanwhile, in a small bowl combine barbecue sauce and orange juice; stir into pork to coat completely. Cook another 2 minutes or until warmed through. If a spicier version is desired, add hot sauce to taste now or at the table. Serve on sandwich or hamburger rolls, preferably whole wheat. Makes 4 servings.

Calories: 173 per serving (245 calories if chops)
Fat: 6 grams per serving (13 grams if chops used)

Orange and raisin bulgur salad

I cup bulgur (uncooked)
2 cups water
2 teaspoons or cubes low-sodium chicken bouillon granules (optional)
1/2 cup raisins
2 oranges
1-1/2 to 2 tablespoons lemon juice
I tablespoon orange juice
1/2 teaspoon cinnamon
I teaspoon sugar (or less to taste, optional)
4 teaspoons olive oil

Cook bulgur in saucepan with water and chicken bouillon granules; bring to a boil, then reduce heat and simmer 15 to 18 minutes until liquid is absorbed and bulgur is just tender. Place raisins in small bowl and cover with water until plump. Meanwhile, peel oranges and cut into sections. Whisk together last five ingredients to make dressing. When bulgur is done, transfer to large bowl, first shaking in strainer and squeezing to remove extra water if necessary. Drain raisins and add to bowl along with orange sections. Whisk dressing again quickly, pour over salad, and toss gently. This can be served immediately but is unquestionably better if covered and allowed to stand at least 30 minutes for flavors to blend. Can be prepared ahead and refrigerated for 1 to 2 days. Makes 4 servings.

Calories: 289 per serving
Fat: 5 grams per serving

Pasta with crab meat

1/2 lb. spaghetti or linguine (uncooked)
4 teaspoons olive oil (or oil of your choice)
1/2 cup onion, chopped
2-3 cloves garlic, minced
8 oz. fresh mushrooms, sliced
20 black olives, sliced
2 tablespoons dried parsley
I teaspoon basil
1/4 teaspoon oregano
I teaspoon lemon juice
2 6-oz. cans crab meat (or imitation crab meat)
1/4 cup walnuts, chopped
3/4 cup evaporated skim milk
Freshly ground pepper to taste

Cook spaghetti or linguine in boiling water according to package directions until just cooked. Drain. Meanwhile, heat oil in large skillet over medium heat. Add onion and garlic; cook, stirring constantly to prevent sticking, until onion is translucent. Add mushrooms, olives, parsley, basil, oregano, and lemon juice; cook 3 minutes, stirring frequently. Reduce heat to medium-low, add crabmeat, walnuts, and evaporated milk; mix well and cook until heated through. Do not allow to boil. Remove from heat and toss with pasta in pan or in serving bowl. Season with pepper to taste and serve. Makes 4 servings.

Calories: 419 per serving
Fat: 14 grams per serving

Vegetarian pizza

> 1 refrigerated pizza crust
> 1 to 1-1/4 cups no-salt-added tomato purée (or tomato sauce)
> 4 teaspoons oregano
> 2 teaspoons basil
> 1 teaspoon garlic powder
> 6 oz. part-skim mozzarella cheese, grated
> 2-3 cups vegetables of your choice, chopped (suggestions: sliced mushrooms, chopped green or red pepper, broccoli flowerets or sliced stems, sliced tomato, zucchini pieces, sliced onion, thinly sliced carrots, chopped spinach)

Preheat oven to 450 degrees. Place crust on cookie sheet. Combine tomato purée with oregano, basil, and garlic powder in a small bowl; spread onto pizza crust. Add vegetables. Sprinkle grated cheese evenly over top. Bake pizza on lowest shelf of oven until cheese is bubbling, about 7 to 15 minutes. Makes 8 servings (slices).

Tip: For extra speed, use vegetables from the grocery salad bar to save chopping time.

Calories: About 190 to 215 per slice
Fat: 7 grams per slice

Mint chicken with fruit

> 4 chicken breasts, skinless, boneless or with bone
> 6 oz. apricot nectar
> 20 oz. canned pineapple chunks, save juice
> 1 teaspoon dried, crushed mint leaves
> 1 medium onion, thinly sliced
> 2 medium carrots, shredded
> 16 oz. mandarin oranges, drained
> 2 tablespoons currants

Preheat oven to 350 degrees. In baking dish, lay chicken breast side up. Mix together apricot nectar, pineapple juice, and mint and pour over chicken. Lay onion slices and carrots over chicken. Bake for 30 minutes. Add fruit on sides of dish and sprinkle with currants. Bake for another 10 minutes or until chicken is done. Makes 4 servings.

> Calories: 404 per serving
> Fat: 5 grams per serving

Turkey chowder

> 2 green onions, sliced, including green stems
> 1/4 cup green pepper, chopped
> 1 cup celery, chopped
> 1 teaspoon margarine
> 24 oz. evaporated skim milk
> 10 oz. frozen corn
> 3/4 lb. cooked turkey, cubed, chopped, or shredded
> 2 cups fresh or frozen carrots, crinkle cut or sliced
> 1/2 teaspoon dried thyme leaves
> 1/8 teaspoon white pepper
> 1 tablespoon fresh parsley, minced

In large quart pan, on low heat, sauté onion, pepper, and celery with margarine until onion is translucent. Add milk, corn, turkey, carrots, thyme, and pepper. Simmer on low heat. Do not bring to a rapid boil. Before serving, sprinkle with parsley. Makes 4 to 6 servings.

> Calories: 367 per larger serving
> Fat: 4 grams per larger serving

Fillet Provencale

10 oz. fresh or frozen chopped spinach
2 green onions, sliced, including green stems
1 clove garlic, crushed or minced
3 oz. fresh mushrooms, sliced
1/4 cup dry white wine or water
1 lb. fresh or frozen white fish fillets
1/4 teaspoon paprika
16 oz. stewed tomatoes
Lemon slices

Prepare frozen spinach according to package directions or steam fresh spinach until tender. In large saucepan, sauté onion, garlic, and mushrooms in wine or water until it has evaporated. Turn heat off. Spread chopped spinach in skillet. Lay fish fillets on spinach. Sprinkle with paprika. Pour stewed tomatoes over fish. Cover tightly and simmer until fish flakes, about 15 minutes. Garnish with lemon slices. Makes 4 servings.

Calories: 150 per serving
Fat: 2 grams per serving

Serving tip: Serve over a bed of brown rice, linguine, or with a baked potato.
Nutritional plus: This recipe is rich in vitamins C and A and low in fat.

Vegetable barley beef stew

1 lb. lean stew beef (less meat can be used if desired)
1 medium onion, chopped
3 cups water
1 bouillon cube
1/4 cup raw barley
16 oz. tomato sauce
16 oz. package frozen mixed vegetables
1-2 bay leaves
2 teaspoons dried oregano
1/2 teaspoon chili powder
1/4 teaspoon pepper
2 cups water

Brown meat and onion in large quart pan. Meat will initially stick to pan but as cooking continues it will become unstuck. Drain off any excess fat. Add 3 cups water and bouillon cube. Bring to a boil. Add barley. Bring to boil again, then cover and simmer for 1 hour. Add tomato sauce, mixed vegetables, seasonings, and 2 cups of water. Bring to a boil and then simmer for 10 minutes. Makes 8 servings.

Calories: 260 per serving
Fat: 9 grams per serving

Chinese New Year crab balls

> 1 lb. crab meat, finely chopped
> 1/2 cup canned water chestnuts, finely chopped
> 1/2 cup whole wheat bread crumbs *
> 1/2 teaspoon white pepper
> 1/2 teaspoon dried mustard
> 1 teaspoon fresh parsley, finely minced
> 1/4 cup scallions (use white and green portions), finely chopped
> 1/2 teaspoon fresh ginger, finely minced
> 4 egg whites
> 2 teaspoons tamari or soy sauce
> 2 teaspoons sesame oil

Preheat oven to 400 degrees. Mix together all ingredients except final 1/2 cup of bread crumbs until well blended. Form into 1-inch balls and roll in bread crumbs. On lightly oiled baking sheet, bake for 12 to15 minutes or until crab balls are crisp and golden brown. Serve with tamari sauce or a mustard dip. Makes 30 crab balls. These can be made and frozen in advance and reheated in the oven or microwave.

Calories: 31 per crab ball
Fat: .8 grams per crab ball

* Whole wheat bread crumbs are easy to make. Toast bread well, until quite dried out, and crumble in food processor or blender.

Artichoke dip

> 2 cups low-fat cottage cheese
> 1/3 cup plain nonfat yogurt
> 1-1/2 teaspoons lemon juice
> 1 teaspoon dried parsley (or 1 tablespoon fresh, chopped)
> 1/2 teaspoon onion powder
> 1 teaspoon curry powder
> 1 14-oz. can artichoke hearts
> 1 10-oz. can water chestnuts

In a food processor, blender, or with electric mixer, blend the first 6 ingredients until smooth. Then add artichokes and water chestnuts and mix until well chopped. Refrigerate for at least 2 hours. Serve cold in a hollowed-out pineapple, melon, cabbage, or pumpernickel bread round. Makes 3 cups.

Calories: 13 per 1 tablespoon serving
Fat: .1 gram per serving

Chocolate mint angel food cake with raspberry sauce

CAKE
3/4 cup cake flour
1/2 cup cocoa powder
3/4 cup sugar
12 egg whites
1-1/2 teaspoons cream of tartar
1/4 teaspoon salt (optional)
1-1/2 teaspoons vanilla extract
1 teaspoon peppermint extract
3/4 cup sugar

RASPBERRY SAUCE
1 10-oz. package frozen raspberries, thawed, reserve juice
1/4 cup sugar
2 tablespoons cornstarch
water

Preheat oven to 375 degrees.

Cake: Sift flour, cocoa, and 3/4 cup sugar two times and set aside. Beat egg whites with cream of tartar, salt, vanilla, and peppermint until stiff enough to form soft peaks but still moist and glossy. Add remaining 3/4 cup sugar, 2 tablespoons at a time, continuing to beat until egg whites hold stiff peaks. Sift about 1/4 cup of flour mixture over whites and fold in. Repeat, folding in remaining flour by fourths. Bake in ungreased two-piece 10-inch tube pan for 35 to 40 minutes or until done. Invert cake over a wine bottle or long-stem soda bottle and cool.

Raspberry sauce: Add enough water to reserved raspberry juice to measure 1-1/4 cups. Mix sugar and cornstarch in one-quart saucepan. Stir in juice and raspberries. Heat to boiling over medium heat. Boil and stir for 1 minute. Cool. Serve with angel food cake.

Calories: 192 per serving
Fat: .8 grams per serving

Pineapple cheesecake squares

CRUST
2 cups graham cracker crumbs
3 tablespoons honey
1/2 teaspoon cinnamon
1/4 teaspoon ground nutmeg
1-1/2 tablespoons vegetable oil

FILLING
1 8-oz. package farmer's style cheese (cream style, not semi-soft),
   room temperature
1 8-oz. package Neufchatel or light cream cheese, room temperature
1/2 cup sugar
5 egg whites
1 teaspoon vanilla
2/3 cup unsweetened pineapple juice

TOPPING
1/4 cup flour
1/4 cup sugar
1 20-oz. can crushed pineapple in juice (reserve juice)

Preheat oven to 350 degrees.

Crust: In food processor or blender or with a fork, blend graham cracker crumbs, honey, cinnamon, nutmeg, and oil together. Press firmly into a lightly oiled 9 x 13-inch baking pan.

Filling: In food processor, blender, or with electric beater, whip together until smooth cheeses, sugar, egg whites, vanilla, and pineapple juice. Pour cheese mixture over crust. Bake 25 to 30 minutes or until center is set. Cool.

Topping: In saucepan, combine flour, sugar, and reserved canned pineapple juice and unsweetened pineapple juice to equal 1 cup. Over medium heat, bring to a boil and stir for 1 minute, until mixture reaches a thick pudding consistency. Remove from heat, fold in pineapple, and cool completely.

Spread pineapple mixture over cheese. Cover loosely and refrigerate about 4 hours. Cut into 24 squares. Makes 24 servings.

Calories: 144 per serving
Fat: 4 grams per serving

Fruit salad ambrosia

I 3-1/4 oz. package noninstant tapioca pudding
I 3-1/8 oz. package noninstant vanilla pudding
I 20-oz. can pineapple tidbits in natural juice (reserve juice)
I II-oz. can mandarin orange sections in lite syrup (reserve juice)
I-1/2 cups (approx.) orange juice
I cup seedless grapes
I cup sliced strawberries

Stir puddings together in saucepan. Combine reserved canned fruit juices and enough orange juice to equal 3 cups. Add to puddings. Cook and stir mixture until it comes to a full boil. Cool. Fold in four fruits. Pour into pretty glass serving bowl. Garnish and refrigerate for several hours. Makes 12 half-cup servings.

Calories: 101 per serving (approximate, depends on fruits used)
Fat: 2 grams per serving

These recipes are used with the permission of the American Institute for Cancer Research (AICR), a nonprofit organization devoted to research and educating the public about cancer and nutrition. These recipes reflect the four basic dietary guidelines recommended by the AICR that help fight diseases like cancer and provide a healthy diet:

• Lower fat intake to no more than 30 percent of your total calories.
• Eat more whole grains, fruits, and vegetables.
• Cut down on pickled, smoked, and salt-cured foods.
• Drink alcohol in moderation if you choose to drink at all.

For more information, you can call the AICR at 1-800-843-8114.

SOURCES

801 Prescription Drugs, FC&A Publishing, Peachtree City, Ga., 1996

1995 USDA Nutritional Data, Internet WWW address <http://www.rahul.net/cgi-bin/fatfree/usda/usda.cgi> retrieved on Oct. 23, 1997

A Guide to Losing Weight, American Heart Association, 7272 Greenville Avenue, Dallas, TX 75231

A Modern Herbal, Dover Publications, Inc., New York, 1981

A Patient's Guide to Migraine Prevention & Treatment, National Headache Foundation, 428 West Saint James Place, Chicago, IL 60614-2750

A Sweetpotato Sampler: The Sweetpotato as Food, Internet WWW address <http://www4.linknet.net/S_POTATO/faq_1.htm> retrieved on Oct., 16, 1997

A-Z of Companion Planting, HarperCollins Publishers, New York, 1993

Acta Obstetricia et Gynecologica Scandinavica (78,2:177)

Addictive Behaviors (20,4:509)

Adverse Reactions to Food Additives, American Academy of Allergy, Asthma and Immunology, Internet WWW address <http://www.aaai.org/patpub/resource/publicat/tips/tip13.html> retrieved on March 11, 1997

Age Page — Constipation, National Institute on Aging, P.O. Box 8057, Gaithersburg, MD 20898-8057

Alcohol & Alcoholism (27,4:359)

All About Fat and Cancer Risk, American Institute for Cancer Research, 1759 R St., N.W., Washington, DC 20069

Allergic Diseases, Saul Rosen, Ph.D., Internet WWW address <http://www.niaid.nih.gov/publications> retrieved on Sept. 19, 1997

Allergies: What They Are, What You Can Do About Them, The CIGNA HealthCare Report and The Rose Resource, Rose Medical Center, 4567 E. 9th Ave., Suite 020, Denver, CO 80220

Allergy Relief, Naturopathic Medicine, Emily Kane, N.D., American Association of Naturopathic Physicians, Internet WWW address <http://www.healthy.net/library/articles/naturopathic/art.allergies.ek.htm> retrieved on Sept. 10, 1997

Alternative and Complementary Therapies (2,1:46)

Alternative Medicine: The Definitive Guide, Future Medicine Publishin Puyallup, Wash., 1993

Alternative Therapies in Health and Medicine (2,6:73)

American Council for Headache Education, 875 Kings Hwy., Suite 200, Woodbury, NJ 08096-3172

American Family Physician (41,1:150; 44,4:1419; 47,5:1183; 48,8:1461; 49,6:1423; 50,3:633; 50,6:1309; 51,6:1527; 51,8:1861,1997; 52,3:965; 55,1 and 55,7:2455,2507)

American Health (January/February, 1997)

American Heart Association News Releases No. 96-4396 (March 15, 1 and No. 96-4454 (Sept. 15, 1996)

American Institute for Cancer Research Newsletter (39:4; 49:7; 49:10; anc

American Journal of Cardiology (79,2:120)

American Journal of Epidemiology (142,4:404; 143,3:240; 144,5:496; 14 and 146,4:294)

American Journal of Obstetrics and Gynecology (173,3:881)

American Journal of Psychiatry (154,3:426)

American Journal of Public Health (84,5:788)

American Journal of Respiratory and Critical Care Medicine (151,5:1

Anaesthesia (45,8:669)

Annals of Epidemiology (6,1:41)

Annals of Internal Medicine (115,7:505; 116,5:353; 119,7:599; 120S,1: 125,2:81; 125,5:353; 126,5:372; and 126,7:497)

Annals of Medicine (29,2:95)

Annals of the New York Academy of Sciences (570,1:291)

Annals of the Rheumatic Diseases (50:463)

Appetite (26,1:71)

Apricot, Internet WWW address <http://food.epicurious.com/db/

dictionary/terms/a/apricot.html> retrieved on Oct. 28, 1997

Archives of Dermatology (132,11:7)

Archives of Environmental Health (46,1:37)

Archives of Family Medicine (4,4:304; 4,8:709; 5,7:413; 5,10:593; and 6,4:354)

Archives of Internal Medicine (156,5:521; 156,11:1143; and 156,13:1399)

Archives of Medical Research (27,4:519)

Archives of Ophthalmology (111,1:104; 112,2:222; 113,6:743; 113,9:1113; 113,12:1518; and 114,8:991)

Are You at Risk? Diabetes Risk Test, American Diabetes Association, Internet WWW address <http://www.diabetes.org/ada/risktest.html> retrieved on March 13, 1997

Arteriosclerosis, Thrombosis, and Vascular Biology (17,8:1490)

*Arthritis Today (*10,1:51; 10,3:34; and 10,5:48)

Aviation Space Environmental Medicine (66,6:537)

Battle of the Fibers, Internet WWW address <http://www.nuskin.net/idn/idnproductmag/information.html> retrieved on Oct. 7, 1997

Before You Call the Doctor, Fawcett Columbine, New York, 1992

Behavior Therapy (24,2:177)

Bestways (18,3:61)

Better Nutrition (58,10:64)

*Better Nutrition for Today's Living (*54,2:42)

Bibliotheca Nutritio et Dieta (52:43)

Binge Eating Disorder, U.S. Department of Health and Human Services, National Institutes of Health, Bethesda, MD 20892

Biomedical and Environmental Sciences (9,2-3:144)

Biotechnology Therapeutics (5,3-4:117)

Blood Purification (7:39)

Bod Squad — Combatting Menstrual Bloating, National Women's Health Resource Center, Internet WWW address <http://www.women.com/1996/

sep/960911.qa.bod.html> retrieved on Sept. 22, 1997

Bowes and Church's Food Values of Portions Commonly Used, HarperPerennial, New York, 1989

British Journal of Cancer (73,5:687)

British Journal of Dermatology (130,6:757)

British Journal of Nutrition (62,3:699)

British Medical Journal (281,6240:578; 291,6495:569; 301,6757:905; 310,6981:693; 310,6994:1559,1563; 311,7013:1124; 311,7018:1457; 311,7021:1657; 312,7031:608; 313,7052:253; 313,7069:1362; and 314,7091:1364)

California Avocado Fun Facts, Internet WWW address <http://avoinfo. cyberworks.net/aboutavocados/funfacts.html> retrieved on Oct. 16, 1997

Canadian Journal of Surgery (36,5:453)

Canadian Medical Association Journal (155,7:935)

Cancer (64,11:2347)

Cancer Causes and Control (5,4:326 and 6,6:532)

Cancer Facts and Figures — 1995, American Cancer Society, 1599 Clifton Road, Atlanta, GA 30329-4251

Cancer Facts, National Cancer Institute, National Institutes of Health, Bethesda, MD 20892

Cancer Research (55,2:259)

Carcinogenesis (15,9:1881)

Carpal Tunnel Syndrome, National Institute of Arthritis and Musculoskeletal and Skin Diseases, National Institutes of Health, Bethesda, MD 20892

Cephalalgia (14,3:228)

Chest (74,4:408)

Cholesterol, Fiber and Oat Bran: AHA Recommendation, Internet WWW address <http://www.americanheart.org/heartg/cholf.html> retrieved on Oct. 9, 1997

Chronic Fatigue Syndrome, National Institute of Allergy and Infectious Diseases, Internet WWW address <http://www.niaid.nih.gov/factsheets/

cfs.htm> retrieved on June 13, 1997

Chronic Urticaria, National Jewish Medical and Research Center, Internet WWW address <http://www.njc.org/MSU/09^6MSU_Chronic_Urticaria. html> retrieved on March 14, 1997

Chung Hua Min Kuo Wei Sheng Wu Chi Mien I Hsueh Tsa Chih (18,3:190)

Circulation (86,3:803; 94,1:14; 94,11:2720,3023,3223; and 96,2:412)

Clinical and Experimental Allergy (26,2:216)

Clinical and Experimental Obstetrics and Gynecology (21,3:170)

Columbia University Crohn's Disease Information, Internet WWW address <http://www.columbia.edu/cu/healthwise/0752.html> retrieved on June 24, 1997

Columbus Ledger-Enquirer (Dec. 8, 1996)

Complementary Medicine: Part Two — Herbs for Diabetics, Internet WWW address <http://www.diabetes.com/site/MISC/FSBODY.HTM?TorF=F& FeatureID=45&> retrieved on July 23, 1997

Complementary Medicine: Part Three — Vitamins for Diabetics, Internet WWW address <http://www.diabetes.com/site/MISC/FSBODY.HTM? TorF=F&FeatureID=44&> retrieved on July 23, 1997

Complete Guide to Symptoms, Illness & Surgery, The Berkley Publishing Group, New York, 1995

Complete Guide to Symptoms, Illness & Surgery For People Over 50, The Berkley Publishing Group, New York, 1992

Constipation: What you can do about it, Procter & Gamble, P.O. Box 171, Cincinnati, OH 45201

Constipation in the Elderly, Medical Sciences Bulletin, Internet WWW address <http://pharminfo.com/pubs/msb/constip.html> retrieved on July 11, 1997

Consultant (36,1:124)

Consumer Reports on Health (8,2:21 and 8,3:33)

Crohn's & Colitis Foundation of America Medical Central Library, Internet WWW address <http://www.ccfa.org/library.htm> retrieved on June 25, 1997

Cruising World (21,9:77)

Culpepper Guides, Herbs and Aromatherapy, Bloomsburg Books, London, 1989

Current Medical Diagnosis & Treatment 1997, Appleton & Lange, Stamford, Conn., 1997

Cutis (55,6:332)

Dermatologic Clinics (7,1:43)

Dermatology (191,1:6)

Diabetes Care (16,4:578 and 18,10:1373)

Diabetes Forecast (42,12:18 and 48,9:52)

Diabetes Medicine (11,3:312)

Diabetes Overview, NIH Publication No. 96-3873, The National Diabetes Outreach Program of the National Institutes of Health, 1 Information Way, Bethesda, MD 20892-3560

Diabetes Statistics, NIH Publication No. 96-3926, The National Diabetes Outreach Program of the National Institutes of Health, 1 Information Way, Bethesda, MD 20892-3560

Diarrhea, Mayo Foundation for Medical Education and Research, Internet WWW address <http:www.mayo.ivi.com/mayo/9310/htm/diarrhea.htm> retrieved on July 1, 1997

Did You Know About the Tomato? Internet WWW address <http://www. tomato.org/tips-pgs/facts.htm#anchor110993> retrieved on Nov. 4, 1997

Diet & Nutrition Resource Center — Ask the Mayo Dietitian, Mayo Health Oasis, Internet WWW address <http://www.mayo.ivi.com/mayo/askdiet/ htm/new/qd961202.htm> retrieved on July 21, 1997

Diet, Nutrition & Cancer Prevention: the Good News, Publication No. 87-2878, National Institutes of Health, Bethesda, MD 20892

Dietary Approaches to Stop Hypertension, Internet WWW address <http://dash.bwh.harvard.edu/> retrieved on July 29, 1997

Dietary Guidelines for Healthy American Adults, American Heart Association, Internet WWW address <http://www.amhrt.org/hs96/dietg.html> retrieved on Sept. 24, 1997

Dietary Guidelines to Lower Cancer Risk, American Institute for Cancer Research, 1991

Dieting and Gallstones, NIH Publication No. 94-3677, National Institutes of Health, Bethesda, MD 20892

Digestive Diseases and Sciences (35,5:630)

Diseases & Treatments: Crohn's Disease, Internet WWW address <http://www.medicinenet.com/mainmenu/encyclop/ARTICLE/Art_C/Crohn.HTM> retrieved on June 23, 1997

Diseases of the Hair and Nails, Year Book Medical Publishers, Chicago, 1987

Diverticulosis and Diverticulitis, National Institute of Diabetes and Digestive and Kidney Diseases, Internet WWW address <http://www.niddk.nih.gov/Divertic/Divertic.htm> retrieved on July 1, 1997

Do Your Level Best, NIH Publication No. 95-4016, The National Diabetes Outreach Program of the National Institutes of Health, 1 Information Way, Bethesda, MD 20892-3560

Doctor's Guide to Medical & Other News, Internet WWW address <http://www.pslgroup.com/dg/33452.htm> retrieved on Aug. 15, 1997

Dr. Dean Ornish's Program for Reversing Heart Disease, Random House, New York, 1990

Dr. Hirsch's Guide to Scentsational Weight Loss, Element Books, Inc., Rockport, Mass., 1997

Drugs (8:330)

Drugs & Aging (6,6:465)

Drugs Under Experimental and Clinical Research (14,4:277)

Eat Right to Help Lower Your High Blood Pressure, NIH Publication No. 92-3289, Department of Health and Human Services, National Institutes of Health, Bethesda, MD 20892

Eating Disorders, NIH Publication No. 93-3477, U.S. Department of Health and Human Services, National Institutes of Health, Bethesda, MD 20892

Eggs, American Heart Association, Internet WWW address <http://www.amhrt.org/hs96/eggs.html> retrieved on Sept. 24, 1997

Emergency Medicine (28,11:49, 64)

Encyclopedia of Natural Medicine, Prima Publishing, Rocklin, Calif., 1991

Encyclopedia of Nutritional Supplements, Prima Publishing, Calif., 1996

Environmental Nutrition (15,10:7; 17,2:7; 18,12:3; 19,8:1; 19,9:8; 19,10:7; and 19,11:7)

Epicurious Dictionary, Internet WWW address <http://food.epicurious.com>

European Journal of Clinical Nutrition (48,8:561; 49,4:282; and 50,9:573)

European Journal of Obstetrics, Gynecology, and Reproductive Biology (38,1:19)

Everything You Need to Know About Diseases, Springhouse Corp., Springhouse, Pa., 1996

Experimental Gerontology (30,3-4:299)

Facts About Angina, NIH Publication No. 92-2890, U.S. Department of Health and Human Services, Bethesda, MD 20892

Facts About Arrhythmias/Rhythm Disorders, NIH Publication No. 91-2264, U.S. Department of Health and Human Services, National Institutes of Health, Bethesda, MD 20892

Facts and Fallacies About Digestive Diseases, National Digestive Diseases Information Clearinghouse, Internet WWW address <http://www.niddk.nih.gov/Facts_Fallacies/FACTS.html> retrieved on Sept. 8, 1997

Fast Food Facts, Chronimed Publishing, Minneapolis, Minn., 1994

FDA Consumer (30,7:15; 24,1:24; 26,2:31; 26,5:26; 29,2:19; 30,1:16; and 30,4:23)

FEMS Immunology and Medical Microbiology (13,4:273)

Fertility and Sterility (62,2:313)

Fever Blisters and Canker Sores, NIH Publication No. 92-247, National Institute of Dental Research, 9000 Rockville Pike, Bethesda, MD 20892

Folic Acid, Homocysteine and Atherosclerosis, American Heart Association, Internet WWW address <http://www.americanheart.org/Heart_and_Stroke_A_Z_Guide/folic.html> retrieved on Dec. 18, 1997

Food and Mood: The Complete Guide to Eating Well and Feeling Your Best, Henry Holt and Co., New York, 1995

Food Safety Notebook (5,1:6 and 7,11/12:91)

Food Values of Portions Commonly Used, HarperPerennial, New York, 1989

Food, Nutrition and Health (21,4:6)

From Around the World, International Menus and Recipes to Lower Cancer Risk, American Institute for Cancer Research, Washington, 1991

Gallstones: A National Health Problem, American Liver Foundation, Cedar Grove, N.J.

Garlic Tidbits, Internet WWW address <http://mastermall.com/garlic/ftx2.htm> retrieved on Oct. 16, 1997

Gas in the Digestive Tract, National Institute of Diabetes and Digestive and Kidney Diseases, Internet WWW address <http://www.niddk.nih.gov/Gas/Gas.html> retrieved on July 16, 1997

Gastroenterology (108,1:125)

Geriatrics (48,10:57; 50,4:14; 50,7:14; 51,5:14; 51,9:13; 51,2:21; 51,12:37; and 52,2:27)

Get Hooked On Seafood Safety, DHHS Publication No. (FDA) 92-2258, Department of Health and Human Services, U.S. Food and Drug Administration, 5600 Fishers Lane, Rockville, MD 20857

Griffith's 5 Minute Clinical Consult, Williams & Wilkins, Baltimore, 1996

Guidelines on Diet, Nutrition, and Cancer Prevention: Reducing the Risk of Cancer with Healthy Food Choices and Physical Activity, The American Cancer Society, 1996

Haematologica (80,6:518)

Hair Loss Journal (6,2:1)

Hamilton & Whitney's Nutrition Concepts and Controversies, West Publishing Co., St. Paul, Minn., 1994

Handling/Storage of Tomatoes, Internet WWW address <http://tomato.org/tips-pgs/handle2.htm> retrieved on Nov. 4, 1997

Hautarzt (47,6:459)

Headache (34,10:590 and 37,5:312)

HeadLines (Fall 1996)

Healing With Food, HarperPerennial, New York, 1993

Health News, The News-Times, Internet WWW address <http://www.newstimes.com/archive/feb1797/hee.htm> retrieved on Oct. 23, 1997

Healthy Flavors of the World: Asia, American Institute for Cancer Research, Washington, 1997

Hematology, Marcia Datz, Internet WWW address <http://www.medstudents. com.br/hemat/hemat4.htm> retrieved on July 21, 1997

Herbal Medicine, Beaconsfield Publishers, Beaconsfield, England, 1988

Herbal Prescriptions for Better Health, Prima Publishing, Rocklin, Calif., 1996

Herbcraft, Yerba Buena Press, San Francisco, 1971

Herbs for Health (Spring/Summer 1996)

Herbs of Choice, The Therapeutic Use of Phytomedicinals, The Haworth Press, Binghamton, N.Y., 1994

Hives, American Academy of Allergy, Asthma and Immunology, Internet WWW address <http:// www.aaaai.org/patpub/resource/publicat/tips/ tip10.html> retrieved on March 11, 1997

Holistic Nursing Practice (10,2:30)

How to Buy Fresh Fruits, U.S. Department of Agriculture, Home and Garden Bulletin No. 260, 1994

How to Buy Fresh Vegetables, U.S. Department of Agriculture, Home and Garden Bulletin No. 258, 1994

Human Nutrition: Clinical Nutrition (38,3:215)

Hypothyroidism, Internet WWW address <http://www.clark.net/pub/tfa/ hypobrochure.html> retrieved on July 25, 1997

Immunopharmacology (35,3:229)

Impotence Resource Center, Internet WWW address <http://www.impotence. org/facts.htm> retrieved on March 19, 1997

Indian Journal of Medical Research (98:240)

Indian Journal of Medical Science (49,1:5)

Information About Tinnitus, American Tinnitus Association, P.O. Box 5, Portland, OR 97207-0005

Internal Medicine (33,2:82)

International Archives of Allergy and Applied Immunology (95,2-3:156)

International Journal of Cancer (50,2:223)

International Journal of Epidemiology (24,1:33)

International Journal of Vitamin and Nutrition Research (66,1:19)

Interview with Dr. Linda Bartoshuk, Yale University, New Haven, Conn.

Interview with Gary Deshon, spokesman for Golden Jersey Products, Vero Beach, Fla.

Interview with Professor Peter Bramley, Division of Biochemistry, Royal Holloway Hospital, University of London, Egham, England

Introduction to Coenzyme Q10, Peter H. Langsjoen, M.D., Internet WWW address <http://weber.u.washingotn.edu/~ely/coenzq10.html> retrieved on Feb. 24, 1997

Iron and Heart Disease, American Heart Association, Internet WWW address <http://www.americanheart.org/Heart_and_Stroke_A_Z_Guide/iron.html > retrieved on Dec. 18, 1997

Iron, UCLA Student Health Services, Internet WWW address <http://www.saonet.ucla.edu/health/healthed/vegiweb/resource.frk/2iron&.htm> retrieved on Aug. 18, 1997

Irritable Bowel Syndrome, Internet WWW address <http://www.niddk.nih.gov/IBS/IBS.html> retrieved on July 1, 1997

Irritable Bowel Syndrome: What It Is and What to Do About It, Internet WWW address <http:www.aafp.org:80/patientinfo/bowel.html> retrieved on Feb. 28, 1997

Japanese Journal of Antibiotics (48,3:432)

Journal of the American College of Nutrition (14,5:419 and 16,2:109)

Journal of Advancement in Medicine (8,1:37)

Journal of Agricultural and Food Chemistry (44,3:701)

Journal of Applied Nutrition (46,3:74)

Journal of Clinical Epidemiology (47,1:43)

Journal of Clinical Microbiology (35,6:1300)

Journal of Clinical Pharmacology (30,7:596)

Journal of Clinical Pharmacy and Therapeutics (21:101)

Journal of Ethnopharmacology (29:267 and 39:129)

Journal of Family Practice (37,2:180)

Journal of Food Science (58,6,1407)

Journal of Occupational and Environmental Medicine (38,5:485)

Journal of Optimal Nutrition (3,1:32)

Journal of Oral Pathology and Medicine (20,10:473)

Journal of Pharmaceutical Sciences (76,5:371)

Journal of Reproductive Medicine (36,2:131)

Journal of Rheumatology (21,8:1477)

Journal of the American Academy of Dermatology (31,1:89)

Journal of the American College of Cardiology (28,5:1103 and 29,5:1028)

Journal of the American College of Nutrition (11,2:172; 11,6:694; 12,4:442,349, 384; 13,2:118; 14,2:116,124; 14,3:229; 14,4:317,387; 15,6:630; and 16,2:109)

Journal of the American Dental Association (113,2:262)

Journal of the American Dietetic Association (89,10:1492; 93,10:1106; 94,2:147; 96,9:854; and 96,12:1254)

Journal of the American Geriatric Society (45,6:718)

Journal of the American Medical Association (271,10:751; 273,20:1563; 274,23:1846; 276,24:1957,1984; 277,3:201; and 277,20:1582)

Journal of the Association of Physicians of India (37,10:647)

Journal of the National Cancer Institute (76,4:621; 86,1:33; and 88,25:1706)

Journal of the Royal Society of Medicine (87,1:9)

Leading with his nose, U.S. News Online, Internet WWW address <http:// usnews.com/usnews/issue/970331/31nose.htm> retrieved on Dec. 15, 1997

Lifetime Encyclopedia of Natural Remedies, Parker Publishing Company, West Nyack, N.Y., 1993

Lupus News (13:1 and 71:1)

Macular Degeneration & Nutrition, American Academy of Ophthalmology, Internet WWW address <http://www.eyenet.org/public/faqs/nutrition_faq. html> retrieved on Dec. 9, 1997

Making Bag Lunches, Snacks and Desserts Using the Dietary Guidelines, USDA Home & Garden Bulletin No. 232-9

Managing Unstable Angina, AHCPR Publication No. 94-0604, U.S. Department of Health and Human Services, 2101 East Jefferson St., Rockville, MD 20852

Maintaining Your Digestive Health, Inside Tract, Glaxo Wellcome Institute for Digestive Health, P.O. Box 2032, West Caldwell, N.J., 07007-9711

Maturitas (21, 3:189)

Mayo Clinic Health Letter (15,7:1)

Mayo Health O@sis, Internet WWW address <http://healthnet.ivi.com/mayo/9310/htm/headache.htm> retrieved on July 21, 1997

Meat, Poultry and Fish, American Heart Association, Internet WWW address <http://www.americanheart.org/Heart_and_Stroke_A_Z_Guide/meat.html> retrieved on Dec. 9, 1997

Medical Hypotheses (46,4:400)

Medical Tribune for the Family Physician (35,18:16)

Medical Tribune for the Internist & Cardiologist (34,8:12; 36,1:19; 36,4:1,14; 36,12:8; 36,19:2; 36,21:17; 36,22:6; 36,23:8; 36,23:18; 37,2:2; 37,4:1; and 37,13:8)

Medical Update (20,1:5 and 20,6:5)

Medicinal Research Reviews (16,1:111)

Melatonin, The Anti-Aging Hormone, Avon Books, New York, 1995

Melatonin, Your Body's Natural Wonder Drug, Bantam Books, New York, 1995

Menopause, National Institutes of Health, National Institute on Aging, Internet WWW address <http://www.pueblo.gsa.gov/cic_text/health/other/menopause.txt> retrieved on Aug. 11, 1997

Modern Medicine (63:26)

Mothering (57:85)

Natural Healing Newsletter (7,77:3)

Natural Health (23,1:43 and 23,3:78)

Natural Medicines and Cures Your Doctor Never Tells You About, FC&A Publishing, Peachtree City, Ga., 1996

Natural Prescriptions, Ballantine Books, New York, 1994

Natural Ulcer Remedies? Internet WWW address <http://www.cc.columbia. edu./cu/healthwise/0953.html> retrieved on Aug. 5, 1997

NCRR Reporter (XXI,4:1)

Neurology (44,9:1687 and 49,3:813)

Nippon Eiseigaku Zasshi (50,4:849)

No Time to Cook, American Institute for Cancer Research, Washington, 1990

North American Menopause Society (NAMS), Internet WWW address <http://www.menopause.org/pfaq.htm> retrieved on Aug. 18, 1997

Nutrition 94/95, The Dushkin Publishing Group, Inc., Guilford, Conn., 1994

Nutrition and Cancer (18,1:1; 25,2:205; and 26,2:167)

Nutrition and Diet Therapy Dictionary, Van Nostrand Reinhold, New York, 1991

Nutrition and Health (10,4:285)

Nutrition Research Newsletter (11,7-8:91; 12,10:103; 14,2:23,25,26; 15,6:72; 15,10:109; and 16,2:23)

Nutrition Reviews (53,5:131; 54,8:241,248; and 54,11:S67)

Nutrition Today (29,3:23)

Obstetrics and Gynecology (75,2:244)

Onhealth: Canker Sores, Internet WWW address <http://www.healthnet.ivi. com/bh/cond/ailments/htm/cankers.htm> retrieved on Sept. 5, 1997

Onhealth: Cold Sores, Internet WWW address <http://www.healthnet.ivi.com /bh/cond/ailments/htm/coldsor.htm> retrieved on Sept. 5, 1997

Onhealth: Gum Problems, Internet WWW address <http://www.healthnet.ivi. com/bh/cond/ailments/htm/gumprob.htm> retrieved on Aug. 25, 1997

Oral Surgery, Oral Medicine, Oral Pathology (72,5:559 and 73,6:708)

Osteoporosis, Office of Scientific and Health Communications, National Institute of Arthritis and Musculoskeletal Diseases, Box AMS, 9000 Rockville Pike, Bethesda, MD 20892

Overcoming Impotence, Prentice-Hall, Englewood Cliffs, N.J., 1994

PDR Family Guide to Nutrition and Health, Medical Economics Co., Montvale, N.J., 1995

Pharmacy Times (61,7:32; 61,9:20; 62,1:77; 62,8:67; 62,12:28; and 63,2:43)

Plant Molecular Biology (32,3:565)

Planta Medica (56,1:44)

Postgraduate Medicine (91,2:115; 92,5:63; 98,2:185; 99,3:109; 99,5:280; 100,4:75; and 101,1:181)

Preparing Foods and Planning Menus, U.S. Department of Agriculture, Home & Garden Bulletin, No. 232-8

Present Knowledge in Nutrition, International Life Sciences Institute Press, Washington, 1996

Presse Medicale (23,10:485)

Preventing Foodborne Illness: Escherichia coli 0157:H7, Centers for Disease Control and Prevention, Internet WWW address <http://www.cdc.gov/ ncidod/publications/brochures/e_coli.htm> retrieved on Sept. 26, 1997

Primary Care for Women, Lippincott-Raven Publishers, New York, 1997

Primary Hyperparathyroidism, Internet WWW address <http://204.141.116. 18:3004/> retrieved on May 29, 1997

Proceedings of the National Academy of Sciences USA (91,16:7688 and 94:10367)

Progress in Clinical and Biological Research (1993,380:47)

Prostate (12,2:179)

Psychology and Aging (11,3:487)

Psychopharmacology Bulletin (27,2:145)

Questions and Answers About Psoriasis, National Institute of Arthritis and Musculoskeletal and Skin Diseases, Internet WWW address <http://www. nih.gov/niams/healthinfo/psoriafs.htm> retrieved on March 20, 1997

Recommended Dietary Allowances, National Academy of Sciences, National Academy Press, Washington, 1989

Revista Medica De Chile (123,1:51)

Riding on the Red Road, Internet WWW address <http://sln.fi.edu/biosci/ blood/red.html> retrieved on Nov. 25, 1997

Rosacea Review (Summer-Fall 1993; Fall 1996; and Winter 1997)

Scandinavian Journal of Primary Health Care (13,2:118)

Science (275,5297:218)

Science News (144,10:153; 149,11:170; and 149,18:287)

Science World (52,6:12)

Soy Flour, U.S. Soyfoods Directory, Internet WWW address <http://www.
soyfoods.com/soyfoodsdescriptions/soyflour.html> retrieved on Dec. 23, 1997

Sports Anemia, E. Randy Eichner, M.D., Internet WWW address <http://
www.uokhsc.edu/sections/hemaonco/sports/sprtanem.htm> retrieved on
July 21, 1997

Stomach and Duodenal Ulcers, National Institute of Diabetes and Digestive
and Kidney Diseases, Internet WWW address <http://www.niddk.nih.gov/
StomachUlcers/Ulcers.html> retrieved on July 1, 1997

Stomach Ulcer Relief with Active Manuka Honey from New Zealand, Internet
WWW address <http://www.wave.co.nz/pages/honey/index2.html>
retrieved on Aug. 5, 1997

Stroke (27,5:813)

Super Healing Foods, Parker Publishing Co., West Nyack, N.Y., 1995

Super Life Span, Super Health, FC&A Publishing, Peachtree City, Ga., 1997

Surgery (107,5:549)

Sweet Potatoes, Cooperative Extension Program; College of Agriculture,
Home Economics, and Allied Programs; Fort Valley State University,
Internet WWW address <http://www.ag.fvsu.edu/html/publications/teletips
/lawn%20and%20garden/vegetables/161.htm> retrieved on Oct. 16, 1997

Symptoms, Illness & Surgery, The Berkley Publishing Group, New York, 1995

Tasty No-cal, High Fiber Substitute, USDA Agricultural Research Service,
Internet WWW address <http://www.newswise.com//articles/ZTRIM.
ARS.html> retrieved on Oct. 1, 1997

Tea Garden Selections, Internet WWW address <http://www.annmarie.com/
AMpg2.html> retrieved on Nov. 14, 1997

The American Journal of Clinical Nutrition (37,3:416; 48,6:1387; 49,4:675;
50,3:551; 53,1:126; 53,1S:346S,193S; 54,5:909; 54,6S:1310S; 56,2:455; 56,4:684;
57,2:115,207; 61,2:325; 61,3S:625S; 61,4S:987S; 61,6S:1402S; 62,1:1; 62,6:1212;

62,6S:1448S,1439S; 63,2:170; 63,6:946,954; 64,5:712,761; 64,6:850,866,928; 65,1:136; 65,1S:327S; 65,2:445; 65,4:1027; 65,6:1803,1826; and 66,2:261)

The American Medical Association Encyclopedia of Medicine, Random House, Inc., New York, 1989

The Apricot, San Luis Obispo County Telegram-Tribune, Internet WWW address <http://www.sanluisobispo.com/stories/0597/apricot.html> retrieved on Oct. 28, 1997

The Art of Aromatherapy, Healing Arts Press, Rochester, Vt., 1977

The Arthritis Cure, St. Martin's Press, New York, 1997

The Atlanta Journal/Constitution (May 18, 1993, E4; Sept. 14, 1995, H12; Nov. 16, 1996, F1; and Sept. 10, 1997, D3)

The Banana as Food, AIMS Education Foundation, Internet WWW address <http://www.aimsedu.org/activities/banana/banana3.html> retrieved on Oct. 13, 1997

The Big Book of Health Tips, FC&A Publishing, Peachtree City, Ga., 1996

The CFIDS Chronicle (1,1:12)

The Clinical Investigator (71,8S:5145)

The Diabetes Advisor (4,5:8 and 5,1:14)

The Doctor's Complete Guide to Vitamins & Minerals, Bantam Doubleday Dell Publishing, New York, 1994

The Enchanted World of Sleep, Yale University Press, London, 1996

The Essential Guide to Vitamins and Minerals, HarperPerennial, New York, 1995

The Estrogen Decision, Westchester Publishing Co., Los Altos, Calif., 1994

The Fat Tooth Fat Gram Counter, Workman Publishing, New York, 1993

The Food Chronology, Henry Holt and Company, New York, 1995

The Medical Letter on Drugs and Therapeutics (39:91)

The Harvard Health Letter (17,4:4)

The History of Bananas, AIMS Education Foundation, Internet WWW address <http://www.aimsedu.org/activities/banana/banana2.html> retrieved on Oct. 13, 1997

The Honest Herbal, The Haworth Press, Binghamton, N.Y., 1993

The International Bottled Water Association, Internet WWW address <http://www.bottledwater.org.html> retrieved on Oct. 14, 1997

The Journal of Agriculture and Food Chemistry (44,3:701)

The Journal of Nutrition (110,4:662 and 122,35:604)

The Journal of the American Dietetic Association (96,10:1027)

The Journal of the American Medical Association (227,22:1775; 265,14:1833; 265,22:3014; 272,18:1413; 272,24:1942; 273,16:1249; 273,11:897; 275,6:447; 276,21:1747; 276,22:1790; 276,24:1957; 277,6:472; and 277,10:776)

The Journal of Urology (155:432 and 155:839)

The Lancet (1,8285:1317; 2,8604:189; 342,8878:1007; 344,8929:1089; 345,8943:170; 346,8974:541; 347,9004:781; 347,8499:426; 347,8993:19; 348,9026:539; 348,9036:1186; 349,9066:1675; 349,9067:1715,1776; 350,9070:31; and 350,9081:850)

The Lawrence Review of Natural Products, Facts & Comparisons, St. Louis, Mo.

The Medical Advisor: The Complete Guide to Alternative and Conventional Treatments, Time Life Inc., Alexandria, Va., 1996

The New England Journal of Medicine (332,5:286; 332,13:894; 333,5:276; 334,7:445; 334,18:1156; 334,24:1557; 336,15:1046; 336,16:1117; and 336,17:1216)

The Nutrition Desk Reference, Keats Publishing, New Canaan, Conn., 1995

The Onion with a Number, Internet WWW address <http://wwwtc.nhmccd.cc.tx.us/bluebonnet/education/humanities/info/v3n2/heatherd.htm> retrieved on Oct. 15, 1997

The PDR Family Guide to Nutrition and Health, Medical Economics Co., Montvale, N.J., 1995

The Physician and Sports Medicine (20,4:51; 21,5:27; 22,8:30; and 23,6:13)

The Ripe Way to Enjoy Avocados, Internet WWW address <http://avoinfo.cyberworks.net/nutrition/theripewaytoenjoy.html> retrieved on Oct. 16, 1997

The Satiety Index, Rick Mendosa, Internet WWW address <http://www.mendosa.com/satiety.htm> retrieved on July 22, 1997

The Thyroid Society, Internet WWW address <http://houston-interweb.com/thyroid/faq/29.html>retrieved on July 31, 1997

The University of Arizona Health Science Center, Tracy W. Gaudet, M.D., Internet WWW address <http://www.ahsc.arizona.edu/opa/answers/apr97.htm> retrieved on Sept. 8, 1997

The Wall Street Journal (May 11, 1994, B9)

Therapeutische Umschau (51,7:502)

Thyroid Disease in the Elderly, Internet WWW address <http://www.clark.net/pub/tfa/elderlybrochure.html> retrieved on July 25, 1997

Tijdschrift Voor Gerontologie En Geriatrie (27,3:97)

Time Life Medical Advisor, Time-Life Books, Alexandria, Va., 1996

Tinnitus Family Information, American Tinnitus Association, P.O. Box 5, Portland, OR 97207-0005

Total Health (16,5:46)

Trans Fatty Acids, American Heart Association, Internet WWW address <http://www.amhrt.org/hs96/tfa.html> retrieved on Sept. 24, 1997

Treatment for Eczema/Atopic Dermatitis, National Jewish Medical and Research Center, 1400 Jackson St., Denver, CO 80206

Tufts University Diet & Nutrition Letter (13,6:2)

U.S. Pharmacist (18,9:100; 20,4:41; and 21,5:19)

Understanding Angina, American Heart Association, 7272 Greenville Avenue, Dallas, TX 75231-4596

University of Iowa Family Practice Handbook, Mark A. Graber, M.D. and Rhea J. Allen, M.D., Internet WWW address <http://vh.radiology.uiowa.edu/Providers/ClinRef/FPHandbook/Chapter04/01-4.html> retrieved on July 15, 1997

Urinary Tract Infections in Adults, Publication No. 91-2097, National Institute of Diabetes and Digestive and Kidney Diseases, National Institutes of Health, Bethesda, MD 20892

USDA Nutrient Values, Internet WWW address <http://www.rahul.net/cgi-bin/fatfree/usda/usda.cgi> retrieved on Dec. 5, 1997

Vestnik Oftalmologii (108,4-6:13)

Vitamin C, The Common Cold and The Flu, Berkley Books, New York, 1981

Voprosy Meditsinskoi Khimii (41,4:33)

Voprosy Pitaniia (3:21)

What Everyone Needs to Know About Exercise-Induced Asthma, Allergy and Asthma Network/Mothers of Asthmatics, Inc., 3554 Chain Bridge Road, Suite 200, Fairfax, VA 22030-2709

What is an Allergic Reaction?, American Academy of Allergy, Asthma, and Immunology, Internet WWW address <http://www.aaaai.org/patpub/resource/publicat/tips/tip5.html> retrieved on March 11, 1997

What is Non-Insulin-Dependent Diabetes?, American Diabetes Association, Diabetes Information Service Center, 1660 Duke Street, Alexandria, VA 22314

What is the difference between a sweet potato and a yam?, North Carolina Cooperative Extension Service, Leaflet No. 23-A, September 1993, Internet WWW address <http://www.ces.ncsu.edu/depts/hort/hil/hil-23-a.html> retrieved on Oct. 16, 1997

What You Need to Know About Diabetes, American Diabetes Association, Diabetes Information Service Center, 1660 Duke Street, Alexandria, VA 22314

What You Need to Know About Periodontal (Gum) Diseases, NIH Publication No. 94-1142, National Institute of Dental Research, P.O. Box 54793, Washington, DC 20032

What You Should Know About Asthma and Food, International Food Information Council (IFIC) and the Division of Allergy, Asthma and Immunology, Scripps Clinic and Research Foundation, Internet WWW address <http://ificinfo.health.org/brochure/asthma.htm> retrieved on July 28, 1997

What Your Doctor May Not Tell You About Menopause, Warner Books, New York, 1996

Why Do I Have Gas?, National Institute of Diabetes and Digestive and Kidney Diseases, Internet WWW address <http://www.niddk.nih.gov/llgas/gas.htm> retrieved on July 16, 1997

WORLD Headquarters of the International Foundation for Functional Gastrointestinal Disorders (IFFGD), Internet WWW address <http://www.execpc.com/iffgd/> retrieved on July 24, 1997

World of Herbs, Crescent Books, New York, 1990

Zentralblatt Fur Hygiene und Umweltmedizin (191,2-3:241)

RECIPE SOURCES

Apricots

"Orange-Apricot Cookies," *Making Bag Lunches, Snacks and Desserts Using the Dietary Guidelines,* USDA Home & Garden Bulletin No. 232-9

"Garden Couscous Salad," *Celebrate Good Health,* American Institute for Cancer Research, Washington, 1989

"Raisin Apricot Oatmeal Bars," *Celebrate Good Health,* American Institute for Cancer Research, Washington, 1989

Avocado

"Guacamole Dip," traditional

"California Guacamole — Diabetic Diet," California Avocado Commission, 1251 E. Dyer Road, Suite 200, Santa Ana, Calif. 92705-5631

"Citrus Salad with California Avocados," California Avocado Commission, 1251 E. Dyer Road, Suite 200, Santa Ana, Calif. 92705-5631

"California Avocado Tacos," California Avocado Commission, 1251 E. Dyer Road, Suite 200, Santa Ana, Calif. 92705-5631

Banana

"Baked Fruit Alaska," *Celebrate Good Health,* American Institute for Cancer Research, Washington, 1989

"The Banana Bread of Kings," submitted by Shari L. Bart as seen on Veggies Unite! <http://www.vegweb.com>

"Fruity Oatmeal Cookies," *Celebrate Good Health,* American Institute for Cancer Research, Washington, 1989

"Baked Banana," *Preparing Foods and Planning Menus,* USDA Home and Garden Bulletin No. 232-8

Broccoli

"Broccoli Soup," *Preparing Foods & Planning Menus,* USDA Home and Garden Bulletin No. 232-8

"Chicken Divan," *Be Your Best: Nutrition After Fifty,* American Institute for Cancer Research, Washington, 1988

"Italian Chicken Stir-Fry," *No Time to Cook,* American Institute for Cancer Research, Washington, 1990

Garlic

"Sopa de Ajo (Cuban Garlic Soup)," by Bill Wood, courtesy of Dr. Gaston Jones

"Cauliflower — Northern Italian Style," *No Time to Cook,* American Institute for Cancer Research, Washington, 1990

"Baked Vidalia Onion," *Vidalia Onion Cookbook,* FC&A Publishing, Peachtree City, Ga.

Grape juice

"Fruit Juice Cubes," *Making Bag Lunches, Snacks & Desserts Using the Dietary Guidelines,* USDA Home & Garden Bulletin, No. 232-9

Legumes

"Three-Bean Chili," *Be Your Best: Nutrition After Fifty,* American Institute for Cancer Research, Washington, 1988

"Quick 'n Hearty Bean Soup," *No Time to Cook,* American Institute for Cancer Research, Washington, 1990

Oat bran

"Currant Bran Muffins," *Be Your Best: Nutrition After Fifty,* American Institute for Cancer Research, Washington, 1988

"Half-the-Fat Carrot Cake," *Celebrate Good Health,* American Institute for Cancer Research, Washington, 1989

Soy

"Surprise Zucchini Brownies," *Celebrate Good Health,* American Institute for Cancer Research, Washington, 1989

Spinach

"Spinach and Lentil Soup," *From Around the World, International Menus and Recipes to Lower Cancer Risk,* American Institute for Cancer Research, Washington, 1991

"Spinach Pita Pizzas," *Celebrate Good Health,* American Institute for Cancer Research, Washington, 1989

Tomatoes

"Salsa," *Making Bag Lunches, Snacks and Desserts Using the Dietary Guidelines,* USDA Home & Garden Bulletin No. 232-9

"Pasta Ruffles and Beef," *Be Your Best: Nutrition After Fifty,* American Institute for Cancer Research, Washington, 1988

"New England Casserole," *Be Your Best: Nutrition After Fifty,* American Institute for Cancer Research, Washington, 1988

"Fresh Tomato Chutney," *From Around the World, International Menus and Recipes to Lower Cancer Risk,* American Institute for Cancer Research, Washington, 1991

Yogurt

"Curry Vegetable Dip," *Diabetes Forecast* (48,9:52)

"Madras Vegetable Stew," *From Around the World, International Menus and Recipes to Lower Cancer Risk,* American Institute for Cancer Research, Washington, 1991

"Potatoes with Mustard-Tarragon Stuffing," *No Time to Cook,* American Institute for Cancer Research, Washington, 1990

INDEX

A

AMD (age-related macular degeneration), 275

Acidophilus, 82. *See also* Lactobacillus acidophilus

Age-related macular degeneration (AMD), 275

Alcohol
  cancer and, 46
  congestive heart failure and, 66
  for angina, 19
  gout and, 28
  headaches and, 115-116
  high blood pressure and, 131
  high cholesterol and, 136
  impotence and, 140
  insomnia and, 149
  irritable bowel syndrome and, 149
  menopause and, 169
  osteoporosis and, 181
  to prevent heart disease, 121
  ulcers and, 213

Alcoholism, 8-9, 122, 307, 311, 324-325

Alfalfa, 155

Allergies, 9-12, 32-33, 110, 193
  canker sores and, 52
  arthritis and, 27

Alpha tocopherol. *See* Vitamin E

Alzheimer's disease, 9, 13-15, 203

Anemia
  arthritis and, 25
  copper and, 304
  hair loss and, 109
  iron-deficiency, 15-18, 309
  manganese and, 313
  restless legs syndrome and, 154

Angina, 18-21, 68, 335

Anise, 105, 123, 168

Anorexia nervosa, 87, 94

Antacids, 18, 307, 309, 312, 316

Anticoagulants, 71, 201

Antihistamines, 11, 30

Antioxidants, 146, 319, 331
  for alcoholism, 8
  for arthritis, 24
  for atherosclerosis, 35, 119

Antioxidants *(continued)*
  for cancer, 41, 330
  for high cholesterol, 134
  sources of, 238, 256, 259-260
  to prevent cataracts, 55

Appetite loss, 87, 93-94, 106, 299, 339

Apples
  health benefits of, 232-233

Apricots, 234
  health benefits of, 234-235, 317
  recipes, 235-237

Arginine, 58, 63

Aromatherapy, 185, 198, 222-223

Arrhythmias, 22-23
  CoQ 10 for, 68
  magnesium deficiency and, 311
  magnesium overdose and, 312
  potassium deficiency and, 318

Arthritis, 23-29, 287, 307

Aspartame, 115

Aspirin, 106, 201-202, 307

Asthma, 29-34

Atherosclerosis, 35-36, 39, 119
  angina and, 19
  attitude and, 38
  garlic for, 251
  high blood pressure and, 127
  impotence and, 139
  macular degeneration and, 158

Avocado, 238-242
  consumer tips for, 240-241
  health benefits of, 238-239, 326
  recipes, 241-242

B

B vitamins. *See* Vitamin B

BPH (benign prostatic hyperplasia), 185

BRAT diet, for nausea and vomiting, 177

Bacteria
  E. coli, 84-86, 290
  H. pylori, 190, 211-213, 252
  Lactobacillus acidophilus, 51, 60, 217-218, 290
  Salmonella, 290
  Vibrio vulnificus, 8

Bacterial infections
  cranberry juice for, 214

Bacterial infections
  garlic for, 252
  in the mouth, 87
  yogurt for, 290

G

GBE (ginkgo biloba extract). *See* Ginkgo
GERD (gastroesophageal reflux disease).
 See Heartburn and indigestion
GLA (gammalinolenic acid), 27
Gallbladder disease, 101-102
Garlic, 46, 251-255
 consumer tips for, 253
 for colds, 65
 for E. coli infection, 86
 for fungal infections, 217
 for high blood pressure, 126
 for high cholesterol, 136, 141
 for ulcers, 213
 health benefits of, 252-253
 recipes, 254-255
Gas, 83, 104-105, 123
Gastritis, 106
Gastrointestinal cancer
 green tea for, 43
Genistein, 271
Germander, 124
Ginger
 for arthritis, 28-29
 for atherosclerosis , 38
 for headache, 111, 113-114
 for menopause, 168
 for nausea and vomiting, 175-176
 for sore throat, 64
 to prevent motion sickness, 170-171
Gingivitis, 207
Ginkgo
 for PMS, 184
 for Alzheimer's disease, 13-14
 for asthma, 31-32
 for cerebral insufficiency, 162
 for headache, 111, 112
 for leg pain, 155
 for memory loss, 162, 163
 for menopause, 168
 for Raynaud's disease, 188
 for varicose veins, 219
Ginseng
 for chronic fatigue syndrome, 59
 for diabetes, 74
 for impotence, 141-142
 for menopause, 168
 for stress, 197
Glaucoma, 107-108
Glucosamine sulfate, 25-26
Glutamine, 210

Glutathione
 for cancer, 47, 252
 for glaucoma, 107
 to prevent cataracts, 56-57
Gluten, 83
Goiter, 205
Goitrogens, 206
Goldenseal, 51, 64, 124, 209
Gout, 27
Grape juice, 121, 255-257
 health benefits of, 256
 recipes, 257
Grapefruit, 258-259
 consumer tips for, 259
 health benefits of, 258-259
Grapeseed extract. *See* Pycnogenol
Green tea
 health benefits of, 43, 199, 213, 259-261
Gum massage, 209
Gurmar, 74

H

H. pylori, 190, 211-213, 252
HDL cholesterol, 35-36, 121, 133-134, 136, 138
Hair loss, 108-109, 320
Hay fever, 11
Headache, 109-116
 iron-deficiency anemia and, 16
Hearing loss, 117
Heart attack, 117-122
 garlic for, 251
 grape juice for, 256
 magnesium for, 311
Heartburn and indigestion, 122-125
 asthma and, 34
 gastritis and, 106
 water for, 287
Hemochromatosis, 310
Hemorrhoids, 125
Herpes simplex, 60
High blood pressure, 68, 126-132, 140, 311
 Coenzyme Q10 for, 67
 fat and, 140
 magnesium deficiency and, 310
High cholesterol, 133-138
 atherosclerosis and, 35
 avocado for, 239
 chromium for, 302
 gallbladder disease and, 102
 garlic for, 252